Practical Concepts in Human Disease

Practical Concepts in Human Disease

Harmon C. Bickley, D.D.S., Ph.D.,
Associate Professor, Department of Pathology, College of Medicine, University of Iowa, Iowa City, Iowa

THE WILLIAMS & WILKINS COMPANY / BALTIMORE

Made in the United States of America

Library of Congress Cataloging in Publication Data

Bickley, Harmon C
    Practical concepts in human disease.
        1. Pathology. I. Title. [DNLM: 1. Disease
QZ40 B583p 1974]
    RB25.B582   616   73-19650
    ISBN 0-683-00912-5

Composed and Printed at the
Waverly Press, Inc.
Mt. Royal and Guilford Aves.
Baltimore, Md. 21202, U. S. A.

foreword

Human pathology is the science in which other sciences are brought to focus on the illness of man. It is the study of disease (dis-ease), the lack of that feeling of ease that prevails when all of the parts of our bodies are in correct working order. To the student of a health profession it is the science that leads immediately and directly into the clinical arts; it is an orientation, a language course and the means of transition between subjects that serve as background and those that are to be practiced. To others it can be a fascinating insight into how the human body is injured and the limited, but critical, ways in which it can respond.

Today we are witnessing a growing need for pathology instruction suitable not only for the health service practitioner but also for the perceptive layman troubled by the increasing subordination of the values of life to those of technology. Quite in contrast to the aspiring pathologist, these individuals should be taught in a single course the broadest possible scope of disease fundamentals, but yet not be burdened with detail. Very few courses exist for this purpose and none of the standard texts emphasize this approach.

Another compelling reason for developing new courses and new texts is that our outlook on human disease is daily becoming more mature and inclusive. We now see the potential for disease not only in a person's body but also in his mind, his environment and his social situation. Neurotic people experience more disease than the well adjusted, poor people more than the affluent. All of this must be considered in a course in abnormal human biology. Perhaps the traditionalist might object that a course of this scope transcends the limits of the science of pathology. But whether or not such a course is to be called "pathology," its first aim should be to awaken the student's interest in disease as a significant component of contemporary culture, relevant to the lives of all of us and not just to the study of medicine.

For many reasons, then, it would seem that this is the time for a significant revision of method and intent in the teaching of pathology. It is a science that continues to become interesting to more and more people. Very few of these will ever become practicing pathologists, but then very few who study chemistry become professional chemists. Add to this the fact that pathology deals with matters of more direct personal concern, and it seems that we are witnessing a real, if not critical, need for practical instruction in human pathology for the non-pathologist, indeed, perhaps even for the non-health professional.

These are some of the premises that account for the idiosyncrasies of this text. It is intended to cover material generally considered "core" in the subject of pathology with a few non-traditional subjects added for good measure. Introductory but comprehensive, the content was selected on the hypothesis that concerned and educated members of a modern society should be familiar with a perspective of human disease but that mastery of the subject will vary with the degree of active involvement assumed by each. It is only from such a broad base of enlightened individuals that we will be able to generate an effective means of limiting, and perhaps reversing, the continued deterioration of our surroundings as a medium for life.

H. C. B.

To my wife, Christy
(who did the index)

and my children:
Susan
Margaret
Elizabeth
David

contents

Part 1

systems of defense

chapter 1
PRINCIPLES OF IMMUNOLOGIC DEFENSE

THE CONCEPT OF BIOLOGIC SELF

LEARNING OBJECTIVE

To be able to compare and contrast substances that the body treats as "self" and "foreign," mentioning the following:

  a) size and chemical nature of molecules that qualify for scrutiny
  b) coupling of recognition to reaction
  c) sources of foreignness
  d) four essential features of biologic self

1. Why Discriminate between Self and Non-Self?

We function throughout our entire lives with the single store of genetic information given us at the time of our conception. This information is coded into a molecular sequence in the genetic material of our cells and contained in the nucleus. Aside from the possibility of minor cytoplasmic genes we have no other archive in which to store it and it is never replenished. Most of the material that constitutes our bodies at birth as well as most of what is added later during growth and maturation will have a structure specified in detail by our genetic plan (genome). It is the master blueprint for all protein that goes into the composition of our bodies.

Although the proteins that make up any one human body are similar in structure to their counterparts in other individuals (and even in other forms of life), most of them are unique in certain small details of composition and shape. It is the aggregate effect of all this uniqueness that begins to define an individual. One of the reasons why people, or whole species, look different, act differently, and are different is because difference starts at the level of molecular structure. Conversely, the fact that most of these molecules can be identified as part of a single individual qualifies them as a component of his biologic "self."

To be considered for classification as either self or foreign the molecule must be large; those having a molecular weight of several thousand provoke the strongest reactions as non-self while small molecules and ions are simply overlooked. In this same regard the chemical nature of the molecule is also important. Proteins, polysaccharides and protein-polysaccharides are most effective whereas simple lipids are disregarded.

From the standpoint of immunologic defense the strategy of preserving the human body is based on the precept that *self-molecules are to be conserved and non-self destroyed.* The reason for this is not simply that foreign molecules might not function as well as native molecules; in fact, in instances in which an individual is born with a developmental defect they may work even better. A higher reason is that nature uses a mechanism for preserving biologic integrity that is based on an absolute dichotomy of native vis-a-vis alien. Native or self material is tolerated whereas foreign or non-self material *automatically* provokes a reaction that leads to its own destruction.

By way of analogy, consider a person's motive for installing a fire protection system. He wants an immediate and automatic response when fire breaks out. To actuate his sprinkler system he selects a mechanism sensitive to heat; thus the presence of heat is the criterion by which fire is detected and a corrective measure instituted. In like manner the body employs foreignness as a criterion of threat or disintegration and uses its detection as a means of triggering some kinds of corrective reactions. This is shown diagrammatically in illustration 1-1. There are, of course, many valid reasons for considering most foreign material a threat. But in the study of disease it is important to realize that foreign material is *automatically* construed as a threat (whether or not it is truly

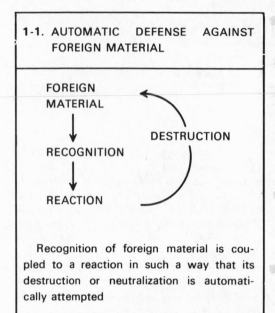

1-1. AUTOMATIC DEFENSE AGAINST FOREIGN MATERIAL

FOREIGN MATERIAL

RECOGNITION

REACTION

DESTRUCTION

Recognition of foreign material is coupled to a reaction in such a way that its destruction or neutralization is automatically attempted

threatening), because it is precisely the quality of foreignness that triggers the mechanism of defense.

2. Where Do We Encounter Foreign Material?

The concept of foreignness, at least from the biologic standpoint, is more complex than it first appears. In fact, there are at least 4 different kinds of foreignness that must be taken into consideration if one is to understand the body's "attitude" toward non-self. These are listed in Illustration 1-2 and discussed in turn below.

Exogenous Material

In the normal individual, if a macromolecule is to be accepted as native, its structure must have been specified by the genome. It is obvious, then, that molecules specified by an alien genome will always appear foreign and if discovered within the body will be rejected. This first kind of foreignness is not difficult to understand because it complies with the usually accepted meaning of the word. For the most part, of course, such extrinsic materials are associated with invading microorganisms and the reaction they provoke is generally appreciated as "host resistance."

Somatic Mutation

A second kind of foreignness, somewhat more subtle than the first, is the kind that arises as a result of the introduction of "error" into the genome. If the genetic information of one or more somatic cells undergoes mutation, the protein structure specified by the mutated gene will be different. This new protein now becomes just as liable to rejection as if it belonged to another life system. In effect, a somatic mutation has actually generated an internal source of foreignness. One cannot help but wonder to what extent this might be held responsible for the phenomenon of biologic aging.

Altered Native Protein

The third kind of foreignness is that resulting when a native protein is changed after it has been normally synthesized. This often occurs when such a protein forms a complex with a drug or other small molecule and the complex presents a slightly altered shape. Although the protein is native, the complex is foreign-appearing and will be rejected. The small molecule is said to be acting as a *hapten*.

Ectopic Material

Our fourth and final category of non-self is, strictly speaking, not even foreignness, but that of the appearance of valid native material in an abnormal location. To understand why this should be so undesirable one must consider that the body must be partitioned into inviolable compartments to function properly. Escape of

1-2. SOURCES OF FOREIGNNESS (OR NON-SELF)

1) EXOGENOUS MATERIAL

2) SOMATIC MUTATION

3) ALTERED NATIVE PROTEIN

4) ECTOPIC NATIVE MATERIAL

1-3. MACROMOLECULES THAT QUALIFY AS SELF
1) NATIVE
2) SPECIFIED BY AN UNMUTATED GENOME
3) UNDENATURED
4) IN NORMAL POSITION WITHIN THE BODY

material from these compartments cannot be tolerated. Indiscriminate communication cannot be permitted, for example, between the inside and the outside of cells. Also, material from various organs must not be allowed to mix, since each requires a particular array of highly specialized proteins and other large molecules to carry out its unique role in metabolism. There is reason to believe that the body treats material that is out of place, i.e. *ectopic* material, just as it would alien material. The reaction that it provokes leads to its disposal and prevents its interfering with active molecules that must be present in the circulation in order to function normally. Returning to our first example, the structures found within the interior of a cell would not operate properly if liberated into the extracellular space. In such a location they would be simply debris. Insofar as the body is concerned they would be effete material, worn out and no longer useful. This treatment is not reserved for cell contents, however. It would also be used in the case of organ-specific material discovered out of place. Consider, for example, that if the protein found normally in the lens of the eye was to be intercepted circulating in the blood stream it would appear quite foreign and elicit a defense reaction. All ectopic material, then, is treated as if it was non-self .

In summary, it now appears that in order to be part of an individual's biologic self (at least in a functional sense), a material must demonstrate the four qualities listed in illustration 1-3. Each type of foreign material will later be seen to give rise to a different kind of disease. For the present, make sure that you are aware of the differences among these four kinds of foreign material.

Additional Reading

Boss, J. H. et al. Patterns of naturally occurring circulating antibodies to rat tissue antigens in the rat. Path. Microbiol. 31:1, 1968
Burnet, M. Self and Not-self. Melbourne Univ Press, Victoria, Australia, 1969
Sharp, G. C. Autoantibodies: Friend or Foe? Am. J. Med. Sci. 259:365, 1970

THE LYMPHORETICULAR SYSTEM AS SENTINEL OF BIOLOGIC SELF

LEARNING OBJECTIVE

To be able to describe the lymphoreticular system and explain the concept of adaptive immunity, mentioning the following:
   a) **components of the lymphoreticular system**
   b) **basis of lymphoreticular function**
   c) **instruction and selection theories of specific reaction**

1. Components of the Lymphoreticular System

To sustain life an individual must persist as "self." But it is important to realize that the maintaining of biologic self is by no means effortless. Quite to the contrary, it is known to be an energy-consuming, incredibly demanding task. Translated into thermodynamic terms, it requires that a focus of extremely improbable order persists in a far more casually ordered environment. It simply cannot be done without the mediation of a system of hard-working cells, which, in turn, must apply significant amounts of energy in carrying it out. In higher animals, this self-maintaining system of cells is the *lymphoreticular system* and its function is called *adaptive immunity*.

An authoritative description of the lymphoreticular system is difficult today, because no one is exactly sure at this writing what would have to be included. Its components are widely distributed throughout the body, and, indeed, even the limits of its function are still to be determined with precision. Since the lymphoreticular system must include all structures associated with recognition and reaction to foreign material, most authorities would probably include at least those components listed in illustration 1-4.

Because of its indefinite status no further attempts will be made to define this system and we will concentrate on what is known of its functions.

2. Functions of the Lymphoreticular System

It must be fully appreciated that adaptive immunity is absolutely essential; the lymphoreticular system must continue to function if a person is to go on living.

The operation of the lymphoreticular system seems to be based on the orientation of an amazingly sensitive recognition mechanism to a limited number of molecular configurations which are accepted as self and the rejection of all others. Those recognized as self are tolerated whereas those failing to be recognized provoke an immune response and are said to be antigens.

**1-5. FUNCTIONS OF THE
LYMPHORETICULAR SYSTEM**

Interrelated abilities to:

1) RECOGNIZE

2) REACT TO

3) REMEMBER

   foreign material

(Note: Although not precisely correct we will not attempt to differentiate between the terms, immunogen and antigen.)

Once it has elicited an immune response, an antigen is remembered and future encounters are usually met with an enhanced ability to react. In many instances, immunologic memory is of life-long duration; however, in others it deteriorates if the time elapsing between the first and second exposures is protracted. In summary, it might be said that the lymphoreticular system is in the very special position of having to remember what is normally part of the body and, using this as a point of reference, determine what is foreign or out of place. If the lymphoreticular system has never "seen" the material, then it must be considered foreign, whether or not it has actually come from outside the body, and an appropriate reaction must be set in motion to preserve the conditions necessary for life.

The function of the lymphoreticular system (adaptive immunity) may be defined as the coordinated abilities to, 1) recognize, 2) react to and 3) remember foreign material (Illustration 1-5).

3. Recognition of Non-Self, Instruction or Selection?

From the very first, the most enigmatic aspect of immunity has been the stage of recognition. How is the lymphoreticular system able to recognize an antigen and then summon a response that is specific for that particular

---

**1-4. COMPONENTS OF THE
LYMPHORETICULAR SYSTEM**

1) CENTRAL LYMPHOID TISSUE
   thymus, bone marrow, Peyer's patches

2) PERIPHERAL LYMPHOID TISSUE
   lymph nodes and spleen

3) LYMPH VESSELS

4) PHAGOCYTES: HISTIOCYTES, RETICULAR CELLS AND SINUSOIDAL LINING CELLS
   at least to the extent that they participate in the collection and processing of antigens

molecule? It is generally conceived that the specificity of the response must be vested in the synthesis of a protein with a structure complementing that of the antigen; however, the means by which the responding cell manages to elaborate just the right protein for each antigen is not understood.

Theories proposed to explain this are of two major categories (Illustration 1-6). The first and older is a collection of ideas known as the *Instruction Theories.* Briefly, these hold that information necessary to permit the immunocompetent cell to respond is brought to the cells by the antigen. The cell, in responding, constructs an antibody (a specific complementary protein) using the antigen as a template. A corollary of these theories is that any immunocompetent cell could react to any antigen since the information for doing so is provided by the antigen itself.

The second category of major theories of immunity is the group known as the *Selection Theories.* These hold that immunocompetent cells exist within the body in small groups called *clones.* Each clone has the potential for synthesizing one specific protein or, at most, a limited group of such proteins. Recognition consists of the antigen's selectively stimulating only the clone that has genetic information that would allow it to synthesize the exact protein required for the response. It is not clear how the antigen is able to select or stimulate a clone; however, some kind of receptor system is usually postulated. The advantage of the Selection Theories is that they do not conflict with

the "central dogma" of molecular biology, i.e. that all information for protein synthesis is contained within the nucleus of the cell and transcribed in the synthetic process through the mediation of RNA. Of the two categories of theories the latter appears to better explain phenomena observed in the study of immune responses. The matter is still one of controversy, however, and neither group of theories is completely sufficient at this time.

Additional Reading

Haurowitz, F. Evolution of selective and instructive theories of antibody formation. Coldspring Harbor Symposia on Quantitative Biology 32:559, 1967
Henry, C. et al. Peyer's patches: immunologic studies. J. Exp. Med. 131:1200, 1970
Silverman, M. S. The macrophage in cellular and humoral immunity. J. Reticuloendoth. Soc. 8:105, 1970

DUAL COMPONENT IMMUNITY

LEARNING OBJECTIVE

To be able to compare and contrast the humoral and cellular systems with regard to:
- a) dependence on antibody synthesis
- b) mediation by the sensitized lymphocyte

It may now be stated with some assurance that the whole immunologic faculty of the human body consists of at least 2 separate and quite distinct types of responses. Although many synonyms are used for these (Illustration 1-7), the most generally accepted terms are *humoral immunity* and *cellular immunity.* More recently, it has come to light that the 2 are mediated by separate cellular systems which, although interdependent in many respects, maintain separate identity. The population of cells mediating humoral immunity has come to be known as B-cells, whereas those responsible for cellular immunity are termed T-cells. Each is identified by a characteristic surface antigen.

1-6. INSTRUCTION AND SELECTION THEORIES

1) INSTRUCTION

information for antibody synthesis is brought to the responding cell by antigen

2) SELECTION

antigen selects and stimulates clone that has information for antibody synthesis

1-7. TWO COMPONENTS OF ADAPTIVE IMMUNITY

1) HUMORAL IMMUNITY
   immediate
   thymus-independent
   B-cell response

2) CELLULAR IMMUNITY
   delayed
   tuberculin
   bacterial
   thymus-dependent
   T-cell response

1. Humoral Immunity

Humoral immunity is, in many ways, the more classic and completely understood. This is the response that usually comes to mind when one thinks of immunologic phenomena. It is almost always signaled by the appearance in the serum of a specific globulin (antibody) and this antibody can be observed to form a complex with its provoking antigen either in the body or in a test tube. The fact that the response can be elicited only after antibody is synthesized and available in the serum is it responsible for features of this response that allow it to be clearly distinguished from cellular immunity. The term "humoral" refers to the necessary presence of antibody in the serum.

2. Cellular Immunity

The second type of immune response is known as cellular immunity. This response does not seem to be mediated by circulating antibody and, in fact, can even be detected in some patients suffering from a complete inability to produce antibodies. In the cellular response, lymphoid tissue reacts to an antigen by "sensitizing" lymphocytes instead of synthesizing antibodies. The term *sensitize* is usually used to describe the change occurring in responding lymphocytes, although the actual nature of this change is not understood. These cells leave the peripheral lymphoid tissue in which sensitization occurs, enter the blood stream and are broadcast throughout the body. Upon encountering the antigen that provoked their sensitization, a very few of these cells can cause a grossly visible reaction by undergoing a series of changes and marshalling other cells to the area. This whole process results in an attack on both the antigen and the tissue in which it is contained.

It is important to realize that no antibody has yet been detected in the cellular immunologic response. The sensitized lymphocyte is the mobile agent of recognition in this response and carries the specificity on (or within) its membrane. The cellular response is mediated solely by lymphoid cells.

The dual-component quality of adaptive immunity is summarized diagrammatically in Illustration 1-8.

Additional Reading

Cooper, M.D. et al. The two-component concept of the lymphoid system. Birth Defects, Original Article Series IV, 7 Feb, 1958
Culliton, B. J. Immunology: Two immune systems capture attention. Science 180:45, 1973

1-8. DUAL-COMPONENT IMMUNITY

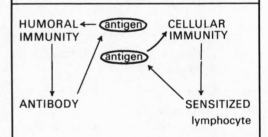

Adaptive immunity consists of at least two component systems. Antigens interact with one or the other eliciting either an antibody or sentized lymphocyte. These react specifically with the antigen that provoked them

ANTIBODIES AND HUMORAL IMMUNITY

LEARNING OBJECTIVE

To be able to discuss the following aspects of humoral immunity:

a) antibody, immunoglobulin, gamma globulin

b) characteristics and functions of each of the 5 major classes of immunoglobulins (G, A, M, D and E)

1. Antibodies and Immunoglobulins

Antibodies are the agents of reaction in the humoral response. Although the term *antibody* is adequate in reference to their biologic role, they are classified chemically as *immunoglobulins*.

Immunoglobulins are a group of proteins distinctly different from others in that they have a characteristic structure of two heavy and two light polypeptide chains. Although they all share this structure, they occur in a variety of types which differ principally in size, composition and the antigenic characteristics of their heavy chains. Illustration 1-9 is a diagram of an immunoglobulin molecule. Note that the antigen combining sites are at one end (N-terminal), whereas the other remains free to engage in reactions that will determine the pharmacologic properties of the complex.

Immunoglobulins (antibodies) are synthesized by plasma cells which develop from a kind of lymphocyte. Most antibodies circulate in the blood and nearly all are found in the gamma electrophoretic fraction of serum. This has given rise to the almost synonomous term, "gamma globulin."

The prevailing concentration of circulating immunoglobulins at any given time is the result of a number of controlling factors; however, in an immunologically competent human being, the most important of these is antigenic stimulation. The rate of immunoglobulin synthesis in germ-free animals has been shown to be 1/50 to 1/300 normal whereas this same rate in hyperimmunized animals may be 5 to 10 times normal. Thus, at the very least, there may be a surprising 500-fold difference in the rate of

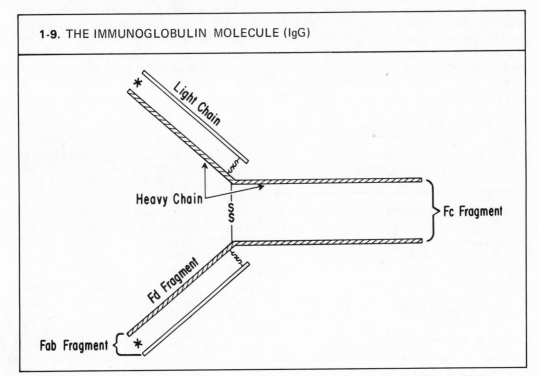

1-9. THE IMMUNOGLOBULIN MOLECULE (IgG)

Light Chain

Heavy Chain

Fd Fragment

Fab Fragment

Fc Fragment

(Reproduced from Richerson, H. B. Immunoglobulins and disease. J. Iowa Med. Soc. 58:935, 1968.)

antibody synthesis in germ-free and high-pathogen environments.

2. The Major Classes of Immunoglobulins

Five major types or classes (isotypes) of immunoglobulins can be distinguished in a single individual and each may ultimately prove to be a heterogeneous group of subtypes. In man and in most higher animals, the 5 major classes are those listed in Illustration 1-10. These designations were proposed through the World Health Organization and are now widely accepted. As more information becomes available, it appears that these major classes of immunoglobulins are the products of different subsystems within the humoral system and each mediates a somewhat different kind of immunologic defense. We will briefly consider each of the major classes in turn.

IgG System

IgG is present in the highest concentration of all immunoglobulins (approximately 12 mg/ml or about 3/4 or all circulating gamma globulins). It is probably the most important in resistance to infection. The adult human body contains about 1 gm of IgG per Kg of body weight. Approximately half of this is intravascular, the remaining being dispersed in interstitial fluid. IgG is the only immunoglobulin that is actively transported across the placenta. The mother's IgG serves as the

---

1-11. IgG SYSTEM
1) DIVALENT MONOMER 150,000 M.W.
2) 3/4 OF ALL Ig IN BODY
3) ABOUT 1/2 INTRAVASCULAR AND CIRCULATING AND 1/2 IN INTERSTITIAL FLUID
4) PLACENTAL TRANSFER
5) FORMED LATER THAN IgM: LASTS LONGER
6) FOUR SUBCLASSES: ALL BUT ONE FIX COMPLEMENT

principal agent of immunologic defense in the newborn. IgG is formed later than IgM in the primary immunologic response, but persists longer than any other immunoglobulin. Its half life in the human body is about 23 days. IgG is known to consist of 4 subclasses in the human and all but 1 of these is fixed complement (complement is a system of proteins that propel the reaction resulting from the formation of the antigen-antibody complex, a subject to be taken up later).

IgA System

IgA occurs in both serum and secretory forms. The latter is the principal immunoglobulin of external fluids such as saliva and differs from the former in that it occurs as two or three basic IgA molecules linked together by a product of an epithelial cell. This linking molecule is known as the *secretory component* or *secretory piece.* Secretory IgA will be considered in more detail later. Serum IgA probably functions as a simple neutralizing antibody within the blood stream. IgA neither fixes complement nor crosses the placenta. It is probably not involved in allergy, at least in the offensive sense. (Allergy is one of the 4 types of diseases that takes origin in the immunologic systems and will be discussed in detail later.)

1-10. MAJOR CLASSES (ISOTYPES) OF IMMUNOGLOBULINS
IgG – Immunoglobulin G
IgA – Immunoglobulin A
IgM – Immunoglobulin M
IgD – Immunoglobulin D
IgE – Immunoglobulin E

Features of the IgA system are summarized in Illustration 1-12.

IgM System

IgM is the largest of the immunoglobulins (almost 3 times the size of any of the others). It is the first immunoglobulin synthesized in the primary immunologic response, but remains for a comparatively short time. The IgM system is the most resistant to immunosuppression and the last to fail in advanced age. IgM does fix complement (IgM and IgG are the only 2 of the 5 isotypes that have been shown to do so) but does *not* cross the placenta. Elevated IgM levels in the newborn indicate that the infant has responded to antigenic stimulation *in utero* and produced antibodies of its own. This usually signifies its having sustained an intrauterine infection (usually viral). Features of the IgM system are summarized in Illustration 1-13.

IgD System

Virtually nothing is known of the biologic function of IgD other than the very rudimentary fact that it does have antibody activity. The IgD system is a comparatively recent discovery and this immunoglobulin is present in the serum in such small quantities that its study has proven most difficult (Illustration 1-14).

IgE System

IgE will be discussed further in the subject covering allergy; however, for now it should be known that this is the only one of the 5 isotypes that is decidely *cytophilic,* i.e. although some may be found circulating in serum, most will be fixed to cells in certain definite locations. (A word of caution should be inserted here about a possible source of confusion. Although IgE is cytophilic, it is in no way associated with cellular immunity or the sensitized lymphocytes.) The IgE system may represent an important subsurface defense facility that regulates vessel permeability and the output of glands that are situated in such a way as to wash mucous membrane surfaces with their secretions. In this role, IgE reactions may regulate the outpouring of secretory IgA onto these surfaces. IgE does *not* fix comple-

---

1-12. IgA SYSTEM

1) MONOMER (serum): DIMER OR TRIMER (secretory)

2) SALIVA, TEARS, COLOSTRUM, URINE, NASAL, BRONCHIAL AND G.I. FLUIDS

3) SURFACE PROTECTION

4) DOES NOT:
   cross placenta
   fix complement
   participate in allergy

1-13. IgM SYSTEM

1) FIRST Ig TO APPEAR AND FADE: PENTAMERIC: 900,000 M.W.

2) MOST RESISTANT TO SUPPRESSION: LAST TO FAIL IN SENESCENCE

3) NO PLACENTAL TRANSFER: PRESENCE IN NEWBORN IS SIGN OF INTRAUTERINE INFECTION

4) DOES:
   fix complement

1-14. IgD SYSTEM

1) RECENTLY DESCRIBED: LITTLE KNOWN

2) VERY SMALL SERUM CONCENTRATION

3) HAS ANTIBODY ACTIVITY

1-15. IgE SYSTEM

1) CYTOPHILIC Ig

2) REGULATES:
   vessel permeability
   mucosal gland secretion

3) CAN ELICIT FIRST STAGES OF ACUTE INFL. RESP.

4) RESPONSIBLE FOR MANY ALLERGIES

---

ments, but acts primarily through the histamine release mechanism and the production of SRS-A, both of which will be discussed later. IgE is *not* passed across the placenta. It is strongly implicated in certain kinds of allergy (anaphylaxis and atopy) to be taken up in a later subject. Features of the IgE system are summarized in Illustration 1-15.

Additional Reading

Putnam, F. W. Immunoglobulin structure: variability and homology. Science 163:633, 1969

Waldmann, T. A. Disorders of immunoglobulin metabolism. N. Engl. J. Med. 281:1170, 1969

Richerson, H. B. Immunoglobulins and Disease. J. Iowa Med. Soc. 58:935, 1968

LOCAL IMMUNITY, A SPECIAL KIND OF HUMORAL DEFENSE

LEARNING OBJECTIVE

To be able to describe the function of secretory IgA as an agent of surface protection. To list the structures of the body in which it operates and discuss its relationship with circulating immunoglobulin

Immunoglobulin-A, already briefly described, has some additional qualities that have proven particularly significant. It has been mentioned that this immunoglobulin is found in 2 forms, serum and secretory. Secretory IgA is the principal antibody of exocrine fluids. Saliva, tears, urine, colostrum and fluids of the nasal and bronchial mucosa, gastrointestinal tract and genital urinary tract all contain this form of IgA as their most prominent immunoglobulin.

The lymphoid tissue synthesizing most of the IgA in these external secretions is found in proximity to the gland or tissue where the secretion originates. In the parotid, for example, it is seen as a conspicious inclusion within the gland substance; in the gastrointestinal tract it is found in diffuse distribution beneath the epithelium. This lymphoid tissue releases its IgA in "both directions," some of it entering the circulating blood and the rest being taken up by the glandular epithelial cells to be modified into a secretory product. The gland cell is thought to form a conjugate of 2 or 3 IgA molecules by adding another molecule that joins them. This latter molecule, a product of the gland cell, is called the *secretory component* or *secretory piece.* Its function is thought to be to stabilize the immunoglobulin against degradation by bacterial or digestive enzymes and to help in the transport of IgA across the gland cell membrane. It is quite clear that secretory IgA bathes mucosal surfaces and can react with bacterial, viral or other antigen that provoke its synthesis. What is not clear is whether this is essential to the defense of these surfaces. IgA deficiency states have been described; however, in many cases there is a compensatory hyperplasia of lymphoid tissue producing other classes of immunoglobulins.

It now seems quite certain that in the healthy individual secretory IgA mediates a kind of immunologic defense that is independent of systemic immunity and may even be confined to a limited area of mucosal surface. Local immunity in a segment of the gastrointestinal tract, for example, is provoked by and reacts against only antigens traversing that segment (Illustration 1-16). It does not show up as either circulating antibodies or antibodies secreted onto any other surface. The most apparent benefit of local surface immunity is resistance to the penetration of pathogens that use the surface as a portal of entry or toxins that poison surface tissue.

The phenomenon of local immunity has recently proven of critical importance in achiev-

1-16. SEGMENTAL REACTION OF GASTROINTESTINAL TRACT (IgA)

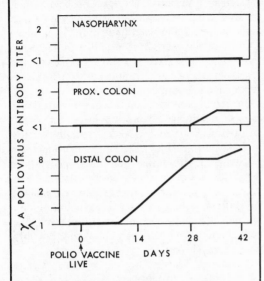

Secretory IgA poliovirus antibody response in the nasopharynx and portions of the colon following local immunization of the distal colon with live-attenuated polio vaccine

(Reproduced from Ogra, P. L. and Karzon, D. T. The role of immunoglobulins in the mechanism of mucosal immunity to virus infection. Pediat. Clin. N. Amer. 17:385, 1970.)

ing immunologic protection against influenza and cholera, diseases that have long resisted control by more conventional immunization techniques.

Additional Reading

Feldman, B. H. et al. Local immunomechanism of the urinary tract. Invest. Urol. 8:575, 1971
Ogra, P. L. and Karzon, D. T. The role of immunoglobulins in the mechanism of mucosal immunity to virus infection. Pediat. Clin. N. Amer. 17:385, 1970
Waldman, R. H. Immune Mechanisms on Secretory Surfaces. Postgrad. Med. 50:78, 1971

CHEMICAL MEDIATORS OF HUMORAL IMMUNOLOGIC REACTIONS

LEARNING OBJECTIVE

To be able to discuss the pharmacologic properties of antigen-antibody complexes formed with each of the 5 major classes of immunoglobulins and describe the following 2 mediator mechanisms in detail:
  a) the histamine release mechanism
  b) the complement system

Just as important as the recognition of foreign material is the ability of the body to cope with it once it has been detected. To assure that non-self material is destroyed as rapidly as it can be discovered antigen-antibody (Ag-Ab) complexes are coupled to inflammatory reactions through a variety of chemical mediators. In fact, these mediators are so much a part of both immunity and inflammation that it is difficult to decide where they should be discussed. They will be mentioned here and once again in the subject of inflammation, using a somewhat different emphasis.

In foregoing sections we have examined the recognition mechanism of humoral immunity; we must now look briefly at the way in which the reaction that follows is made the absolutely automatic outcome of antigen-antibody complex formation. Although the picture is far from clear, it appears that in the case of

1-17. REACTIONS PROVOKED BY Ig COMPLEXES

IgG

fixes complement through which it is coupled to the acute inflammatory response

IgA

neutralizing antibody, apparently not coupled to any reaction

IgM

fixes complement, coupled to acute inflammation

IgD

nothing known of properties of complex

IgE

coupled to histamine release mechanism and other mediators of acute inflammation

1. The Histamine Release Mechanism

Histamine is the only one of the chemical mediators of humoral immunity that exists in its active form before the reaction begins. It is released from cells and cell-like reservoirs (mast cells, platelets and even neutrophils) following the union between antigen and a molecule of cytophilic IgE fixed to the surface of the reservoir. Its release can also be brought about secondary to complement fixation.

In its action as local hormone, histamine causes arteriolar dilatation, increased capillary permeability and, when the reaction occurs in association with the lungs, bronchiolar constriction. Histamine does not persist long within tissues because it is easily diffusible and quickly degraded by ubiquitous amine oxidases. An inflammatory reaction mediated only by histamine would be simple and short-lived; the best and most familiar example would probably be *urticaria* (hives).

Histamine usually acts in concert with a more obscure substance known as SRS-A (the so-called slow reacting substance of anaphy-

humoral immunity we are dealing with 2 principles:

1) The character of the reaction will be determined by the class of immunoglobulins participating in the complex. (Reactions associated with each major class of immunoglobulins are described in Illustration 1-17.)
2) The ensuing reaction is caused by the release or activation of intermediates that are usually pre-formed and available as inactive precursors. These intermediates act as "local hormones" in that they are produced and act in the same area. We will return to the concept of the local hormone in our discussion of inflammation. For now we will look at only 2 of the now numerous chemical mediator systems, the *histamine release mechanism* and the *complement system.*

1-18. COMPLEMENT FIXATION SEQUENCE

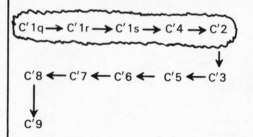

The eleven proteins that make up the complement system form nine "activated" components when fixed in a definite sequence: the encircled group represents the "barrier" sequence: very little pharmacologic effect is noted until after fixation of C'3

1-19. PHARMACOLOGIC EFFECTS OF COMPLEMENT COMPONENTS

component	action
C'3 and C'4	IMMUNE ADHERENCE adherence between antigens and cells is enhanced
C'3	OPSONIZATION phagocytosis and intracellular killing of bacteria is promoted
C'3 and C'5	ANAPHYLATOXIN histamine is released
C'3 and C'5, 6, 7	CHEMOTAXIS neutrophils are attracted
Entire sequence	MEMBRANOLYSIS enzymatic destruction of cell wall of certain bacteria and plasma membrane of alien cells

laxis) as well as the kallekrein-kinin system which will be mentioned again in the next subject.

2. The Complement System

Since complement is such an important component of humoral immunity, we must take an appropriate amount of time to review this rather complex subject.

Complement is the term used in reference to a group of 11 serum proteins that normally circulate as inactive precursors. Each of these proteins is fixed in a definite sequence to IgG and IgM antigen-antibody complexes and, depending upon the number of proteins fixed, can give rise to up to 9 extremely versatile agents with very different pharmacologic actions.

Although complement is usually activated by fixation to IgG and IgM complexes, the formation of active complement can be brought about directly by certain kinds of chemicals, most notably the endotoxins of gram-negative bacteria. There may be a defensive need to activate complement directly but it frequently leads to a distressful situation such as severe shock (generalized circulatory collapse).

The normal fixing of complement by IgG and IgM complexes actually provides several modes of reaction as possible outcomes of 1 immunologic event. The sequence of activation and a brief description of the effect of each of the 9 activated components is diagrammed in Illustration 1-18 and briefly described in Illustration 1-19.

Additional Reading

Orange, R. P. and Austen, K. F. Chemical mediators of immediate hypersensitivity. Hosp. Pract. 6:79, 1971
Ruddy, S. et al. The complement system of man. N. Engl. J. Med. 287:642, 1972

CELLULAR IMMUNITY AND THE SENSITIZED LYMPHOCYTE

LEARNING OBJECTIVE

To be able to discuss in detail the role of the sensitized lymphocyte in cellular immunity, including
   a) discrimination of cellular immunity
   b) the sequence of events following an encounter between the sensitized lymphocyte and its antigen
   c) the hypothetical "tissue surveillance" function of cellular immunity

1. Strategy of the Cellular Immunologic System

We have seen that the antibody (immunoglobulin) serves as the agent of specificity in humoral immunity and that, upon encountering its antigen and forming a complex, any one of a variety of reactions can ensue, the quality of which is determined by the type of immunoglobulin participating in the complex. In somewhat this same way, the sensitized lymphocyte functions as the agent of specificity in cellular immunity, but the similarity is only vague at best. Cellular immunity is very different from its humoral counterpart and an appreciation of this difference is essential to the proper understanding of many disease states. Three prominent qualities of cellular immunity are listed in Illustration 1-20 and compared to the same qualities in the humoral immunologic response.

2. The Cellular Immunologic Reaction

A large number of sensitized lymphocytes is formed when an antigen is brought into contact with immunocompetent cells of the cellular immune system; this happens as the antigen becomes entrapped in peripheral lymphoid structures (lymph nodes and spleen). Once formed, sensitized lymphocytes are released from these structures and distributed widely throughout the body where eventually only a very few of them will manage to come in contact with the antigen that provoked their generation.

Upon encountering their antigen a very small number of these cells can initiate a reaction that is rapidly expanded through another of the many examples of biologic amplification. They do this by undergoing a series of changes during which they proliferate and form a group of similarly committed cells at the site of antigen recognition. In the course of the reaction they also marshall other cells to active participation by elaborating a whole series of chemical mediators that will be discussed in more detail later.

1-20. CELLULAR IMMUNITY (AS COMPARED TO HUMORAL)

1) MORE DISCRIMINATING

2) MORE ABLE TO REACH SEQUESTERED AREAS OF BODY

3) REACTION IS AMPLIFIED LOCALLY AND TENDS TO REMAIN MORE CONFINED

The object of a cellular immunologic reaction is, of course, the same as that of a humoral reaction, to rid the body of alien material and preserve the integrity of native tissue. The meeting between the sensitized lymphocyte and its antigen is complicated and poorly understood; however, a reaction that results seems to include a variety of means of eliminating the antigen as a threat. Lymphocytes attack the antigen directly or, unfortunately, even native tissue containing the antigen. They proliferate and release mediators that direct macrophages and perhaps other kinds of cells to join in the attack. The effect is (usually) the destruction of the antigen or at least its neutralization at the center of a granuloma (a lesion to be discussed later).

3. Antigen Recognition by the Sensitized Lymphocyte

Far less is known about recognition in cellular immunity than about the same step in humoral immunity. No immunoglobulin (at least in the usual sense) has yet been isolated from a cellular reaction and at this writing it is not at all clear how recognition is even accomplished. However it manages to recognize its antigen, the discrimination of the sensitized lymphocyte probably exceeds that of the antibody. Many examples of cross reactivity can be pointed out in humoral reactions, but the cellular system seems remarkably free of confusion. Add to this the ability of the lymphocyte to wander actively throughout most tissues and it can be seen that the possibility for recognition, of even the most subtle change, is greater in cellular immunity than in humoral immunity. The difference is analogous to that between the National Guard and the FBI. The former deals with gross violations of order while the latter detects and apprehends threats to national integrity that are far more subtle.

4. The Tissue Surveillance Function of Cellular Immunity

Because of its exquisitely developed discrimination and its ability to wander just about anywhere in the body, many authorities postulate a tissue surveillance service as part of the function of the cellular immune system.

Although the picture is neither clear nor

1-21. INCIDENCE OF MALIGNANCY DURING NORMAL LIFE SPAN

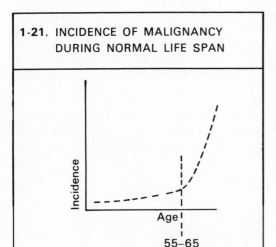

CHEMICAL MEDIATORS OF CELLULAR IMMUNE REACTIONS

LEARNING OBJECTIVE

To be able to compare and contrast the general quality of the mediators of cellular immunity with those of humoral immunity, outlining the role of chemical mediators in the cellular immune response and *briefly* describing the actions of:

    a) migration inhibitory factor
    b) mononuclear cell chemotactic factor
    c) blastogenic factor
    d) transfer factor

complete, it is at least conceptually helpful to think of the cellular immune system as having evolved as a means of ridding the body of dangerously deviant cells or of native structural material that is no longer self-conforming. This function could be particularly important in that it is a means of destroying transformed cells that might otherwise go on to form a life-threatening cancer. Support for this concept is drawn from the well known increase in the incidence of malignancy seen with advancing age (Illustration 1-21).

But, whatever its part in tissue surveillance, it is clear that cellular immunity also protects us against certain kinds of invading pathogens. Curiously, these pathogens are mostly higher microbes such as mycobacteria (the bacterium of tuberculosis, for example) and fungi. The action of cellular immunity against higher pathogens may have developed in parallel with the tissue surveillance mechanism at a time when animals were becoming complex to a degree that some mechanism was needed to monitor the condition of highly specialized and strongly isolated tissues as well as cope with new forms of pathogenic organisms.

Additional Reading

Keast, D. Immunosurveillance and cancer. Lancet, 710, Oct 3, 1970

Mackaness, G. B. Cell mediated immunity to infection. Hosp. Pract. 5:73, 1970

Schlossman, S. F. and Yaron, A. Immunochemical studies on the specificity of cellular and antibody-mediated immune reactions. Ann. N. Y. Acad. Sci. 169:108, 1970

Just as humoral immunity depends upon mediators for its reactions so does cellular immunity depend upon similar agents. In the latter case, however, the origin and function of mediators is quite different. We have seen that the mediators of humoral immunity are either pre-formed or exist as latent systems within the

---

1-22. CHEMICAL MEDIATORS OF CELLULAR IMMUNE REACTIONS

1) **MIGRATION INHIBITORY FACTOR (MIF)**
    prevents migration of macrophages from a capillary tube *in vitro*, function *in vivo* probably relates to lymphocyte control of macrophage

2) **MONONUCLEAR CELL CHEMOTACTIC FACTOR**
    attracts macrophages

3) **BLASTOGENIC FACTOR**
    promotes cell proliferation

4) **TRANSFER FACTOR**
    transfers specific sensitivity, originally described as an agent of transfer between animals

blood. We have also seen that these agents are activated following immune complex formation. Quite in contrast, *mediators of cellular immune reactions are products of the sensitized lymphocyte and are not elaborated until this cell encounters its antigen.* They are produced only where and when they are needed. It may be assumed, therefore, that they are produced sparingly and must be very labile so as to restrict the range of their actions to the immediate area of antigen encounter.

Upon recognizing its antigen the sensitized lymphocyte becomes a veritable factory of special hormone-like products. The list of those described to date is long and confusing so rather than present the entire catalog a few examples are cited in Illustration 1-22.

Additional Reading

Lawrence, H. S. and Valentine, F. T. Transfer factor and other mediators of cellular immunity. Am. J. Path. 60:437, 1970

PRIMARY AND SECONDARY PATTERNS OF IMMUNOLOGIC RESPONSE

LEARNING OBJECTIVE

To be able to compare and contrast the primary and secondary responses in the humoral and cellular immunologic systems mentioning the following:
   a) immunoglobulin patterns in the primary and secondary humoral responses
   b) morphologic changes in peripheral lymphoid tissue in both types of response
   c) the "second-set" response

By and large it is the character of the antigen that determines which of the major systems (humoral or cellular) will respond. Many antigens, of course, are very complex and elicit reactions from both; others are noted for being highly selective. For example, a small molecule (hapten) forming an antigenic complex with a native tissue protein will elicit a predominately cellular reaction whereas pneumococcal polysaccharide causes a nearly pure humoral reaction.

On first exposure, an antigen will cause a *primary response* and, on subsequent exposures, a *secondary response.* The 2 differ in that the former takes longer to reach a peak and, with respect to the humoral system, is characterized by a different relative rate of synthesis of IgM and IgG. The difference will be discussed in detail below but we must first examine the way in which the antigen is introduced to lymphoid tissue.

All reactions, primary or secondary, humoral or cellular, begin within peripheral lymphoid tissue.

1. Immunization and Primary Reaction

The first steps in the primary reaction are comparable in both the humoral and cellular responses and can be described as follows:
1) An antigen, having gained access to tissue, drains through lymphatic vessels or is carried in the blood stream to an organized lymphoid structure. In the lymph system this would be a node; in the blood stream, the spleen.
2) The antigen is taken up by a cell which initiates the reaction. The first cell to ingest the antigen is still a matter of controversy but is known to be some kind of phagocyte.
3) Lymphocytes are caused to undergo proliferation and transformation to plasma cells (humoral response) or sensitization (cellular response).
4) In the humoral response the plasma cell (or precursor) produces antibody that is carried by circulating lymph into the blood stream. In the cellular response the sensitized lymphocyte is, itself, released into the lymph and later seen as the typical small lymphocyte in circulating blood.

Germinal centers such as are found in the cortical area of the lymph node are known to be involved in the humoral response. These germinal centers are occupied by the cell line

1-23. DIFFERENTIAL IMMUNOGLOBULIN SYNTHESIS IN PRIMARY AND SECONDARY IMMUNOLOGIC RESPONSES

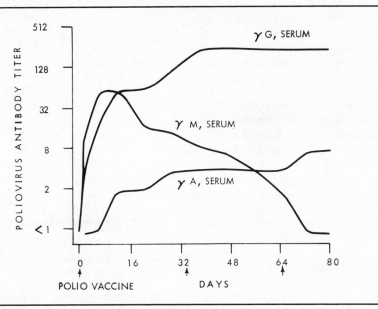

(Reproduced from Ogra, P. L. and Karzon, D. T.: The role of immunoglobulins in the mechanism of mucosal immunity to virus infection. Pediat. Clin. N. from Amer. 17:385, 1970.)

1-24. IMMUNIZATION

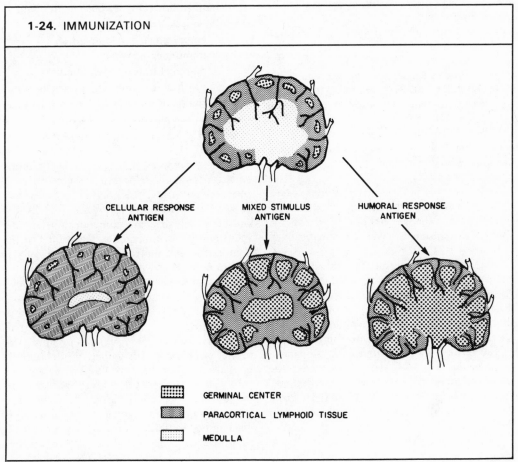

(Reproduced from Bickley, H. C. Immunity and oral disease: A synopsis of the science of immunity. J. Am. Dent. Assn. 79:368, 1969.)

derived from Peyer's patch tissue (in the human). In cellular immunity, the primary response takes place in paracortical tissue where thymus or theta-carrying lymphocytes are found. If an organism responds to an antigen with the humoral response, germinal centers are seen to enlarge and selected lymphocyte undergo development to plasma cells which are known to produce the specific immunoglobulins. These plasma cells become crowded into the medullary portion of the responding node where they continue to manufacture and release their antibodies.

In a cellular response, the selected lymphocyte is thought to undergo a kind of transformation during which it assumes the appearance of a very primitive cell which then proliferates and becomes a much larger clone of committed, sensitized lymphocytes. In this case, paracortical tissue enlarges compressing the medulla. These changes are shown diagrammatically in Illustration 1-23.

With regard to its manifestations in peripheral blood the primary humoral response will be characterized by:

1) The early appearance of IgM and IgA antibodies.
2) The somewhat later appearance of IgG antibodies (in 1 study IgG was detectable only after the 18th day following antigen exposure and then only in very small amounts).

Upon re-exposure by the same route per a comparable dose of the same antigen the body manifests a secondary humoral response. This is characterized by:

1) A sharp rise in IgG shortly after exposure.
2) A slight but much less pronounced response of the IgM and IgA systems.

These 2 patterns are shown diagrammatically in Illustration 1-24.

From the foregoing it can be seen that IgG-secreting cells appear to be the principal "memory cells" of the humoral system. They store the immunologic history of the individual and are responsive for his not "forgetting" the antigen. This ability to remember immunologic exposure is known as *anamnesia*. A comparable phenomenon can be demonstrated in the cellular immune system with the "second-set" response where a second graft of tissue from the same donor is rejected more quickly than the first.

Additional Reading

Bandilla, K. K. et al. Immunoglobulin classes of antibodies produced in the primary and secondary responses in man. Clin. Exp. Immunol. 5:627, 1969
Rowley, M. J., and MacKay, I. R. Measurement of antibody-producing capacity in man. Clin. Exp. Immunol. 5:407, 1969

THE DEVELOPMENT OF IMMUNOCOMPETENCE

LEARNING OBJECTIVE

To be able to describe the development of the dual component immunologic system in the human and discuss the immunologic status of the human fetus and newborn mentioning the following:

  a) embryologic development of immunocompetence
  b) maternal transfer of antibodies
  c) synthesis of antibodies by the neonate
  d) the significance of IgM in cord serum

1. Embryologic Development

In the developing embryo, all cells mediating both types of immunity are thought to have a common precursor, the primitive reticular cell of bone marrow. From this stage, the cells that will eventually become immunocompetent develop along 1 of 2 main lines, 1 leading to the humoral system and the other to the cellular system. Cells that will ultimately carry out the humoral response must migrate from bone marrow to an organized lymphoid structure associated with the gastrointestinal tract, whereas those destined for the cellular system must first spend time in the thymus. The former structure differs among species. In birds it is known to be the bursa of Fabricius (Illustration 1-25), whereas in man it is thought to be Peyer's patch tissue of the ileum. The entire scheme of embryologic differentiation is diagrammed in Illustration 1-26.

chapter 2
INFLAMMATION

INFLAMMATION: ONE WORD WITH MANY MEANINGS

LEARNING OBJECTIVE

To be able to differentiate briefly among the following 3 conventionally recognized types of inflammation:
   a) acute inflammation
   b) chronic inflammation
   c) granulomatous inflammation

One of the most difficult subjects in the entire science of pathology to teach effectively on the first try is inflammation. This is undoubtedly because the term, itself, is far too inclusive. It is conventionally used in reference to a large group of normal reactions provoked by injury or alien material. These include defense mechanisms based on non-immunologic systems as well as some based on both humoral and cellular immunity.

There are many different clinical patterns of inflammation but, according to traditional doctrine, all are reducible to one of 3 basic types (Illustration 2-1). Since much of currently used terminology is soundly anchored in this idea we will use it as the basis for our organization of this subject. These 3 types of inflammation may be contrasted as follows.

1. Acute Inflammation

Acute inflammation is a response of relatively short duration (days or weeks) that most often clears without residual scar. It is manifested as changes in the caliber and permeability of blood vessels followed by an outpouring of fluid and cells called an *exudate*.

2. Chronic Inflammation

Chronic inflammation is a response of longer duration (months or years) in which elements

---

2-1. THREE BASIC TYPES OF INFLAMMATION

1) ACUTE
   short duration (days or weeks), clears without residual scar, consists of vascular changes followed by neutrophil exudate

2) CHRONIC
   long duration (months or years), scar is formed, consists of concurrent acute reaction (late stages) and fibrosis

3) GRANULOMATOUS
   based on action of sensitized lymphocyte, seen in transient and chronic forms, chronic lesion is the characterisitc "granuloma"

---

of an acute reaction and fibrous repair can be seen concurrently and during which a scar is formed at the site of the lesion.

3. Granulomatous Inflammation

Granulomatous inflammation is a response of varying duration now thought based on the action of the sensitized lymphocyte. In its transient form it may leave no scar, whereas in its chronic form it assumes the architecture of the *granuloma*, the healing of which results in scar or a calcific deposit being left at the site of the lesion.

Additional Reading

Jensen, K. D. and Killman, S-A. (ed). Aspects of Inflammation. Baltimore, Williams and Wilkins Co., 1970

PROVOCATION AND CONTROL OF ACUTE INFLAMMATION

LEARNING OBJECTIVE

To be able to discuss the acute inflammatory reaction as a response to injury or the presence of alien material within the body, mentioning the following:

  a) provocation of acute inflammation by injury
  b) provocation through a humoral immunologic reaction
  c) chemical mediation of acute inflammation

---

1. General Features of Acute Inflammation

Acute inflammation is perhaps the most prominent reaction of living tissue to injury. It is distinguished from all other reactions by two microanatomic features:

  1) Characteristic changes in vessels at the inflammatory site.
  2) The outpouring of fluid and cells from these altered vessels. — *Exudation*

Even the earliest medical writers were familiar with acute inflammation. Celsus, in the first century A.D., enumerated its first 4 cardinal signs:

  1) Tumor (swelling).
  2) Rubor (redness).
  3) Calor (increased heat).
  4) Dolor (pain).
  5) Functio laesa (loss of function).

and the fifth was added by Galen in the second century A.D.

Although early physicians were familiar with acute inflammation, they considered it more of a disease than a corrective reaction. John Hunter (1728-1793) was perhaps the first to recognize the acute response as a defense reaction. He championed the concept that the appearance of copious exudate indicated that the body was winning the contest for recovery, the principle of "laudable pus."

With the development of the microscope and histologic techniques, the study of inflammation shifted to microanatomic description and later to combined microanatomic and biochemical analysis. Today, although much more is known about acute inflammatory reactions, many key insights are still hidden and a great deal must yet be learned. This is particularly true of the intricate molecular mechanism through which acute inflammation is initiated, controlled and terminated.

The acute inflammatory response is provoked in 2 ways (Illustration 2-2). Although most injuries would consist of both types of provocation, we will consider each separately.

2. The Relationship of Acute Inflammation to Injury

It has been stated that acute inflammation is a response to injury or alien material. Either injury or a *humoral* immunologic reaction is sufficient to provoke acute inflammation, but in most cases it seems certain that both are

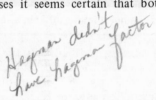

2-2. PROVOCATION OF THE ACUTE INFLAMMATORY REACTION

1) THROUGH INJURY

injury
↓
action of mediators
↓
reaction

2) THROUGH A HUMORAL IMMUNOLOGIC REACTION

antigen-antibody complex
↓
action of mediators
↓
reaction

actually involved. Either may initiate the reaction, but undoubtedly the other adds its influence shortly after the process is underway.

It now seems that even the slightest tissue damage may be adequate to bring about acute inflammation. This remarkable sensitivity is due to the function of native (but not denatured) collagen in the activation of a molecular system that sets off the acute inflammatory response. Since collagen is a component of basement membranes it follows that even the momentary, simple retraction of an endothelial cell would be sufficient to at least initiate an acute response.

The molecular "transducer" that intervenes between injury and the acute inflammatory response is *Hageman factor,* one of the 13 known molecular components of the intrinsic coagulation mechanism. (In the latter scheme it is known as Factor XII.) Hageman factor circulates in the blood as an inactive precursor. In effect, it detects the results of injury (collagen exposure) and converts this "signal" to a complex inflammatory response.

It has been known for some time that Hageman factor activation depends upon its being fixed to some regular crystalline or paracrystalline (anisotropic) surface. Activation, for example, will result from contact with glass, kaolin and other ionic surfaces. This quality of Hageman factor permits its being activated by collagen since the collagen fibril is a crystalline formation made up of the aggregation of tropocollagen monomers. Hageman factor can also be activated by contact with other ionic polymers, deposits of sodium urate (the tophi of gout) and endotoxin. Once activated, Hageman factor serves as the simultaneous activator of a number of molecular systems which it brings together in coordinated activity. These systems serve as the chemical mediators of acute inflammation and initiate each of its subsequent stages. The relationship between injury and acute inflammation is diagrammed in Illustration 2-3.

3. Relationship of Acute Inflammation to Humoral Immunity

Just as injury can bring about acute inflammation by exposing collagen and and activating Hageman factor, some kinds of humoral immunologic reactions can do much the same

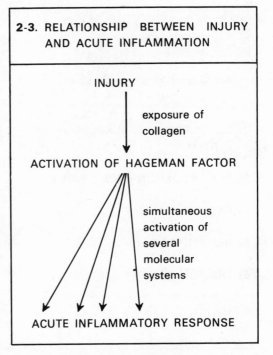

2-3. RELATIONSHIP BETWEEN INJURY AND ACUTE INFLAMMATION

INJURY

exposure of collagen

ACTIVATION OF HAGEMAN FACTOR

simultaneous activation of several molecular systems

ACUTE INFLAMMATORY RESPONSE

through histamine release and the fixation of complement. Bear in mind, however, that it is the *humoral* system that provokes acute inflammation, not the cellular system. The latter appears to mediate granulomatous inflammation and will be considered later.

4. Chemical Mediators of Acute Inflammation

However the acute inflammatory response is provoked (injury or immunity), its progress soon comes under the control of a group of molecular systems known collectively as *chemical mediators.* These have also been termed *local hormones, humoral mediators* and *autacoids.*

Whereas a true hormone is a chemical messenger produced in one place and broadcast to distant tissues through the blood stream, a local hormone or chemical mediator is produced in active form only at the location where it is expected to work. It is prevented from becoming widely disseminated by a very efficient destruction mechanism that simply deactivates it if it diffuses far from the site of its production. Although useful in a particular

2-4. CHEMICAL MEDIATORS OF ACUTE INFLAMMATION

---

1) THE INTRINSIC COAGULATION MECHANISM

2) THE PLASMIN (FIBRINOLYSIN) SYSTEM

3) THE KALLIKREIN-KININ SYSTEM

4) PROSTAGLANDINS

5) HISTAMINE

6) THE COMPLEMENT SYSTEM

place, at a particular time these mediators would be extremely dangerous if distributed in active form throughout the body.

We have already encountered 3 examples of such material in histamine, the complement system, and Hageman factor. In gathering together all of the agents and systems that act as local hormones in the acute inflammatory response one would have to include at least those listed in Illustration 2-4. Very obviously a thorough treatment of the chemical mediation of acute inflammation is beyond the scope of this discussion. The model we will be using here is outlined in Illustration 2-5.

Injury or a humoral immunologic reaction (usually both) causes the activation of several mediator systems including kallikrein-kinin system and complement. These lead to early vascular changes and later to the more profound and sustained vessel alterations associ-

---

2-5. CHEMICAL MEDIATION OF ACUTE INFLAMMATION

INJURY - - - - - - - - - - - - - - - -
(with exposure of native collagen)

ACTIVATION OF   HUMORAL REACTION
HAGEMAN FACTOR   (histamine release)

ACTIVATION OF   BINDING OF
KALLIKREIN   COMPLEMENT
(causing formation of kinin)   (further histamine release)

EARLY STAGES OF ACUTE INFLAMMATION
(preliminary vascular changes)

FORMATION OF: FURTHER ACTION OF
fibrin clot   BOUND COMPLEMENT
plasmin   chemotaxis
additional intermediates   opsonization

LATER STAGES OF ACUTE INFLAMMATION
(sustained vascular changes and exudation)

2-6. LOCAL EFFECTS OF CHEMICAL MEDIATORS OF ACUTE IN-FLAMMATION

---

1) MICROCIRCULATORY DILATATION

2) ENHANCED MICROCIRCULATORY PERMEABILITY *of walls of venules + arterioles*

3) LEUKOTAXIS — *or chemotaxis*

4) PAIN — *caused by action of kinins*

a control of body

ated with exudation. Since mediators are rapidly destroyed if they diffuse far from the inflammatory site, the process is localized as a circumscribed lesion. Local effects of mediators are usually summarized as those listed in Illustration 2-6. A resolution of the acute inflammatory process results when mediators are no longer supplied in active form.

Additional Reading

Gözsy, B. and Kato, L. Balancing Mechanisms in Acute Inflammation. Quebec, Institute of Microbiology and Hygiene, Montreal University, 1970

Kellermeyer, R. W. and Graham, R. C. Kinins: possible physiologic and pathologic roles in man. N. Engl. J. Med. 279:754, 1968

Pike, J. E. Prostaglandins. Sci. Amer. 225:84, 1971

Ratnoff, O. D. et al. The demise of John Hageman. N. Engl. J. Med. 279:760, 1968

Sherry, S. The kallikrein system: a basic defense mechanism. Hosp. Pract. 6:75, 1970

STAGES OF ACUTE INFLAMMATION

LEARNING OBJECTIVE

To be able to describe local tissue changes and other events occurring in the following 6 stages of acute inflammation:

a) injury
b) immediate vasoconstriction
c) vasodilatation and vessel permeability changes
d) exudation and consolidation
e) neutralization of noxious stimulus
f) resolution or repair

Now that we have considered how acute inflammation is provoked and mediated we will look at the phenomenon as a whole. To do so, we must confine our first efforts to the description of the most rudimentary kind of acute lesion. In summoning such an uncomplicated reaction we will need to imagine a simple injury that will produce a correspondingly simple kind of inflammation; a good example would be the mosquito bite. Keep in mind, however, that although this is a very simple inflammatory reaction, the prolongation or exaggeration of any stage would result in a lesion of very different appearance. We are merely using the mosquito bite as an example of a mild injury that elicits a balanced, complete, acute inflammatory lesion. This type of inflammation is said to be acute because of certain features of duration and morphology, i.e.:

1) The whole sequence is of comparatively short duration.
2) The microscopic morphology of tissue changes that occur is typical of this kind of reaction in that they consist mainly of vascular changes followed by the appearance of an exudate containing the neutrophil leukocyte, the hallmark of acute inflammation.

A brief description of the 6 steps of acute inflammation as they might be seen in the mosquito bite are listed in Illustration 2-7 and described below.

1. Injury

With the insertion of the mosquito's proboscis, cells are disrupted releasing their con-

[handwritten margin notes at top: infl. cite becomes consolidated / Clot obstructs cap. draining + blood flow]

2-7. STAGES OF ACUTE INFLAM-MATION

1) INJURY

2) VASOCONSTRICTION

3) VASODILATATION AND PERME-ABILITY CHANGES

4) EXUDATION AND CONSOLIDATION

5) NEUTRALIZATION OF NOXIOUS STIMULI

6) RESOLUTION OR REPAIR

---

tents into the extracellular milieu and a foreign irritant (the mosquito's saliva) is deposited in the area.

2. Vasoconstriction

The first reaction to this injury is the sudden but very transient constriction of arterioles. This is mediated by vascular nerves and is not a prominent part of all responses. *[handwritten: helps c re-establish homeostasis]*

[handwritten margin: sudden tightening of vessels]

3. Vasodilatation and Permeability Changes

Since this is a very complicated step it is discussed in more detail below. Note, however, that it can be biphasic. There is the possibility of an early, transient stage followed by a late stage that is maintained for as long as the need dictates. Within vessels at the site of injury, circulation slows and finally becomes stagnant. A host of changes now begin to affect the normal permeability of the capillary endothelial membrane preparatory to exudation. Concurrently, changes occur at the surface of cells in the area of the lesion.

[handwritten margin: account for redness of area]

4. Exudation and Consolidation

Exudate is a complex of formed elements and solutes that emits from the circulatory system in an area of acute inflammation. It differs from a non-inflammatory effusion (transudate) in that it contains cells. The

presence of cells in a fluid found in tissue spaces or body cavities means that an exudate is involved and is suggestive of inflammation. Consolidation of the developing lesion results from the formation of a fibrin clot which is a prominent part of all acute inflammatory reactions. *[handwritten: leukocytes fibrinogen - forms scab/clot / forms clot]*

5. Neutralization of Noxious Stimuli

The neutralization of noxious material and of cell debris is largely a function of the exudate and its cells. Details of this step will be discussed below.

6. Resolution or Repair

Once irritants and cell debris have been cleared from the area, the fibrin clot that has formed as part of the reaction is digested and chemical mediators sustaining vascular changes are destroyed. Circulation is re-established and the injured area returns to normal. In an injury as innocuous as a mosquito bite, those few cells which have been destroyed are replaced by simple regeneration. If damage had been more extensive or had it included cells or structures that could not regenerate, the defect would be filled in with fibrous connective tissue (scar) in a process called *repair*. This will be discussed in detail later.

The results of the acute inflammatory reaction described above are much the same as those of any other:

a) The elimination of an irritant.

b) Clearing of the debris resulting from the death of cells.

c) The restoration of normal tissue function. The task in this case is a comparatively easy one. The damage is minimal, the injurious stimulus does not persist, the irritant substances are not living, cannot proliferate and would be present only in very small amounts; therefore the degree of tissue change required for an adequate response is minimal. If any of the above would have been more grave, however, as they would certainly have been in most cases of trauma or infection, the response in order to be adequate would have to be distributed over a larger area and "cascade" to greater intensity. The lesion would then appear quite different. Consider, for example, the difference between the mosquito bite and a large, painful boil; both are based on the same 6 steps yet appear almost unrelated.

[handwritten at bottom: exudate dominates c boil. / when 1 stage exaggerated lesion looks different.]

generalization of a. inf - life threatening response (handwritten)

urticaria (hive) - lesion only goes to early-transient stage - vascular phenomenon (handwritten)

don't really see (handwritten)

- prominent (handwritten)

LOCAL FACTORS IN ACUTE INFLAMMATION

LEARNING OBJECTIVE

To be able to organize and discuss a description of changes occurring at the site of the inflammatory lesion (local factors) under the following headings:
   a) biphasic vascular response
   b) function of each type of participating cell
   c) biphasic cellular response
   d) blood sludging

2-9. BIPHASIC VASCULAR CHANGES IN ACUTE INFLAMMATION

1) EARLY-TRANSIENT STAGE
   mediated by histamine and other labile substances, short duration

early kinins (handwritten)

usually preferentially involved (handwritten)

2) LATE-SUSTAINED STAGE
   mediated by kinins, complement and other long-acting substances

---

Acute inflammation gives rise to a lesion that is protective only when it remains confined. The acute inflammatory response is a local reaction consisting of a series of changes happening within a well circumscribed area. As examples of these local factors in acute inflammation, we will consider the 3 listed in Illustration 2-8.

1. Vascular Alterations

An important component of acute inflammation is the alteration of the microvasculature leading to exudation. As mentioned previously, it is known that there is at least the possibility for a biphasic process consisting of the 2 stages listed in Illustration 2-9. Each of these is mediated by a different kind of agent. True early-transient vasodilatation (when present) is undoubtedly caused by short-lived, labile substances, foremost among which is histamine. Whereas histamine is unquestionably the first

mediator in certain kinds of immunologic inflammatory reactions, its general utility in this role is questionable.

In most lesions early and late phases of vascular change blend and are difficult to discriminate as separate phenomena mediated by separate agents.

Long-term vascular changes are undoubtedly promoted by a number of very different agents including kinins and complement. Also frequently mentioned in this role is lysolecithin although its role as part of the mediator system has not been elucidated.

2. Exudation

With the slowing of the circulation at the inflammatory site, and with increased permeability of the microvasculature, the stage is set for exudation and the consolidation of the inflammatory site into a rather strictly circumscribed area of special defense activity. *Exudation* is the outpouring of normally intravascular cells and solutes into the injured tissue. The entire strategy of acute inflammation seems to focus on this step. Cells, immunoglobulins, fibrinogen, complement and a host of other agents that normally circulate in anticipation of just such need are now released into the area of tissue injury.

so they can begin acting (handwritten)

The escape of coagulation factors from their normally intravascular location permits the formation of a clot that serves to knit the entire lesion into a contiguous, scaffold-like structure. Clots also form within minor blood and lymph vessels preventing the escape of fluid from the area. In addition to obstructing circulation and drainage, the fibrin mesh of the clot supports inflammatory cells as they go about their task

---

2-8. LOCAL FACTORS IN ACUTE INFLAMMATION

1) VASCULAR ALTERATIONS - *characteristic sign* (handwritten)

2) EXUDATION
   cells of acute inflammation
   biphasic cellular response

3) BLOOD SLUDGING

---

kinins - causes pain (handwritten)

granulomatous - localization very precise (handwritten)

of purging the tissue of pathogens and debris.

Cells associated with the usual acute inflammatory reaction are listed in Illustration 2-10 and will be discussed in that order below.

Neutrophil

The neutrophil is the definitive agent of acute inflammation. It is normally produced by hematopoietic marrow and is distinguished by its lobulated nucleus and neutral-staining cytoplasm. It is heavily endowed with cytoplasmic organelles called lysosomes and, in fact, its classification as a neutrophil *granulocyte* is based on the presence of these structures in its cytoplasm; the granules that establish the classification are actually lysosomes. Lysosomes are vacuole-like organelles bearing a rich variety of hydrolytic enzymes capable of destroying many kinds of biologic material. Neutrophil lysosomes do not take up stain readily and are said to be neutrophilic.

Neutrophils are directed to an inflammatory site by chemotaxis. This is the phenomenon whereby a cell is attracted by the diffusion of a material from an object or location. The cell, in this case the neutrophil, migrates up the concentration gradient toward the source of attractant. As long as the chemotactic signal persists more neutrophils are drawn to the lesion. The life span of the neutrophil in the lesion is very short and their continued presence is dependent upon sustained chemotaxis. The activation of at least 2 of the components of complement is known to release chemotactic

---

2-10. CELLS OF ACUTE INFLAMMA-TION

1) NEUTROPHIL

2) EOSINOPHIL

3) ERYTHROCYTE

4) LYMPHOCYTE

5) MONOCYTE

---

substances. Therefore, should any substance at the inflammatory site react with 1 of the 2 complement-fixing immunoglobulins (IgG or IgM) it may attract neutrophils and become more readily engulfed and digested because of the "opsonizing" effect of this same complement component. Kinins are also somewhat chemotactic but not to the degree exhibited by complement.

Whereas the neutrophil is a voracious phagocyte it is not considered a macrophage because it does not ingest large particulate debris.

As mentioned above, the neutrophil is thought to be able to release a kinin from an inactive substrate molecule normally found in serum. As long as neutrophils remain at the scene, more and more of this kinin will be formed, supporting the vascular changes leading to exudation.

Eosinophil

The eosinophil is another of the granulocyte series of cells and, like the neutrophil, is manufactured in hematopoietic marrow. It, also, exhibits an abundance of cytoplasmic lysomes but, unlike the neutrophil, these stain a brilliant red with eosin. This affinity for eosin is the basis of the term *eosinophil*. The eosinophil is also distinguished by a lobulated nucleus, but the degree of segmentation is less than that of the neutrophil. The function of the eosinophil is still in dispute; it is rarely seen as a prominent component of inflammatory exudate except in longstanding inflammatory lesions of allergy. Nasal polyps resulting from allergic rhinitis, for example, will almost always contain an abundance of eosinophils. An increase in circulating eosinophils (eosinophilia) is also seen in certain allergies as well as in parasitic infestation.

Lymphocyte

Lymphocytes are not seen in the acute inflammatory lesion until its later stages. They are considered part of the "round cell" infiltrate which also includes macrophages. The term lymphocyte is fast becoming inadequate in view of recent descriptions of many different populations of small lymphocytes as well as the usually recognized medium and large types. Also, there is still some question as to the relationship between the lymphocyte and the macrophage. Some authorities hold that the

monocyte - macrophage found in blood

former can actually change into the latter with proper stimulus. It is generally agreed that the principal function of all lymphocytes is as an agent of immunity. This makes their participation in the acute inflammatory response enigmatic. Lymphocytes are produced in lymph nodes, spleen, thymus and bone marrow. We will not attempt any detailed consideration of the lymphocyte because of the enormous complexity of the subject.

1st not produced hematopoietic marrow

Macrophage

Macrophages are large cells with an oval of indented nucleus. They, also, are found in the round cell infiltrate of the later stages of acute inflammation. They persist longer than the neutrophil and presumably attend to the clearance of debris from the resolving lesion. Blood-borne macrophages or monocytes are the cells that arrive at the inflammatory lesion. They are produced in hematopoietic marrow and probably undergo further maturation after they have reached the inflammatory site. The relationship between the sensitized lymphocyte and the macrophage has been discussed; however, the applicability of this cooperative arrangement to the acute inflammatory response is not known. Tissue macrophages or histiocytes (fixed macrophages) take origin from the blood-borne monocyte. Histiocytes are more prominent in granulomatous inflammation and will be discussed later.

Erythrocyte

The presence of erythrocyte outside an endothelium-lined (vascular) space is the technical criterion of hemorrhage. Hemorrhage by diapedesis (in contrast to hemorrhage by angiorrhexis) is often seen as part of the acute inflammatory response. It is not seen in mild, acute inflammation and suggests that permeability changes have been extreme. Infection with certain endotoxin-producing bacteria can cause hemorrhagic tissue necrosis and an extremely hemorrhagic inflammatory response.

Biphasic Cellular Response

Egress of cells from vascular channels during acute inflammation takes place in 2 stages (Illustration 2-11). The first of these begins immediately after permeability changes take

---

2-11. TWO-STAGE CELLULAR RESPONSE IN ACUTE INFLAMMATION

1) EARLY
   neutrophil predominates in exudate

2) LATE
   mononuclear ("round cells") predominate in exudate

lymphocyte & macrophages

---

effect and is characterized by outpouring of neutrophils. These cells exit from blood channels by phenomenon known as *diapedesis*, i.e. to "step across." Neutrophils penetrate through holes that appear in the capillary membrane as it dilates. These holes or gaps frequently become so large that erythrocytes are forced through passively, resulting in hemorrhage by diapedesis.

Emigration of neutrophils constitutes the first stage of cellular egress in the acute inflammatory reaction. The second stage begins even before the first stage is completed and consists of the gradual appearance of mononuclear cells such as lymphocytes and phagocytic cells of the monocyte series.

Despite the ultimate participation of mononuclear cells, it is worth reiterating that the cell most characteristic of the acute inflammatory response is the neutrophil. The cause of the later appearance of mononuclear cells is not known. They may be attracted to the site or may simply be arrested there in their normal cycle of circulation. Whatever the reason, phagocytes soon become very actively engaged in clearing the area of irritants and tissue debris.

3. Blood Sludging

In conjunction with permeability changes in the capillary endothelial membrane a related change is occurring in blood and tissue cells. The surface of most cells, including those of the endothelium, is predominantly electronegative. Mutual repulsion keeps them from colliding with one another and with the wall of blood

2-12. BLOOD SLUDGING

Substances liberated from the acute inflammatory lesion are presumed to neutralize the normally electronegative surfaces of blood cells and endothelium.

1) LOCAL EFFECTS
   disruption of axial flow
   margination of leukocytes
   → rouleau formation
2) SYSTEMIC EFFECTS
   may contribute to increased ESR
   (discussed below)

[handwritten margin notes: "Cause for Blood Sludging", "also lose repulsion between cells & other cells", "Clear zone of plasma keeps blood cells away from wall from damage", "axial stratification breaks down", "leukocytes stick to walls", "stacking up of erythrocytes"]

vessels. Something happens at the site of inflammation, however, that disrupts this relationship. Mutual electrostatic repulsion determines that normal blood flow in a vessel will be *axially stratified* with a cell-free layer of plasma between the wall and the moving cells. As circulation slows, cells begin to contact the endothelium and shortly thereafter neutrophils begin adhering to the vessel walls preparatory to their emigration. This is called "margination" or "pavementing." Also, erythrocytes are seen to stack up in tiny formations resembling piles of poker chips; these are referred to as rouleau (sing. rouleaux). If the inflammation is extensive, blood drawn at this stage will exhibit a more rapid *erythrocyte sedimentation rate* (ESR).

All of these changes in the normal interrelationship among cells are grouped together under the term *blood sludging*. The reason for blood sludging is not known, but it is thought to result from a change in the normal electronegativity of cell surfaces. Its effects, when added to those of other simultaneous changes in the vessel wall, disrupt the normal pattern of circulation through the injured area and provide the conditions necessary for exudation. The 3 components of blood sludging are summarized in Illustration 2-12.

Additional Reading

Ryan, G. B. The origin and sequence of the cells found in the acute inflammatory response. Aust. J. Exp. Biol. Med. Sci. 45:149, 1967

SYSTEMIC FACTORS IN ACUTE INFLAMMATION

LEARNING OBJECTIVE

To be able to discuss systemic changes in acute inflammation under the following 5 headings:
   a) hormonal changes
   b) fever
   c) leukocytosis
   d) alterations in serum proteins
   e) increased ESR

Although acute inflammation is a localized response to injury or alien material, substances liberated from the site of the reaction elicit a number of supportive changes in organs remote from the inflammatory lesion. Some of these are listed in Illustration 2-13. We will see that many of these are valuable as diagnostic signs of inflammatory disease.

1. Hormonal Changes

Just as important as initiating the acute inflammatory response is the body's ability to control its vigor and extent. A quick review at this point will reveal that, without some checking mechanisms, the acute reaction would continue to expand until it became life-threatening. Before this happens, agents liberated from the lesion itself slow the process. A chemical signal is sent to the pituitary which stimulates the adrenal glands to increase the output of glucocorticoids. Among a host of other actions these interfere with the function of complement, exerting an anti-inflammatory effect.

2. Fever

Fever is elevation of body temperature above the normal value of $37°$ C (± 1) ($98.6°$ F) as part of a disease syndrome. Fever occurs in different patterns as listed in Illustration 2-14.

Not all examples of elevated body temperature qualify as fever. Exercise or high environmental temperature, for example, may cause temporary elevation of the body temperature which subsides when the cause is removed. True fever involves a disturbance of *thermoregulator* function. The thermoregulator is a group of

[handwritten note: KNOW!]

2-13. SYSTEMIC FACTORS IN ACUTE INFLAMMATION

1) HORMONAL CHANGES

2) FEVER

   in severe cases accompanied by malaise and lassitude comprising the "syndrome of being sick"

3) LEUKOCYTOSIS

4) ALTERATIONS IN SERUM PROTEINS

5) INCREASED ESR

2-14. PATTERNS OF FEVER

1) HYPERTHERMIC

   temperatures greater than 105°F

2) SUSTAINED

   temperature continued above normal

3) INTERMITTENT

   daily rise with drop below normal

4) REMITTANT

   daily rise without return to normal

5) SEPTIC

   major diurnal variations, often with chills and sweating

6) RELAPSING

   febrile episodes alternating with periods of normal temperature

cells in the hypothalamus that maintain constant body temperature by monitoring body core temperature (blood, muscle) and surface temperatures (skin, respiratory tract) and regulates heat generation through control of metabolism. In fever the thermoregulator is actually set for a higher temperature, much in the same manner as a thermostat is readjusted to raise the temperature of one's home.

The heat used in raising body temperature in fever is obtained from increased metabolic activity, particularly that of voluntary muscle and liver. A cooling effect to restore temperature to normal when the fever subsides is gained by using the skin surface to radiate heat into the environment. Shivering is used to increase heat production in raising the temperature while cutaneous vasodilitation and sweating increases heat loss from the surface and serves to lower it.

Fever is caused by the action of materials called pyrogens. These are released by damaged tissue and have the effect of resetting the thermoregulator to a higher temperature. The body then increases heat production to comply with the new regulatory signals (sometimes so rapidly that it must shiver to do so).

Fever occurs in 3 stages. Each of these is accompanied by the signs and symptoms listed in Illustration 2-15.

Sustained fever leads to loss of appetite as well as increased breakdown of endogenous protein and fat. Rapid use of stored fat may give rise to ketosis and acidosis.

There is a great deal of controversy about the actual benefit of fever. Since prolonged fever has a debilitating effect and may even cause brain damage one wonders if there can be a commensurate therapeutic value. In support of the beneficial effect of fever, it might be mentioned that induced fevers were once used successfully for the treatment of syphilis and that some present day investigators believe that fevers may impair the replication of virus.

3. Leukocytosis

Leukocytosis is a condition in which there is an increase in the number of circulating leukocytes. It is associated with a number of disease states and manifested as white blood cell counts exceeding 10,000 per cu. mm. The range of normal values for adult leukocyte

2-15. STAGES OF FEVER

1) COLD STAGE

body core temperature is rising, cutaneous circulation diminished to conserve heat, skin feels cold, appears blanched, shivering, teeth chattering,"goose pimples"may appear

(handwritten margin note: mechanism for conserving heat as core temp increases)

2) HOT STAGE

body core temperature is constant at new high level, cutaneous circulation is increased to radiate excess heat, skin feels hot, appears red *cutaneous circulation re-established*

3) DEFERVESCENCE

body core temperature is falling, drenching sweat may occur in response to need for rapid loss of heat from cutaneous surface

(handwritten margin note: fever breaks)

counts are presented in Illustration 2-16. The neutrophil is the cell most commonly overrepresented in leukocytosis. The normal neutrophil lives only a short time and is used in great numbers, particularly during a significant acute inflammatory reaction. In the healthy individual, some neutrophils are circulating, others are adhering to vessel walls and a huge reserve is stored in the bone marrow.

Violent exercise washes neutrophils adhering to vessels back into the circulation causing 1 kind of leukocytosis (sometimes reaching 25,000 cells per cu. mm.) In a somewhat different manner, sympathetic reactions (extremes of anxiety and fright) and inflammation cause leukocytosis by stimulating the release of neutrophils from bone marrow reserves. Sustained use of marrow reserves will result in marrow hyperplasia and an increased rate of neutrophil production (Illustration 2-17).

Continued abnormal rates of production result in the release of immature neutrophils into the circulation. These cells are distinquished by a relatively non-segmented, rod-like nucleus in contrast to the mature neutrophil in which the nucleus is divided into 3 or 4 discrete lobes. The presence of a large number of

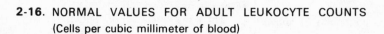

(handwritten note: leukocytosis - usually manifested by ↑ neutrophils)

2-16. NORMAL VALUES FOR ADULT LEUKOCYTE COUNTS
(Cells per cubic millimeter of blood)

	minimum	average	maximum	percent
TOTAL WBC	5,000	7,000–8,000	10,000	100
NEUTROPHILS	3,000	4,000–4,500	7,000	50–70
EOSINOPHILS	50	200	400	1–4
BASOPHILS	0	25	100	0–1
LYMPHOCYTES	1,500	2,000	3,000	25–40
MONOCYTES	−200	400	800	3–8

leukemia = Tumor of white cells, not leukocytosis (handwritten, top left)

"shift to left" - release of immature neutrophils (handwritten, top center/right)

2-17. LEUKOCYTOSIS

1) NORMAL WBC COUNT:
5,000–10,000 cells per cubic mil-limeter of blood (c/mm^3)

2) LEUKOCYTOSIS IS A CONDITION IN WHICH CIRCULATING WHITE CELLS EXCEED 10,000 c/mm^3 (excepting leukemia)

    after strenous exercise —
    sympathetic reactions
    severe pain
    inflammation

rapid circul. washes neutrophils from walls → leukocytosis extremes of light or injection of noripine (handwritten)

(due to Release of marrow reserves (handwritten)

2-18. NEUTROPHIL FORMS

"BAND" OR "STAB" FORM

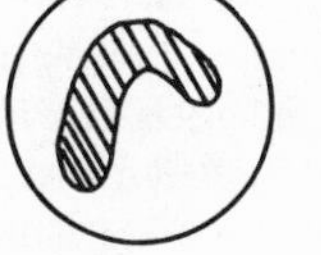

immature / *sign of prolonged inflammation* (handwritten)

curved, rod-shaped nucleus

    intervening stages

MATURE FORM

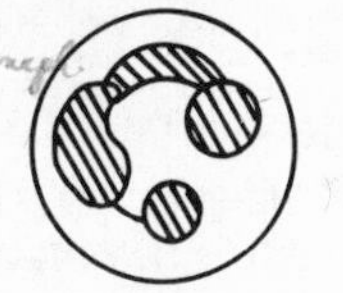

segmented (handwritten)

nucleus has two or more lobes with at least one connected by thread-like filament

---

neutrophils (stab forms or band forms) indicates that the patient has been sustaining a continuing inflammatory reaction for a relatively long time (Illustration 2-18).

Although the neutrophil is responsible for the usual leukocytosis, elevation of circulating levels of other white blood cells is also seen under certain circumstances. Increased numbers of eosinophils, for example, are usually observed in allergic reactions and parasitic infections. A differential blood cell count is required to establish the cell or cells actually responsible for leukocytosis.

Depression of white blood cell count is called *leukopenia*. It is seen as a transient phenomenon in the early stages of inflammation and as a constant characteristic of certain diseases such as typhoid fever, tularemia and many viral infections. Leukopenia may also result from depression or exhaustion of the marrow. Selective depression of the neutrophil count is called *neutropenia* or *granulocytopenia* and, if this condition should reach such an extreme that neutrophils represent only a small fraction of circulating leukocytes, *agranulocytosis*. A summary of conditions in which leukocytosis and leukopenia are regularly seen is presented in Illustration 2-19.

lack of granulocytes (handwritten)

4. Alterations in Serum Proteins

Severe acute inflammatory reactions are often accompanied by significant changes in

---

2-19. CONDITIONS FAVORING LEUKOCYTOSIS AND LEUKO-PENIA

1) LEUKOCYTOSIS
    neutrophil
        infections provoking acute inflammation
    eosinophil
        allergy and parasitic infections
    lymphocyte
        pertussis (whooping cough)
        infectious mononucleosis
    monocytes
        typhoid fever

2) LEUKOPENIA
    very early stages of acute inflammation
    many viral infections
    typhoid fever
    tularemia

protein solutes of the serum. We will examine 2 such changes as listed in Illustration 2-20.

Elevated Gamma Globulins

We have seen in Subject 1 that the factor most significant in determining the rate of antibody synthesis is antigenic stimulation. Sustained infection or other diseases in which there is prolonged exposure to foreign material will result in an increase in circulating gamma globulins (antibodies or immunoglobulins). This is detected by subjecting the patient's serum to electrophoretic separation and assaying the amount of protein in each resulting fraction. Gamma globulins are so termed because they form the slowest migrating class of such proteins. Quantitation of the gamma fraction is an index of antibody concentration in circulating blood. It says nothing of the specificity of such antibodies but merely that the patient has reacted immunologically to a significant antigenic challenge.

Elevated Fibrinogen

Also part of the alteration seen in serum proteins during previous acute inflammation is an elevated concentration of fibrinogen.

5. Increased Erythrocyte Sedimentation Rate (ESR)

Blood drawn from a patient sustaining a severe acute inflammatory response will exhibit a more rapid rate of separation into cells and clear plasma when allowed to stand in a heparinized tube. This phenomenon is known as an increased erythrocyte sedimentation rate or increased *ESR* (Illustration 2-21).

2-21. INCREASED ESR

1) BLOOD DRAWN INTO HEPARINIZED TUBE WILL EXHIBIT INCREASED RATE OF ERYTHROCYTE SETTLING

2) NOT SPECIFIC TO ACUTE INFLAMMATION
   pregnancy
   malignancy
   rheumatic fever

3) EXACT REASON NOT KNOWN
   change in protein components of serum is related and perhaps causative

---

The increased ESR is not pathognomonic of acute inflammation; it is seen in a number of other, essentially unrelated conditions such as pregnancy, malignant tumor and rheumatic fever. It is, however, a valuable adjunctive sign in the diagnosis of a disease based on the acute inflammatory response.

The reason for increased ESR is not entirely understood but it is thought to be referable to changes in blood solutes such as proteins.

Additional Reading

Backwalter, J. A. and Kent, T. H. General Pathology: A Programmed Text. Unit VI. Systemic Manifestations of Inflammation. Department of Pathology, The University of Iowa College of Medicine, Iowa City, 1973

2-20. ALTERATIONS IN SERUM PROTEINS

1) INCREASE IN GAMMA GLOBULINS

2) INCREASE IN FIBRINOGEN

CLINICAL PATTERNS OF ACUTE INFLAMMATION

LEARNING OBJECTIVE

To be able to describe the following patterns of acute inflammation:

* a) purulent (suppurating)
  b) fibrinopurulent or pseudomembranous
  c) serous
  d) fibrinous
  e) hemorrhagic
* f) catarrhal
* g) phlegmonous (cellulitis)

Despite its being based on a number of fundamental steps, acute inflammation occurs in a variety of clinical forms. There is an almost unlimited number of combinations of injurious agents, locations, personal idiosyncrasies and complicating factors that can impart a different quality to each lesion. We have seen that, once the reaction has started, it proceeds in a sequence of more or less definite stages. The duration and severity of each of these changes and hence the character of the fully developed reaction will be dependent on the nature and location of the injury. A cut finger, for example, is a far different challenge to the body than an infected appendix or a broken leg and, although inflammation is instrumental in correcting all 3, each will require a reaction of different quality and intensity. Part of the genius of the body's organization is that it can usually fit the reaction to the need. Taken collectively, acute inflammatory lesions tend to fall into a limited number of morphologic categories. The classification of the lesion is usually based on its location and the composition of its exudate, but in many cases it is impossible to classify each lesion precisely.

The types of acute inflammatory lesions most commonly encountered are listed in Illustration 2-22 and discussed below.

1. Purulent or Suppurating Inflammation

A purulent lesion is one characterized by the accumulation of pus. Pus is a semifluid substance consisting of components listed in Illustration 2-23. *Pus is predominately neutrophils*; it is this abundance of neutrophils

---

2-22. CLINICAL PATTERNS OF ACUTE INFLAMMATION

1) PURULENT (SUPPURATING)

2) FIBRINOPURULENT (PSEUDOMEMBRANOUS)

3) SEROUS

4) FIBRINOUS

5) HEMORRHAGIC

6) CATARRHAL

7) PHLEGMONOUS (CELLULITIS)

2-23. COMPONENTS OF PUS

1) WATER AND SOLUTES

2) DEAD AND DYING NEUTROPHILS

3) NECROTIC TISSUE

4) TISSUE DEBRIS

(white blood cells) that gives pus its whitish color. This enormous concentration of enzyme-rich neutrophils is also responsible for the liquefaction of both necrotic tissue and even some viable normal tissue although the latter is usually more resistant. Dying neutrophils release their lysosomal enzymes into the inflammatory site resulting in the digestion of any susceptible substrate, without regard to origin or importance. Pus formation (suppuration) is elicited by bacteria or irritating substances that are chemotactic. It can be considered an exaggeration of the stage in acute inflammation where neutrophils exit from capillaries by

abscess –
neutrophils
found

transudate –
fluid not provoked
by inflam. process

diapedesis and are attracted to the irritant by a chemotactic signal. The presence of pus implies a strong, sustained chemotaxis. Pus can occur on a surface, within tissue as a well circumscribed pocket or focus (abscess) or in a diffuse pattern throughout tissue.

√ 2. Fibrinopurulent Inflammation

Some agents, notably the diphtheria toxin, are so lethal to epithelium that they result in the denudation of extensive areas of tissue surface. In diphtheria, this occurs primarily in the upper respiratory tract where the entire tracheal surface, for example, may be rendered necrotic. In such cases a fibrinogen-rich, purulent exudate flows out onto the surface. The fibrinogen is converted to fibrin which entraps the exuded cells and the now-solid exudate adheres to the tracheal wall. This membrane-like coating undergoes desiccation and hardening to become the typical diphtheric fibrino-purulent "pseudomembrane." Although irritant gases may cause this kind of inflammation, it is most often seen in association with diphtheria.

KNOW

3. Serous and Fibrinous Inflammation

outpouring of fluid

found mainly in cavities

Serous inflammation is that in which there is outpouring of protein-rich fluid into body cavities. It is the characteristic response of irritated serous surfaces such as the peritoneum or pleura. The true serous exudate contains some inflammatory cells and differs in this respect from the transudate or fluid that leaks into body cavities in non-inflammatory conditions such as hypoproteinemia. The inflammatory exudate also contains more protein and has a high specific gravity.

Occurs between viscera

If the irritation becomes severe, fibrinogen may be included in the serous exudate, and, once outside the vessel, it may form a fibrin coating on the irritated surface. This is termed *fibrinous* or *serofibrinous* inflammation and introduces the possibility of constriction or adhesion should the fibrin organize (be replaced by connective tissue).

can mature & be constrictive

4. Hemorrhagic Inflammation

Infections with extremely virulent organisms such as hemolytic streptococci and meningococci may damage blood vessels and result in

hemorrhage as a complication of the inflammatory process. In such cases, exudate will be characterized by an abundance of red blood cells as well as the usual neutrophils. Also, in the case of gram-negative bacteria that produce a potent endotoxin (such as the meningococcus), there is the additional possibility of the direct and uncontrolled activation of complement at the site of bacterial localization. Since activated complement is chemotactic, neutrophils are attracted and release enzymes that cause additional vascular damage and more hemorrhage.

5. Catarrhal Inflammation

KNOW

Catarrhal inflammation is the pattern of response that results from the superficial infection of mucous membrane surfaces such as the upper respiratory and gastrointestinal tracts. Mucin is a prominent component of the exudate.

abundant liberation of mucous

6. Phlegmonous Inflammation (Cellulitis)

Phlegmonous inflammation or cellulitis is a pattern of acute inflammation in which the reaction spreads rapidly along tissue planes and potential spaces that contain loose fibro-elastic connective tissue (the so-called "cellular" tissue in reference to compartments formed by the loose fibrous reticulation). A common cellulitis is one that occurs in the tissue plane between the dermis and subjacent muscle.

caused by hemolytic streptococci

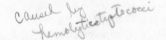

CHRONIC INFLAMMATION

LEARNING OBJECTIVE

To be able to compare and contrast chronic and acute inflammation mentioning the following:
   a) lesions
   b) cell populations
   c) examples of the former
   d) duration

Chronic inflammation is a well recognized reaction, distinctly different in many ways from acute inflammation. One difference, sug-

if fibrinogen present – liquid can clot

injurating = hardening

2-24. CHRONIC INFLAMMATION

1) SOME VESTIGE OF ACUTE RE-
   SPONSE
   usually later stages of exudate

2) SCAR FORMATION
   fibrosis or the process of repair

gested by the term itself, is that the chronic
form persists while the acute form, however
severe, is transitory. The typical picture of
chronic inflammation will be seen wherever an
injurious stimulus is maintained for a considerable length of time; and, further, it is this
persistent kind of injury that causes the
persistent reaction. Chronic inflammation is
found, for example, at the base of a long-standing peptic ulcer, in infections such as osteomyelitis and in other situations where tissue is
subjected to sustained injury. In these common
afflictions where the injury is obvious, chronic
inflammation assumes a very typical microscopic morphology:

1) There is usually some vestige or recurrence of the acute response; hence some
   neutrophils are seen close to the source of
   injury and near the periphery of the
   lesion.
2) A greater number of cells are of the
   "round cell' type (lymphocytes and
   macrophages) and these are seen deeper
   within the lesion.
3) Some degree of fibrosis (repair) has
   occurred, usually at the deepest and most
   mature area of the reaction. The older the
   lesion, the more prominent the accumulation of this fibrous tissue (scar). Since it
   is the process of repair that distinguishes
   chronic inflammation from the acute
   form, we will consider the presence of
   fibrous repair the hallmark of chronic
   inflammation.

In lesions of very long duration, such as some
gastric ulcers, the accumulation of scar may
begin to impede the normal function of the
tissue. Huge deposits of scar around an ulcer at
the pylorus of the stomach, for example, may
obstruct passage of gastric contents into the
duodenum.

GRANULOMATOUS INFLAMMATION

LEARNING OBJECTIVE

To be able to compare granulomatous
inflammation to acute and chronic
inflammation, mentioning the following:
  a) role of the sensitized lymphocyte
  b) the transient granulomatous reaction
     (such as the tuberculin skin test) as
     contrasted with the chronic granuloma
  c) the architecture of the chronic granu-
     loma
  d) pathogenesis examples of infectious
     and non-infectious granulomatous dis-
     ease

Granulomatous inflammation is a process
based on the action of the cellular immunologic
system. It is not a variation of acute or chronic
inflammation but a fundamentally different
process. Like the others, it incorporates the use
of mediators (but in a much different way) and
is seen in a variety of clinical forms.

1. Transient Granulomatous Inflammation

Transient granulomatous inflammation is a
form that resolves without the formation of
scar. It manifests some of the signs of acute
inflammation but tends to be more indurated
and less painful. Perhaps the most familiar and
valid example of transient granulomatous inflammation is the reaction experienced in the
positive tuberculin skin test.

2. Chronic Granulomatous Inflammation

In most instances, the reaction provoked by
a sensitized lymphocyte is adequate and the
noxious cell, microorganism or other substance
is destroyed. In some reactions, however, the
antigenic substance steadfastly resists destruction and may even kill the cells that engulf it.
When this happens, the reaction reverts to a
form that appears to be specialized toward
containing and confining the antigen. This form
of granulomatous inflammation exhibits a very
characteristic microscopic architecture and is
known as a *granuloma*.

The granuloma is so termed because early

action of sensitized lymphocyte

not based on vascular changes arises more in tissue itself

can or cannot have a scar

mediators

Scar tissue

Occurs in 2 forms —

pathologists considered it a granule-sized focus of abnormal enlargement (the suffix oma always refers to swelling enlargement or tumor). The cross-sectional structure of the typical granuloma is shown in Illustration 2-25. Note that the outermost layer is fibrous connective tissue, analogous to the scar seen in non-granulomatous chronic inflammation.

A granuloma usually develops in reaction to higher forms of parasitic microorganisms and not as a response to more common forms of injury. Perhaps the best known example of the granuloma is the tubercle of tuberculosis; however, many other organisms elicit comparable lesions. Some granulomas result from reaction to non-living material such as silica or the unknown antigen of the granulomatous disease, sarcoidosis. The fact that the granuloma can occur as a reaction to either living or non-living agents has prompted the classification of granulomatous diseases into the 2 listed in Illustration 2-26.

[handwritten annotations: lung; usually in form of silica dioxide]

2-25. GRANULOMATOUS INFLAMMATION IN A LYMPH NODE (SARCOIDOSIS)

PERIPHERAL FIBROSIS

LYMPHOCYTES

GIANT CELLS

EPITHELIOID CELLS

NECROTIC CENTER

[handwritten annotations: all granulomas will exhibit at least epithelioid cell.; macrophage; macrophage develop from fusion or nuclear division of macrophage; macrophage; not feature of all but most of T.B. ones]

2-26. CLASSIFICATION OF GRANULOMATOUS LESIONS

1) SPECIFIC (INFECTIOUS) GRANULOMA

reaction to living agent such as tubercle bacillus or fungus

2) NON-SPECIFIC GRANULOMA

reaction to non-living agent such as silica or asbestos

chapter 3
ADAPTATION, WOUND HEALING AND DEGENERATION

SOMATIC CELL REACTIONS (AND NON-REACTIONS)

LEARNING OBJECTIVE

To be able to discuss the reactive potential of the somatic cell including the pathogenesis of degeneration and cell death.

In preceding chapters we have seen how highly specialized defense cells such as lymphocytes, macrophages and neutrophils react to injury or foreign material anywhere in the body. In the present subject, we will consider those few reactions that can be mustered by somatic cells at the site of injury or challenge.

Injurious stimuli range in intensity from the extremely subtle to the extremely severe. Perhaps the most innocuous injury is the simple demand that a cell or tissue increase its rate of function. Under such circumstances, the body is required to *adapt*, i.e. to change responding cell or tissue in such a way that the increased demands are met without exhausting strain or continued damage. Some injurious stimuli are so overwhelming or persistent (or unusual) that none of its repetoire of responses is adequate to equip the body to continue. Under these circumstances, cells or tissues are challenged beyond their ability to respond and begin to degenerate and die. It is precisely these 2 kinds of response (depicted in Illustration 3-1) and their sequellae that will concern us in this discussion.

Additional Reading

Adolph, E. F. Physiological adaptations: hypertrophies and superfunctions. Am. Scientist 60:608, 1972

3-1. ADAPTIVE RESPONSES OF CELLS OR TISSUES

1) OVERTAXATION OR SUBLETHAL IRRITATION

↓

ADAPTATION
   hypertrophy
   hyperplasia
   metaplasia

2) OVERWHELMING, PERSISTENT OR UNUSUAL INJURY

↓

DEGENERATION

↓

DEATH OF CELLS OR TISSUE

CELL AND TISSUE ADAPTATION: HYPERTROPHY, HYPERPLASIA AND METAPLASIA

LEARNING OBJECTIVE

To be able to describe each of the following kinds of adaptive responses defining the term used and citing examples of each:
  a) hypertrophy
  b) hyperplasia
  c) metaplasia

1. Hypertrophy

Hypertrophy (defined in Illustration 3-2) is one means by which an organ or tissue can adapt to increased functional demand. Instead of more cells being added, each cell is made larger. Hypertrophy is typical of organs that have no capacity for reproducing their component cells.

When the heart wall thickens in response to athletic activity, the increased myocardial substance is due not to an increase in the number of myocardial fibers (heart cells) but rather to an increase in the size of each component fiber. Another prominent example of hypertrophy is the increase in the size of the remaining kidney following unilateral nephrectomy. Each kidney is made up of about 1 million nephrons which are never replaced when lost. Although there is no possibility for an increase in their number, each nephron of the remaining kidney enlarges in an effort to accommodate increased functional demands.

For purposes of instruction, it is convenient to set rigid specifications for the definition of hypertrophy. However, the student must bear in mind that this exact definition is not always honored in the clinic. The term, *benign prostatic hypertrophy,* for example, although universally used to refer to enlargement of the prostate associated with advanced age, is actually inappropriate in that the condition is an example of a mixture of hypertrophy and hyperplasia.

2. Hyperplasia

When a tissue or organ increases the number of its component cells as a response to

---

3-2. HYPERTROPHY

Increase in the size of an organ or tissue *without* an increase in the number of its component cells

Examples

1) HEART WALL OF THE ATHLETE

2) ENLARGEMENT OF THE REMAINING KIDNEY AFTER UNILATERAL NEPHRECTOMY

3-3. HYPERPLASIA

Increase in the size of an organ or tissue *due to* an increase in the number of its component cells

Examples

1) BREAST CHANGES IN PREGNANCY

2) THICKENING OF THE EPIDERMIS IN THE FORMATION OF A CALLOUS

---

increased functional demands, the reaction is called *hyperplasia* (Illustration 3-3).

Increase in the size of the breast in pregnancy, for example, is caused by rapid proliferation of secretory epithelium and duct cells. A second example of hyperplasia is seen in the increase in the thickness of skin over an area of constant abrasion or pressure. On microscopic examination, this proves to be due to an increase in the keratin layer and to increased numbers of cells in the prickle cell layer of the epidermis. These changes are called hyperkeratosis and acanthosis respectively and represent a form of hyperplasia. Their combination gives rise to an adaptive lesion known as a *callous.*

Again, as in the case of hypertrophy, the term hyperplasia cannot always be used with precision because many tissue changes are made up of both hypertrophy and hyperplasia. The enlargement of the uterus in pregnancy, for example, is due to an increase in both size and number of its component units.

3. Metaplasia

Metaplasia (Illustration 3-4) is seen as a response to various situations, each of which is caused by a somewhat different stimulus.

Metaplasia Secondary to Chronic Irritation

Certain kinds of epithelium when chronically irritated undergo a change to the more resistant stratified squamous epithelium. This is seen commonly in respiratory epithelium, but may also occur in transitional epithelium or in the epithelium of the pancreatic or biliary duct system; it has not been described in the gastrointestinal tract. It is now well known that, in the development of a particular kind of cancer of the respiratory tract, the first change is metaplasia of the highly specialized, pseudostratified, columnar epithelium to the more resistant stratified squamous epithelium. The cancer that later develops is characteristically of the squamous cell type.

Vitamin A Deficiency

For some unknown reason, a deficiency of vitamin A causes metaplasia of various epithelia to the stratified squamous type. This is seen primarily in the eye, but other tissues, including respiratory and ductal epithelium, are also affected.

Myeloid Metaplasia of Spleen or Liver

On occasion there is a change in the specialization of the spleen or liver to hematopoietic tissue. This usually occurs in response to an increased demand for blood cells and is also termed "extramedullary hematopoiesis," since it represents blood cell production occurring outside of its normal location in the medulla of the bones of the axial skeleton.

Additional Reading

Gross, R. J. Hypertrophy versus hyperplasia. Science 153:1615, 1966

3-4. METAPLASIA

Change from one adult type of tissue to another

Examples

1) CHANGE OF RESPIRATORY EPITHELIUM TO STRATIFIED SQUAMOUS SECONDARY TO CHRONIC IRRITATION

2) VITAMIN A DEFICIENCY

3) MYELOID METAPLASIA OF SPLEEN OR LIVER IN EXTRAMEDULLARY HEMATOPOIESIS

CELL AND TISSUE INVOLUTION (ATROPHY AND DEGENERATION)

LEARNING OBJECTIVE

To be able to define atrophy and cite at least 3 situations in which it is seen. To be able to explain cellular degeneration using fatty degeneration of the liver and accumulation of lipofuscin pigment as examples

When an injurious stimulus is persistent or unusual, it may surpass the ability of a cell or tissue to adapt. This leads to morphologic changes that signal deterioration and such changes are usually classified as *degeneration*. Before we consider degeneration, we must say something about a slightly different kind of situation, that leading to *atrophy*.

1. Atrophy

Atrophy (defined in Illustration 3-5) results from any of a number of influences that restrict nourishment, stimulation or function of a tissue. A representative collection of such conditions is included in Illustration 3-5.

Atrophy is not always pathologic; in certain situations the reduction in the size of an organ comes about as part of a normal developmental process. An example would be involution of the thymus following puberty.

The concept of atrophy must not be confused with that of hypoplasia in which a structure fails to reach its normal adult size or aplasia in which it fails to grow after organogenesis.

2. Degeneration

Degeneration is an ill-defined term used in reference to a variety of retrograde changes in cells. Degeneration of any kind is usually manifested as an accumulation of abnormal material within a cell. Although it would be desirable to spend a suitable amount of time discussing the mechanism of each type of degeneration, we will restrict our attention to their simple morphologic classification. Bear in mind, however, that more is known about each degenerative process than can be mentioned here and that the changes one sees are evidence of an underlying condition and not its cause.

The nature of the material that accumulates within a cell in degeneration will depend upon a number of factors, foremost among which are the quality of the injury and the type of cell responding. We will use the 2 very common patterns of degeneration listed in Illustration 3-6 as our examples.

Fatty Degeneration of the Liver

Injury to liver parenchymal cells produced by either direct chemical damage, dietary insufficiency or anoxia causes the intracellular accumulation of fat. This condition is called *fatty degeneration* and is seen as a diffuse and quite prominent change in alcoholism and childhood protein starvation (kwashiorkor). It is reversible if not severe, but often progresses to a more serious disease, *fatty nutritional*

3-5. ATROPHY

Decrease in the size of an organ or tissue that had previously been of normal adult size

Examples

1) STARVATION

2) INTERRUPTION OF NERVE SUPPLY TO AN EXTREMITY

3) CONSTANT PRESSURE ON THE SKIN OVER A BONY PROMINENCE

4) ENDOCRINE IMBALANCE

5) SENESCENT OR ARTERIOPATHIC CHANGES

6) AS PART OF A NORMAL DEVELOPMENTAL PROCESS

3-6. INTRACELLULAR DEPOSITS AS EVIDENCE OF DEGENERATION

The following two are used as examples of this phenomenon

1) FATTY DEGENERATION OF THE LIVER

2) ACCUMULATION OF LIPOFUSCIN PIGMENT IN MYOCARDIAL FIBERS AND NEURONS

cirrhosis. Cirrhosis is a condition in which there is diffuse scar formation within liver parenchyma; it ensues only after longstanding fatty degeneration. Both of these conditions will be taken up again in Chapter 19.

Pigment Degeneration of the Heart and Brain

The aging of myocardial fibers and neurons results in the accumulation of a perinuclear, membrane-bound material known as *lipofuscin pigment*. Although the exact nature of this material is not known, it is presumed to be the residue of a lifetime of intracellular digestion. Pigment degeneration of heart and nerve cells is not reversible, but neither is it acutely toxic. It would seem that this condition represents a microscopic stigma of advanced age and may, at worst, act as a kind of cellular impediment.

Additional Reading

Lieber, C., et al. Alcoholic fatty liver. N. Engl. J. Med. 280:705, 1969

3-7. NECROSIS

The death of a part of a living organism

Clinical Patterns

1) SIMPLE NECROSIS (CELL DEATH OR NECROSIS WITHOUT INFARCTION)

2) NECROBIOSIS

3) COAGULATION NECROSIS AND THE INFARCT

4) CASEOUS NECROSIS

5) LIQUIFACTION NECROSIS

6) FIBRINOID NECROSIS

7) GANGRENE

8) GUMMATOUS NECROSIS

CELL AND TISSUE DEATH (NECROSIS)

LEARNING OBJECTIVE

To be able to define necrosis, describe the 8 clinical patterns presented and discuss the pathogenesis of each. Also, to be able to list the fates of the necrotic area.

Necrosis is the death of a part of a living organism. Tissue changes occurring after somatic death are not termed necrosis because all parts of the body undergo comparable deterioration. Necrosis occurs in a number of distinct clinical patterns (Illustration 3-7). As was true of degeneration, such changes are not the cause but rather the effect of an underlying failure of the cell or tissue to compensate for intense or unusual damage. Just as in the foregoing learning objective, we will settle for a more conventional, morphologic description of the patterns of necrosis since these are still in common use.

1. Simple Necrosis (Cell Death)

Cell death occurs in a series of stages that are distinguishable as morphologic changes in the stained microscopic section (Illustration 3-8). Again, bear in mind that a great deal of systematic knowledge underlies these simple terms and that they are used only as a convenient means of designating the stage of cell death encountered.

Many instances of cell death occur as a result of incipient (but not absolute) circulatory insufficiency. In the liver, this is seen as necrosis of hepatocytes surrounding the central vein (centrilobular necrosis); in the kidney, it is manifested as selective necrosis of tubular epithelial cells (acute tubular necrosis). In both cases, should the patient survive, necrotic cells

---

3-8. STAGES OF SIMPLE NECROSIS (CELL DEATH)

1) OCCULT DEGENERATION

   degenerative changes have begun but have not yet become morphologically apparent

2) CLOUDY SWELLING

   cell enlarges, cytoplasm becomes finely granular

3) HYDROPIC DEGENERATION

   cytoplasm is coarsely granular and begins to show vacuolation

4) PYKNOSIS

   nucleus becomes shrunken and stains much darker than normal

5) KARYORRHEXIS

   fragmentation of nucleus

6) KARYOLYSIS

   dissolution and disappearance of nucleus

---

are regenerated and no permanent lesion results. For this reason, simple necrosis is also referred to as *necrosis without infarction* (an infarct is a lesion consisting of necrotic tissue).

2. Necrobiosis

The death of a part of a living body *in a normal process* is termed *necrobiosis*. Examples of this pattern of necrosis are the cornification and sloughing of the outer layers of the skin as well as the normal sloughing of the endometrium in menstruation.

3. Coagulation Necrosis

Coagulation necrosis is a pattern resulting from the sudden, complete or near-complete ischemia of tissue with a single blood supply. It is most often seen as the result of vascular obstruction in the kidney and heart. The tissue retains the outline of its architecture, but cellular detail is lost. The resulting lesion is usually well circumscribed and walled off from normal contiguous tissue by an area of inflammation; such a lesion is called an *infarct*.

4. Caseous Necrosis

Caseous necrosis is the pattern seen in tuberculosis, leprosy and some varieties of mycotic infection. It is formed at the center of the active granuloma in these diseases, presumably the result of the combined necrotizing effect of the infectious agent and the host reaction. It is described as "caseous" because of its resemblance to cottage cheese.

5. Liquefaction Necrosis

Liquefaction of necrotic tissue is seen principally in the brain. When brain substance is rendered necrotic for any reason it usually liquifies, leaving a fluid-filled cavity. Another kind of liquefaction necrosis occurs in the abscess where a large collection of neutrophils causes indiscriminate digestion of tissue.

6. Fibrinoid Necrosis

Fibrinoid necrosis is the pattern found typically in mesenchymal auto-immune disease. It is thought to represent a focus of altered collagen. In the conventionally stained microscopic section it appears as a pink (eosinophilic), refractile, homogeneous deposit of amorphous material and seems to be located primarily (but not exclusively) within or around the wall of blood vessels.

7. Gangrene

Gangrene is ischemic necrosis with superimposed saprophytic (putrifying) infection. It is seen in many varieties depending upon the structure affected, the cause of the original necrosis and the type of organism predominating in the infection.

8. Gummatous Necrosis

Gummatous necrosis is found at the center of the gumma, a destructive granulomatous

---

3-9. FATES OF THE NECROTIC AREA

---

1) WILL CAUSE DEATH IF EXTENSIVE OR INVOLVING ESSENTIAL TISSUE
     brain
     myocardium

2) WILL SLOUGH IF AT OR NEAR SURFACE

3) MAY BE WALLED OFF AND NEUTRALIZED BY CHRONIC INFLAMMATORY BARRIER

4) MAY BE CLEARED AND DEFECT REPLACED WITH SCAR

5) MAY BE CALCIFIED

CELL AND TISSUE REPLACEMENT (REGENERATION AND REPAIR)

LEARNING OBJECTIVE

To be able to discuss the classification of somatic cells into labile, stable and permanent with reference to their ability to regenerate and define *regeneration* and *repair*, explaining each step of the latter in some detail

---

Somatic (body) cells of the adult can be roughly classified into 3 categories as regards their ability to reproduce (Robbins, Boyd). These are listed and described with examples in Illustration 3-10. This classification of normal somatic cells of the adult will be used as a basis for our discussion of regeneration and repair.

lesion of tertiary syphilis. It is called a gumma because it resembles rubber in consistency.

9. Fates of the Necrotic Area

The necrotic area is not a welcome passenger in the body. Judging from the variety of its fates, it is usually noxious and strongly provocative of a corrective response. Fates of necrotic tissue are listed in Illustration 3-9 and should be made part of your working knowledge.

The clinical patterns of necrosis mentioned in this learning objective represent characteristic changes in tissue that are seen as part of certain specific diseases or as a result of a particular kind of severe or unusual injury. They are not diseases in themselves, nor are they the cause of the disease (except when the physical presence of necrotic material leads to interference or obstruction). We have done little more than take this opportunity to gather them together for collective inspection. Each will be encountered in a latter chapter in context with the syndromes in which they occur. In many cases, they will be seen to be highly pathognomonic of the disease with which they are associated.

3-10. CLASSIFICATION OF NORMAL SOMATIC CELLS BY MITOTIC ABILITY

(after Boyd, Robbins)

1) LABILE
    reproduce as part of their normal function
      lymphoid tissue
      gastrointestinal epithelium
      marrow
      epidermis

2) STABLE
    can be stimulated to reproduction
      fibrous tissue, bone, liver
      renal tubular epithelium

3) PERMANENT
    cannot reproduce
      mature nerve cells
      myocardial fibers
      renal glomerular structures

1. Simple Regeneration

Since they do retain the capacity for reproduction, cells in the first 2 categories (labile and stable) can be replaced by *simple regeneration*, i.e. fatally damaged cells can be replaced by replication of their intact neighbors. However, when tissue composed of permanent cells are damaged they are nearly always replaced by fibrous scar. The latter process is known as *repair* (Illustration 3-11).

2. Repair

Repair is more complex than regeneration. It occurs in 3 principal clinical situations as listed and described in Illustration 3-12. All of these share the same fundamental sequence of microscopic and chemical events. In all 3 the process of repair proceeds from fibrin clot to granulation tissue to mature scar (or bony callous) in the manner diagrammed in Illustration 3-13. The sequence of morphologic and clinical changes detectable in the repair of a simple, incisional wound of soft tissue is listed in Illustration 3-14 and described below.

1) An incision is made and the wound edges reapposed and sutured.
2) Hemorrhage from severed blood vessels fills the defect and the blood clots. The surface of the clot becomes dessicated, forming the *eschar* or scab.
3) An acute inflammatory exudate forms and the wound site is cleared of microorganisms and tissue debris. At approximately this stage, the edges of the wound

contract slightly, probably because of the rounding up of cells at its periphery, a change preparatory to mitotic division.
4) Macrophages move into the area and remove extravasated erythrocytes and any remaining debris.
5) Capillary buds from adjoining vessels grow into the wound site. At the same time, fibroblasts migrating along the fibrin scaffold enter the wound and begin to proliferate.
6) With capillary circulation re-established, fibroblasts begin to elaborate tropocollagen, the monomeric, molecular precursor of collagen fibrils. Tropocollagen mole-

---

3-12. REPAIR

1) WOUND HEALING

2) FRACTURE HEALING

3) ABERRANT REPAIR

3-13. THE PROCESS OF REPAIR

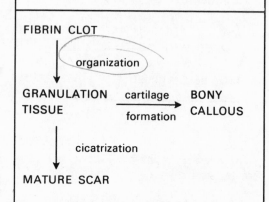

The vertical component of this diagram depicts the healing of a soft tissue wound while the horizontal component shows that of a fracture

---

3-11. REGENERATION AND REPAIR

1) REGENERATION
    replacement of necrotic cells with normal cells of the same type

2) REPAIR
    replacement of necrotic cells or other tissue elements with fibrous connective tissue

3-14. WOUND HEALING BY FIRST OR PRIMARY INTENTION

1) INCISIONAL WOUND

2) HEMORRHAGE, HEMOSTASIS, CLOT FORMATION

3) ACUTE INFLAMMATION

4) CONTRACTION OF WOUND EDGES

5) CLEARANCE OF BLOOD PIGMENT AND OTHER DEBRIS

6) INGROWTH OF CAPILLARY BUDS

7) FIBROBLAST PROLIFERATION, MIGRATION INTO CLOT SCAFFOLD

8) SYNTHESIS AND AGGREGATION OF TROPOCOLLAGEN

9) RE-EPITHELIALIZATION

10) MATURATION AND CONTRACTION SCAR

in the extracellular milieu. It results in the formation of strong (covalent) bonds that cross-link the component molecules into a stressworthy feltwork of interconnected collagen fibers. These countless strong crosslinks cause the contraction of repair tissue into a dense, relatively avascular, fibrous patch called a scar or *cicatrix.*

8) Cicatrization (collagen maturation and scar contraction) proceeds while the epithelial covering grows over the defect, displacing the eschar and the process of healing is essentially complete. Maturation continues, however, and the scar, at first pink and friable, slowly becomes white and tough, gaining approximately 85 per cent of the strength of the undamaged skin. During cicatrization most of the cells and blood vessels disappear and the formerly delicate, vascular granulation tissue becomes the dense, homogeneous, mature scar.

3. Collagen Kinetics in Repair

A key to the understanding of the repair process is an appreciation of the kinetics of

cules associate in a pattern of quarter-length overlap to form collagen fibrils which knit the severed edges of the wound together (Illustration 3-15). At this same stage, capillaries begin to course toward the surface of the wound where they form loops that will nourish the epithelial covering, soon to grow over the defect. The tissue filling the defect at this stage is known as *granulation tissue.* Granulation tissue is young, vascular connective tissue. It has several interesting and distinctive features that will be discussed further.

7) The newly formed collagen of the granulation tissue now begins a process of *maturation.* Maturation consists of a series of chemical events that take place

3-15. COLLAGEN KINETICS IN WOUND HEALING

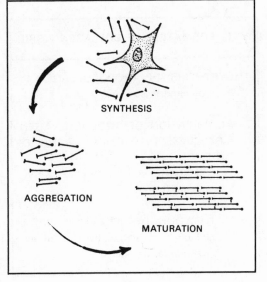

SYNTHESIS

AGGREGATION

MATURATION

collagen. Three steps in the elaboration of the collagen fibril are listed in Illustration 3-16 and described below.

Synthesis of the Tropocollagen Molecule

The first step in the formation of collagen is carried out within fibroblasts as synthesis of the tropocollagen molecule. Tropocollagen synthesis is dependent upon availability of Vitamin C (ascorbic acid). Vitamin C-deficient animals are said to be scorbutic (suffering from scurvy). They cannot synthesize collagen and hence cannot heal wounds. Scurvy is a very complex disease and will be considered again as a nutritional deficiency.

Fibril Formation

Formation of the collagen fibril is a process similar to the growth of a crystal. Tropocollagen molecules aggregate spontaneously in the extracellular milieu to form the fibril which is the first architectural level of the collagen fiber. No known (spontaneously occurring) condition interferes with this step.

Maturation of Collagen

The maturation of collagen is actually a series of chemical events that takes place outside the cell. It leads to the formation of an intricate system of strong bonds within and

---

3-17. A PORTION (N-TERMINAL) OF THE TROPOCOLLAGEN MOLECULE

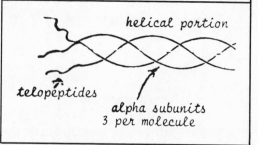

helical portion

telopeptides

alpha subunits
3 per molecule

3-18. MATURATION OF COLLAGEN

1) AS CLOSER FIT IS ACHIEVED BETWEEN TROPOCOLLAGEN MOLECULES WITHIN FORMING FIBRIL SHORTER INTERMOLECULAR DISTANCES PERMIT FORMATION OF STRONG COVALENT BONDS

2) MATURATION BONDS FORM BETWEEN PEPTIDE CHAINS WITHIN A SINGLE MOLECULE AND BETWEEN ADJACENT MOLECULES

3) ALL MATURATION BONDS ARE FORMED BETWEEN TELOPEPTIDES AT THE N-TERMINAL END OF PARTICIPATING MOLECULES

3-16. FORMATION OF COLLAGEN FIBRIL

1) SYNTHESIS OF TROPOCOLLAGEN
   inhibited in scurvy

2) AGGREGATION OF TROPOCOLLAGEN MOLECULES INTO FIBRIL ARCHITECTURE
   no known spontaneous or experimental disease

3) MATURATION OF COLLAGEN FIBRIL
   inhibited in osteolathyrism, an experimental disease

---

between tropocollagen molecules. These bonds form through interaction of small peptides located at the N-terminal end of each molecular unit (Illustration 3-17). The effect is to knit the mass of collagen into a highly compact matrix of high tensile value (Illustration 3-18). A laboratory disease called *experimental lathyrism* or *osteolathyrism* can be induced in animals by the simple feeding of certain chemicals. In this disease there is a near complete arrest of collagen maturation. As would be expected, these animals manifest multiple signs of collagen failure; muscle attachments pull away from bone, arteries rupture and wound healing is inadequate.

4. Granulation Tissue

Granulation tissue is the intermediate between clot and scar. It is remarkable in many respects, not the least of which is its appearance. It is called "granulation" tissue because, distributed over its uncovered surface, one sees a scattering of tiny red granules that are actually capillary loops. These loops form in anticipation of nourishing the slowly creeping borders of epithelium that will eventually meet to close the last trace of the defect caused by the incision.

In addition to qualities already mentioned, granulation tissue is also fragile, highly vascular, easily injured and copiously hemorrhagic when damaged. It is very resistant to infection (for reasons not completely understood) and often anesthetic since it lacks innervation in its early stages of development. Granulation tissue and its successor the cicatrix are compared in Illustration 3-19.

5. Healing by Primary and Secondary Intention

The uncomplicated incisional wound is said to heal by "first intention" or "primary intention." These terms were undoubtedly coined because the scar appears to be acting like a simple adhesive, bonding the cut edges together.

A wound that creates a hole or void in tissue is said to heal by "second" or "secondary" intention, because the scar seems to fill the defect as well as act as a bonding agent. In actual fact, both processes are identical but the latter takes longer because there is a need to synthesize more repair tissue. The 2 situations are compared in Illustration 3-20.

6. Fracture Healing

The healing of a fracture (hard tissue wound) differs from soft tissue healing, principally in its outcome. Breaking of the bone leads to hemorrhage from the marrow cavity into the periosteum causing it to distend the fracture site. A clot forms and undergoes organization to become the soft tissue splint for the

3-19. GRANULATION TISSUE AND THE CICATRIX

granulation tissue	cicatrix
YOUNG, VASCULAR CONNECTIVE TISSUE	MATURE SCAR
COLLAGEN IMMATURE EASILY DAMAGED BLEEDS EASILY, COPIOUSLY	COLLAGEN VERY MATURE HIGH TENSILE STRENGTH
ANESTHETIC IN EARLY STAGES	INNERVATED
HIGHLY CELLULAR AND VASCULAR	RELATIVELY ACELLULAR AND AVASCULAR
MANY MONONUCLEAR INFLAMMATORY CELLS HIGHLY RESISTANT TO INFECTION	FEW INFLAMMATORY CELLS
UNDERGOES MATURATION TO BECOME CICATRIX	DOES NOT REMODEL

3-20. HEALING BY PRIMARY AND SECONDARY INTENTION

1) PRIMARY INTENTION
   healing together of the two edges of an incisional wound

2) SECONDARY INTENTION
   filling of a defect with repair tissue

developing union. This fibrous splint (provisional callous) does not mature, but undergoes metaplasia to cartilage which subsequently ossifies forming the bony callous. Under favorable conditions, the bony callous remodels completely to assume the normal form of the intact bone (Illustration 3-21).

As in soft tissue wounds, the process of the repair of fractures is comparable, regardless of the specifications of the wound. The success of its outcome, however, will depend to a large extent on the form of the fracture. A variety of different kinds of fractures are listed and briefly described in Illustration 3-22.

7. Aberrant Repair

Finally, we must consider the third important situation in which we see fibrous tissue replacing a fibrin clot, the multiple and adverse occasions of aberrant repair (disorderly repair). Aberrant repair, as we will use the term in this discussion, is any occasion upon which repair is

---

3-22. FRACTURES

1) SIMPLE: bone breaks but edges remain in good apposition

2) GREENSTICK: bone cracks but does not break

3) DISPLACED: bone breaks and edges are displaced

4) COMPRESSION: bone is crushed or compacted

5) COMMINUTED: bone breaks and edges are fragmented

6) COMPOUND: bone breaks and one edge is forced through skin

7) MARCH: bone fails because of too rapid remodelling

8) PATHOLOGICAL: bone fails because of lesion

3-21. FRACTURE HEALING

FRACTURE
↓
PROVISIONAL CALLOUS
(granulation tissue followed by cartilage)
↓
BONY CALLOUS
↓
REMODELLING

Formation of provisional callous is analogous to granulation tissue in soft tissue wound

Formation of callous is analogous to scar

In uncomplicated fracture callous will remodel completely

3-23. ABERRANT REPAIR
Examples

1) ORGANIZATION OF EXUDATE ON SURFACE OF VISCUS
    adhesions
    constriction

2) ORGANIZATION OF THE EXUDATE OF LOBAR PNEUMONIA
3) KELOID

DEPOSITS AND INFILTRATIONS

LEARNING OBJECTIVE

To be able to discuss the following specific phenomena as examples of the appearance of deposits and infiltrations in the body:
a) urolithiasis and cholelithiasis
b) gout
c) amyloidosis (primary, secondary, heredofamilial and local)
d) pathologic calcification (mechanism of dystrophic and metastatic calcifications)
e) cholesterolosis

either unwarranted or works to the detriment of the patient's health. Several examples are listed and briefly described in Illustration 3-23.

Of the examples presented, the keloid is different enough to warrant discussion. A keloid is actually an example of a hypertrophic or exaggerated scar. Individuals from certain areas of Africa and Asia tend to form keloids as part of their normal healing process, even when the wound is uncomplicated. Because the propensity for forming keloids is inherited, they are seen almost exclusively in members of the black race. Although cosmetically undesirable in contemporary western culture, they are considered appropriate as decoration or adornment for body surfaces among certain African tribes.

Additional Reading

Bornstein, P. The crosslinking of collagen and elastin and its inhibition in osteolathyrism. Am. J. Med. 49:429, 1970
King, G. D. Keloid scars: analysis of 89 patients. Surg. Clin. N. Amer. 50:595, 1970
Ross, R. Wound Healing. Sci. Amer., 220:40, 1969
Schwartz, P. L. Ascorbic acid in wound healing. J. Am. Dietetic Assn. 56:497, 1970

Extracellular deposits are seen as the accumulation of amorphous material or the formation of crystalline masses within tissues. Either condition is usually a sign of an underlying disorder, often a metabolic disorder. The variety of human stones and infiltrating materials is truly impressive and an entire catalog is beyond the scope of this discussion. We will, however, single out a few of the most common of these manifestations of disease as our examples.

Again, the student must bear in mind that a great deal more is known of this subject than can be presented here. Also, we will be using an admittedly archaic system of classification (deposits and infiltrations) in an effort to collect a few of these conditions under a single heading.

1. Human Stones

A variety of true crystalline stones often form in hollow organs that contain or conduct fluid. Although seen most often in the gallbladder and urinary outflow tract they are also frequently found in salivary gland ducts.

Urinary stones vary in composition, the most common being formed of oxalate or phosphate salts. Gallstones are most often formed of cholesterol, usually mixed with calcium salts and bilirubin.

Acute distress caused by the presence of a stone is usually referable to obstruction or inflammation. In addition, there is the possibility for stricture or other irreversible damage to affected structures.

Stone formation is termed *lithiasis* and a prefix is employed to specify location. Nephrolithiasis, for example, would mean a stone in the kidney, whereas cholelithiasis refers to one or more stones in the gallbladder. The nature of the defect signaled by the presence of a stone varies with its location and composition. Specific examples will be encountered in subsequent subjects (Illustration 3-24).

2. Gout

Gout is a complex disease based on an inherited enzyme deficiency. In gout, deposits of crystalline sodium urate form in and around various joints as well as, less prominently, in kidneys and other tissue. The joint deposits are called *tophi* and are truly pathognomonic of gout. Gout is not a rare disease, being second only to non-specific degeneration as a cause of arthritis.

The metabolic defect that leads to clinically apparent gout is thought to be based on an over-production of urate rather than its source being the breakdown of body tissue or the digestion of food. There is no doubt that the immediate cause of tophus formation is the high concentration of urate in the blood and body fluids (hyperuricemia) resulting from a deficiency of one or more of the enzymes that control urate concentration in the normal individual.

Because these enzymes are deficient from birth, gout is actually a congenital disease. However, early in its course, during the phase

---

3-25. GOUT

1) URATE ACCUMULATES IN BODY BECAUSE OF AN INHERITED TENDENCY TO OVERPRODUCE THIS ION

2) DEPOSITS OF SODIUM URATE ACCUMULATE IN JOINTS (TOPHI), KIDNEYS AND OTHER AREAS

3) ARTHRITIS USUALLY APPEARS AFTER THE AGE OF 40

4) DISEASE IS PAINFUL AND DISABLING BUT NOT FATAL

---

when tophi are building, the patient is essentially free of distress. It is only in its later stages that the typical severe arthritis is experienced. The first attack usually occurs after the age of 40 and most often affects the great toe first in a series of joints. Gouty arthritis is caused by the tophus and occurs in repeated acute attacks followed by symptom-free periods. Attacks are characterized by red, swollen, exquisitely painful joints. But despite these attacks and the resulting destruction of articular cartilage, most patients with gout lead an essentially normal life and usually die of unrelated causes (Illustration 3-25).

3. Amyloidosis

Amyloidosis is a condition in which a waxy, "lardaceous" material infiltrates the liver, spleen and other organs causing enlargement (but rarely failure) of the affected part. The infiltrating material is called *amyloid* because its affinity for certain stains resembles that of starch. Its avidity for the dye, congo red, forms the basis for its identification.

The etiology of amyloidosis has recently been firmly established as a disturbance of immunoglobulin metabolism; however, details of the development of this condition remain to be worked out. Amyloid, itself, is known to consist largely of the light chains of the immunoglobulin molecule.

Many attempts have been made to establish a

3-24. HUMAN STONES

1) STONE FORMATION CALLED LITHIASIS
   nephrolithiasis = kidney stone
   cholelithiasis = gallstone

2) SIGN OF METABOLIC DISORDER OR OTHER PREDISPOSING CONDITION
   chronic infection
   abnormal rate of hemolysis

new and more valid classification of the patterns of amyloidosis, but the one that has proven most serviceable is one of the very earliest, a classification based on the presence or absence of an associated disease or hereditary pattern. In this system, amyloidosis is divided into the 4 clinical patterns listed and described in Illustration 3-26. Primary amyloidosis is that pattern in which no other disease is found to be causing amyloid deposition; secondary amyloidosis is seen as the sequel of a number of diseases, most of which are listed in Illustration 3-27.

With the advent of the electron microscope, it was discovered that the ultrastructure of amyloid is actually quite complex, consisting of fine, rigid, non-branching fibrils embedded in a protein-polysaccharide matrix. Further, it soon became apparent that this same structure prevails regardless of the clinical pattern in which the amyloid occurs. The mechanism of amyloid deposition has eluded explanation. The fibril that characterizes amyloid is apparently unrelated to other fibrous proteins of the body such as collagen, elastin or fibrin and its matrix is also unique in many respects.

One particularly intriguing aspect of amyloidosis is that it occurs quite often in advanced age, particularly in the heart. The condition (when sought) is a surprisingly frequently concomitant of aging and may some day lead to a better understanding of this phenomenon.

4. Pathologic Calcification

Practically all hard tissue of the body consists of a single basic crystalline structure, hydroxyapatite. On occasion, hydroxyapatite will also form under circumstances that are deleterious to the patient's health. This phenomenon is known as pathologic calcification.

Critical to an understanding of pathologic calcification is appreciation of the fact that both serum and extracellular fluid are supersaturated with respect to calcium, the most prominent component of hydroxyapatite. In response to agents regulating calcium homeostasis (Illustration 3-28), various cells of the body are causing calcium to be "forced" into solution against a prevailing concentration that would favor its being deposited out. Thus, there is a distinct tendency for hydroxyapatite crystals to form and grow in the normal human body.

3-26. CLINICAL PATTERNS OF AMYLOIDOSIS

1) PRIMARY
   no other disease is associated with amyloid deposit

2) SECONDARY
   associated with a number of chronic diseases

3) LOCAL
   produced by a tumor

4) HEREDOFAMILIAL
   occurs in related groups

3-27. DISEASES COMPLICATED BY AMYLOIDOSIS

1) CHRONIC INFECTIOUS DISEASES
   tuberculosis
   leprosy
   syphilis
   osteomyelitis
   bronchiectasis

2) PROBABLE INFECTIOUS DISEASES
   Reiters syndrome
   Whipple's disease

3) CHRONIC INFLAMMATORY DISEASES
   rheumatoid arthritis and other connective tissue diseases
   regional enteritis
   ulcerative colitis

4) NEOPLASMS
   Hodgkin's disease
   multiple myeloma
   renal cell carcinoma
   medullary carcinoma of thyroid
   others

5) DIABETES MELLITUS

3-28. CALCIUM HOMEOSTASIS

1) PARATHYROID HORMONE
   raises blood Ca^{++}

2) CALCITONIN
   lowers blood Ca^{++}

3) CALCIFEROL (Vit. D)
   raises blood Ca^{++}

3-29. PATHOLOGICAL CALCIFICATION

1) ELEVATION OF BLOOD CALCIUM LEVEL

   causes

   METASTATIC CALCIFICATION

   Deposition of solid calcium salts within normal tissue in a hypercalcemic animal

2) EXPOSURE OF NUCLEATING TEMPLATE (SUCH AS MIGHT OCCUR IN NECROSIS)

   causes

   DYSTROPHIC CALCIFICATION

   Deposition of solid calcium salts within necrotic tissue in a normocalcemic animal

---

Normal blood calcium levels, although supersaturated as described above, are said to be in the "metastable" range of saturation. In this range crystal formation will not occur spontaneously. In order to initiate the formation of a hydroxyapatite crystal, either an actual crystal of hydroxyapatite or a nidus of the right kind of organic material (collagen works well) is needed to act as a nucleation "seed." Given an appropriate organic template, hydroxyapatite crystals will form and grow in the normocalcemic body. Another mechanism that will cause the formation of such crystals is hypercalcemia. When the concentration of calcium and body fluids is raised above the normal metastable level, spontaneous crystal formation occurs without need for a nucleating template.

From the foregoing it can be seen that there are 2 major factors that can lead to pathologic calcification. These are listed in Illustration 3-29. In the first of these (metastatic calcification), the blood calcium level is elevated to the point where spontaneous crystal formation occurs, whereas in the latter (dystrophic calcification), crystal formation is initiated by the exposure of an appropriate nucleating template, even though the concentration of calcium in body fluids remains normal.

Metastatic calcification occurs in cases where the patient sustains severe or long-standing hypercalcemia (Vitamin D intoxication or a functioning tumor of the parathyroid), whereas the latter is most often seen in the healed tubercle.

5. Cholesterolosis

Cholesterolosis is a condition in which cholesterol and other fats are deposited in

---

3-30. CHOLESTEROLOSIS

1) ABNORMAL DEPOSIT OF CHOLESTEROL WITHIN TISSUES
   xanthoma
   mucosa of gallbladder
   atherosclerosis

2) ATHEROSCLEROSIS AND ITS COMPLICATIONS ARE THE MOST IMPORTANT CAUSE OF DEATH IN THE U.S. TODAY
   cerebrovascular accident
   coronary heart disease
   peripheral vascular insufficiency

---

abnormal locations. The most common examples of cholesterolosis are listed in Illustration 3-30. Cholesterol found within a cluster of macrophages in the dermis is known as a xanthoma. These are often found on the eyelids (xanthoma palpebri). Cholesterol deposited beneath the mucosa of the gallbladder appears as tiny white specks on the bile-stained mucosa (strawberry gallbladder).

But the most common and, by far, the most important form of cholesterolosis is atherosclerosis. In atherosclerosis, cholesterol and other fats are deposited within the intima of the aorta and its main muscular branches (coronary, cerebral, renal, carotid and others). The deposit begins as a yellowish, subendothelial streak which eventually broadens to become a plaque. Growth of the plaque causes it to impinge upon the media leading to inflammation and fibrosis. Confluence and calcification of fibrotic plaques renders the affected artery stiff and unyielding, hence the process that began as a soft fatty deposit in the artery ends as profound sclerosis.

Atherosclerosis and its complications can be predicted to cause the death of 40 per cent of American males living today. Such complications include the cerebrovascular accident (intracranial hemorrhage or cerebral infarction), coronary heart disease (angina pectoris and myocardial infarction) and peripheral vascular insufficiency, manifested as gangrene of the distal-most segments of the lower extremities in severe forms.

Since atherosclerosis and its complications are such an important cause of chronic disease and death they will be mentioned repeatedly in this and subsequent discussions.

Additional Reading

Cohen, A. S. Amyloidosis. N. Engl. J. Med. (3 parts) 227:522, 574, 628, 1967
The Exquisite Pain, The Sciences 8:19, 1968
Gordon, T. and Kannel, W. B. Predisposition to atherosclerosis in the head, heart and legs. JAMA 221:661, 1972
Glenner, G. E. et al. The immunoglobulin origin of amyloid. Am. J. Med. 52:141, 1972
Howell, D. S. Current concepts of calcification. J. Bone J. Surg. 53A:250, 1971
Kleeman, C. R. et al. The clinical physiology of calcium homeostasis, parathyroid hormone and Calcitonin (2 parts) California Med. 114: (3 and 4) 1971
Lonsdale, K. Human stones. Sci. Amer.: 104: 1968

BIOLOGIC AGING

LEARNING OBJECTIVE

To be able to discuss the changes of senescence occurring at each of the following levels:
   a) molecular level
   b) cellular level
   c) physiologic senescence
   d) the relationship between the aging and immunity

Biologic aging is a complex pattern of physical decline manifested by all forms of life that do not renew themselves totally through regular mitosis. Although the rate of aging varies among animal groups, the common outcome is death. Aging has been attributed to many different kinds of things, but the only point that enjoys near-universal agreement is that the root of it all must be the deterioration of large, information-carrying molecules. Since life is so critically dependent upon the precise form and fit of large molecules and since such molecules are so vulnerable to distortion, aging must be based ultimately on the accumulation of battered protein and genetic material that fails to function properly and cannot be repaired. The whole effect is analagous to clinkers accumulating in a fire. Or, in another sense, it is like the generalized loss of critical detail such as one sees when a photograph is taken of a photograph of a photograph.

1. Senescence

The collection of changes that occur in a person as a result of advancing age are known as senescence. Most of these changes are disabling to some degree and will lead eventually to incurable disease. Senescence is detectable in many different processes through the body at the molecular, cellular and gross physiologic levels (Illustration 3-31).

Molecular Senescence

As mentioned above, the most fundamental change associated with aging is probably the distortion of critical macromolecules. This has been demonstrated as the gradual accumulation of unwanted crosslinks in collagen, a change that presumably renders it refractory to normal

---

3-31. BIOLOGICAL AGING

1) AT THE MOLECULAR LEVEL

2) AT THE CELLULAR LEVEL

3) PHYSIOLOGIC SENESCENCE

4) RELATIONSHIP BETWEEN AGING AND IMMUNITY

---

enzymatic degradation and remodeling. The application of this same principle to other kinds of large molecules is postulated. It might be imagined that the effect of unwanted crosslinks in genetic material would be far more profound.

Cellular Senescence

Normal, diploid human cells explanted from an embryo into tissue culture will give rise to approximately 50 generations of progeny before they stop reproducing and begin to die. This same type of cell taken from an adult will double only 20 times whereas comparable cells from an individual suffering from progeria (a syndrome of premature senescence) may reproduce only 5 times. Many authorities interpret this to mean that there is an inviolable limit to the reproductive allotment of normal, diploid human cells. Once a person uses this up his body begins to fail for want of cell replacement and death results from the exhaustion of the most poorly endowed or consistently abused cell type. As we will see, this concept becomes particularly intriguing when applied to immunocytes.

Other examples of senescence at the cellular level include the strong possibility that irreplaceable structures are gradually lost (such as neuron or nephron units) or perhaps rendered less efficient in their operation by the gradual accumulation of ingestible material such as lipofuscin pigment. Also, there is the possibility that a number of cells with very subtle genetic changes accumulates throughout life. These altered cells would live at the expense of their neighbors but contribute little or nothing to the support of the body.

Physiologic Senescence

There is very obvious deterioration of blood vessels in advancing age, a decrement that seems to affect arteries more than veins or lymphatic vessels. There may also be a slowing of the rate of diffusion between intravascular and extravascular space, a phenomenon known as the emergence of a "histohematic barrier." It is also apparent that there is generalized involution of the elastic component of all tissues, a change that particularly affects the function of the lung. Numerous other examples of senescence at the physiologic level could be cited.

Aging and Immunity

The precise role of immunologic failure in the process of aging is not known; however, there is good reason to suspect that immune capability diminishes with age. Burnet has put forth a comprehensive theory of aging emphasizing immunologic deterioration. Briefly it is made up of the following:

1) The average lifespan ("mean time to failure") is characteristic of a species and has evolved as a genetically determined quality of each biologic group. The individual is, therefore, genetically programmed to exist long enough to best serve the needs of his group.
2) The program is mediated by a biologic clock, the basis of which is the limit to the number of times a cell can proliferate in the euploid state (Hayflick Limit).
3) Tissues differ in the time taken to use up their quota of cells. That system, vital to life, which first exhausts its quota will be the one to initiate aging.
4) Exhaustion of the cellular immune system is the critical mediator of aging in mammals and probably in other vertebrates as well.
5) With exhaustion of the cellular immune system, an organism loses the capacity to deal with cellular anomalies arising by somatic mutation. In effect, an essential immunologic tissue surveillance mechanism is lost and this leads to the appearance of cancer and autoimmune phenomena. These, of course, lead ultimately to the death of the individual.

Although other factors prevail in the over-all

picture of aging, the incidence of malignancy is seen to increase sharply with the onset of senescence. It begins to appear that immunologic scrutiny of body tissue gradually comes to a stop in very old age. In the fullness of what ever time is set as the need of his species, an animal finds that its ability to sort self from non-self is spent. Nature, after all, has little interest in the individual.

Additional Reading

Comfort, A. Biological theories of aging. Hum. Dev. 13:127, 1970

Goldstein, S. The biology of aging. N. Engl. J. Med. 285:1120, 1971

Guthried, R. D. Senescence as a selective trait. Persp. Biol. Med. 12:313, 1969

Hayflick, L. Aging under glass. Exp. Geront. 5:291, 1970

Warren, S. Radiation and aging. Bull. N. Y. Acad, Med. 17:1355, 1971

chapter 4
ABNORMALITIES OF THE IMMUNOLOGIC SYSTEMS

MAJOR CATEGORIES OF IMMUNOLOGIC DISEASE

LEARNING OBJECTIVE

To be able to outline general differences among the following 4 kinds of diseases that take origin in the immunologic systems:

a) immunologic deficiency
b) allergy
c) autoimmunity
d) immunoproliferative disease

In the first chapter we saw that immunologic systems are not only protective but actually indispensable. On occasion, however, these systems will give rise to disease; when this happens the disease will be one of the 4 kinds listed in Illustration 4-1.

The important difference between these and any other kind of disease is their source. When immunologic systems are the seat of disease, defense capabilities of the body are seriously diminished. The situation is analogous to a corrupt police department in that the agency reponsible for protection becomes the perpetrator of mischief. The purpose of this learning objective is to gain a brief overview of these 4 categories of immunologic disease. Each is described (as it affects both the humoral and cellular immunologic systems) in Illustration 4-1. Take time now to study and compare them before considering them individually in detail.

4-1. MAJOR CATEGORIES OF IMMUNO-LOGIC DISEASE

1) IMMUNOLOGIC DEFICIENCY
congenital or acquired, permanent or transitory inability to synthesize immunoglobulin or sensitize lymphocytes in response to antigen challenge

2) ALLERGY
immunologic response to an *exogenous* antigen that is inappropriate or damaging and not shown by all members of a species

3) AUTOIMMUNITY
immunologic response to an *endogenous* antigen that is inappropriate or damaging and not shown by all members of a species

4) IMMUNOPROLIFERATIVE DISEASE
unprovoked proliferation of lymphoid cells sometimes accompanied by the synthesis of large amounts of essentially functionless immunoglobulin

IMMUNOLOGIC DEFICIENCY

could be
deficiency of
a. inability to synthesize
immunoglobulin
b. paucity of lymphocytes
d. deficiency of complement

LEARNING OBJECTIVE

To be able to define immunologic deficiency
and describe each of the following categories of
this condition mentioning specific clinical
examples:

  a) congenital *or acquired*
  b) secondary   *permanent or*
  c) iatrogenic   *transient*
  d) senescent
  e) stress-induced

Immunity and inflammation are our most
critical means of defending tissues against
certain deterioration. Fortunately, the complete absence of one or more of these faculties
is seen only rarely, and then usually as a
congenital defect. The partial, transitory, acquired deficiency of immunity or inflammation, however, is surprisingly common. In fact,
the frequency with which an otherwise normal
person is likely to experience some kind of
temporary impairment of a defense system is
now known to be far greater than suspected.
Such alterations of defense mechanisms can be
caused by a variety of previously unsuspected
agents ranging from emotional disturbance to
general anesthesia. Before beginning our examination of immunologic deficiency, we must
look briefly at the over-all phenomenon of
immunologic unresponsiveness.

All literature on immunology emphasizes the
fact that the inevitable result of exposing an
antigen to an immunocompetent cell is an
immunologic reaction. Yet, it is apparent that
any mature human body contains an abundance
of both. Lymphoreticular cells constantly encounter a variety of potentially excellent
antigens in the molecules of the body's own
tissue. Why, then, is immune attack on one's
own tissue more the exception than the rule?
Why does the lymphoreticular system usually
fail to respond while literally immersed in
antigens? The answer is not known but the
phenomenon itself has been called "immunologic unresponsiveness" or "immunologic tolerance."

One fact seems certain, most of the components of immunologic unresponsiveness are
acquired, not genetically determined. The body
actively "learns" what is self and what is
foreign; it does not inherit this knowledge
passively. The basis for self-recognition is not
understood but the conditions of its operation
can be described very concisely: *all potential
antigens present during the time of the development of immunologic competence will be
accepted as self.* And not only is the acceptance
of self antigens learned, but it can be demonstrated that by intervening in this process one
can actually alter a developing individual in
such a way that he will learn to accept
completely foreign material. For example; if a
representative sample of tissue (say a sus-
pension of spleen cells) is taken from a
newborn animal of a highly inbred strain of
mouse (strain A) and injected into a newborn
animal of another, different but also inbred
strain (strain B), then, even after the recipient
animal (B) reaches full maturity, it will continue to accept grafts of most tissues from
members of strain A. Strain A antigens were
present in B during the onset of immunologic
maturity and are therefore confused with native
antigens. He accepts both his own and strain A
antigens as self.

To reiterate, then, immunologic self determination is conditioned and not a part of the
information with which we start life. Immunologic tolerance, in one sense, is more specific
than immunologic rejection, since it involves
recognizing and ignoring comparatively few of a
multitude of antigens.

With this as background, we must now
examine a representative variety of those
situations in which immunologic deficiency
states can be detected (Illustration 4-2).

1. Congenital Immunologic Deficiency

On occasion, a patient is detected who
manifests a full or partial deficiency of either or
both immunologic systems at birth (Illustration
4-3). These patients, although rare and not
representing a numerically significant health
problem, are nonetheless interesting as "experiments of nature." Their importance to the
clinical immunologist (aside from their innate
importance as human beings in need of help)
has been immense in that he is actually able to
observe the effects of complete ablation of

any type; abnormal def. could result or congenital basis

Occurrence of certain disease syndromes E congenital

4-2. KINDS OF IMMUNOLOGIC DEFICIENCY DISEASES

1) CONGENITAL
deficiency present from birth, hereditary or teratologic - *developmental defect in genetically normal individual*

2) SECONDARY
resulting from some other disease or injury, particularly viral infections, lymphoid neoplasms and severe burn injury

3) (IATROGENIC)
intentional or unintentional suppression of immunologic responses as part of a therapeutic regimen

4) SENESCENT
immunologic decline in advanced age

5) STRESS-INDUCED
sustained, severe physical or emotional stress

4-3. CONGENITAL IMMUNOLOGIC DEFICIENCY

1) HUMORAL

2) CELLULAR

3) PARTIAL OR COMPLEX DEFICIENCIES INVOLVING A PART OR PARTS OF ONE OR BOTH OF THE ABOVE

---

some component of the immune systems and can deduce its normal function in health.

Congenital Humoral Immunity

A congenital deficiency confined strictly to the humoral system is even more rare than a complex deficiency, but not unknown. As would be expected, it is manifested as a lack of circulating gamma globulin. The term agammaglobulinemia, although literally meaning a total absence of gamma globulin, has been recommended for use in describing any such condition, from total absence to a clinically significant deficiency. Other authors prefer to use the term, hypogammaglobulinemia, for the latter. Since a deficiency of immunoglobulin production can affect any stage in the complex scheme of immunocyte maturation it can occur in a bewildering variety of single and combined defects, ranging from complete dysgenesis of the immunoglobulin-producing system to the partial deficiency of a single immunoglobulin or complement component. The usual agammaglobulinemic patient requires both gamma globulin and antibiotic therapy and even then may be bothered with recurrent sepsis. The most conspicuous result of agammaglobulinemia is severe pneumococcal infection. Also notable are recurrent infections involving other pyogenic bacteria such as streptococci and staphylococci. Strangely enough, although patients suffering from an immunologic deficiency confined to the humoral system are very susceptible to infections with pyogenic cocci, they cope normally with most viral and fungal infections. Thus, the protection from infectious disease afforded by a healthy humoral immunologic response is apparently directed primarily toward relatively few pathogens, foremost among which are the extracellular pyogenic cocci.

Congenital Deficiencies of Cellular Immunity

Just as was seen in the case of the humoral system, congenital deficiencies of cellular immunity also occur spontaneously. Quite in contrast to the humoral deficiency, in which pyogenic infections are prominent, cellular deficiency predisposes the patient to infection with the tubercle bacillus, yeasts, fungi and a host of organisms that normally live in complete harmony with the body's defenses (commensal organisms). In fact, one of the most useful signs of cellular immunologic deficiency is infection with the commensal fungus, *Candida albicans.* The condition is called *chronic mucocutaneous candidiasis* and is easily observed as a slightly elevated, whitish plaque growing on the pink surface of oral or vaginal

ablation - complete absence of humoral + cellular systems

KNOW usually lives in harmony E body until chronic irritation or skin cancer RASH

mucosa. The patient with cellular immunologic deficiency also exhibits a decidedly greater propensity to contract cancer and to experience its recurrence following surgery. This is undoubtedly because cellular immune mechanisms protect the body against transformed cells which might otherwise grow out into a dangerous tumor.

Congenital deficiencies of the humoral and immunologic systems are briefly compared in Illustration 4-4.

2. Secondary Immunologic Deficiency

disorders mediating tissues [?] immunol [?]

Both humoral and cellular immunologic responses are depressed in many diseases (Illustration 4-5). Such depression is most conspicuously associated with infectious diseases of viral etiology as well as in cancer primary to the lymphoreticular system (lymphoma and lymphocytic leukemia). In the latter, altered lymphoid cells produced by the cancer displace normal cells, causing a severe impairment of function. Also, it has been repeatedly shown in both humans and experimental animals that uremia depresses homograft rejection presumably through its effect on cellular immunity.

3. Iatrogenic Immunologic Deficiency

Iatrogenic immunologic deficiency, like any iatrogenic disease, is that caused by treatment.

ABLATION

4-4. CONGENITAL DEFICIENCIES OF HUMORAL AND CELLULAR SYSTEMS

1) HUMORAL SYSTEM *↑ capacity to [?] autoimmune*
   recurrent URT infections with extracellular, pyogenic pathogens *recurrent pneumonia + bronchitis*

2) CELLULAR SYSTEM
   { recurrent infections with mycobacteria, yeasts, fungi and commensal organisms
   inability to confine certain viral infections
   increased susceptibility to primary and recurrent cancer

current [?] first infection / humoral intact

4-5. SECONDARY IMMUNOLOGIC DEFICIENCY

1) OCCURS AS AN UNTOWARD EFFECT OF CERTAIN KINDS OF DISEASES

2) MOST SUCH DISEASES AFFECT THE LYMPHORETICULAR SYSTEM DIRECTLY
   certain virus infections
   lymphoma and leukemia

4-6. IATROGENIC IMMUNOLOGIC DEFICIENCY

1) INTENTIONAL IMMUNOSUPPRESSION *therapeutic strategy to control inflamm disease*
   anti-inflammatory steroids
   antimetabolites — *imuran — prevents mitotic division*
   local irradiation — *too dangerous*
   heterologous antilymphocyte
      serum — *prepared against human lymphocyte (hyperimmune)*

2) UNINTENTIONAL IMMUNOSUPPRESSION
   inhalation anesthesia
   control of inflammatory disease

Illustration 4-6 lists the 2 varieties of iatrogenic immunologic deficiency that we will mention as examples.

Intentional Suppression of Immunity

Despite its hazards, it is sometimes necessary to induce a deficiency of immunologic defenses. When an organ, such as a kidney or a heart, is transplanted the recipient will usually reject the graft, if his cellular immune system is left intact. Such intentional immunosuppression can be accomplished in a number of ways; those in routine use are listed in Illustration 4-6. The term, *heterologous antilymphocyte*

Tubercle bacillus - PPD
* patient's inability to reject grafts - principle confirmation of cellular immun. deficiency — Not by humoral

Cold sore - labile lesion caused by Herpes virus (lip)

gradual decline of immunological competence (handwritten margin note)

zeros in on lymphocytes (handwritten margin note)

serum, refers to hyperimmune serum generated in a horse or goat against human lymphoid cells. This serum is injected into a human graft recipient (or other patient in whom immunologic responses are to be suppressed) and its antibodies coat lymphoid cells, impairing their function. A horse or goat is used because humans share a number of cell surface antigens in common, but very few with lower animals. These animals react strongly to human tissue antigens and make excellent "factories" for antibodies specific against human cells. Although the methods listed are reasonably serviceable, resorting to non-specific immunosuppression to permit retention of an allogeneic graft is, in one sense, exchanging one immunologic disorder for another. It is far from the ideal means of prolonging graft acceptance, its primary shortcoming being the necessity to diminish *all* immunologic capability to permit the tolerance of only a *few* unacceptable antigens. This has been criticized as a "shotgun" or "blunderbuss" solution. Ideally one would induce a selective tolerance for only those graft antigens that the recipient recognizes as alien. Although beyond current technology, this is potentially possible and its accomplishment is certain to open up a new era in organ transplantation.

Unintentional Immunosuppression

side effect of treatment (handwritten margin note)

In addition to the intentional suppression of tissue defenses, there are many instances in which this happens unintentionally as an expected or unexpected complication of the use of a drug or anesthetic. Since the action of most drugs on tissue defense systems is not known, it would be impossible to cite every agent that can act as an immunosuppressant. In fact, some degree of toxicity to tissue defense systems probably results from the use of most drugs and drug-like agents, even beverage alcohol. Recent research has disclosed that inhalation anesthetics are conspicuous for their ability to inhibit inflammation and immunity, even though they are never used primarily for that purpose. These same agents have been shown to inhibit cell migration and suppress exudate formation in experimental peritonitis.

4. Immunologic Deficiency of Senescence

The precise role of gradual immunologic

failure in biologic aging is not known: however, there is a good reason to suspect that immune capability diminishes with age. Perhaps the most conspicuous effect of this deficiency is a greatly increased liability to cancer. In Illustration 4-7, it can be seen that, after the age of 65 to 70, the incidence in cancer increases sharply. The reason is not yet known, but the definite and predictable characteristics of the phenomenon suggest that a great deal could be learned from its further study. Although other factors may prevail in aging, it is no coincidence that cancer increases sharply with the onset of senescence, while the mass of lymphoid tissue is severely diminished. *appearance of cancer indicates failure of immune system* (handwritten margin note)

5. Stress-Induced Immunologic Deficiency

Physical stress such as might result from surgery or an extensive burn is known to depress tissue defense systems, a phenomenon probably mediated by the secretion of endogenous adrenocorticosteroids. This is particularly unfortunate in that both of these categories of patients, as well as others subjected to traumatic injury, frequently experience wound infections and septicemia.

There is growing evidence that immunologic deficiency can also be caused by certain kinds of emotional stress. The picture is far from

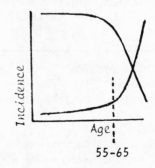

4-7. IMMUNOLOGIC   DEFICIENCY   IN   ADVANCED AGE

Lower curve depicts the incidence of malignancy in man as a function of age while the upper represents an estimate of concurrent immunocompetence.

4-8. STRESS-INDUCED IMMUNOLOGIC DEFICIENCY

1) PHYSICAL STRESS
    increased secretion of adrenal steroids following severe burn, major surgery or other serious stress

2) EMOTIONAL STRESS
    more chronic but comparable to above, mediated through

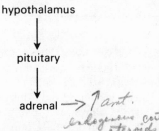

hypothalamus

↓

pituitary

↓

adrenal → ↑ amt.
endogenous cortico steroids

diminished resistance to infection and neoplastic disease

person suppresses own immunolog. responses.

clear as regards either the type of stress or the means by which it acts, but most clinicians and investigators would support the general conclusion that there is real physical hazard in sustained emotional disturbance. Again, although it is not well understood, the hypothalamus has been shown to be involved in the regulation of immunologic responses and may be the route through which the emotional status of an individual comes to modify his tissue defenses. This is represented diagrammatically in Illustration 4-8. Even the earliest of medical records include comments to the effect that certain kinds of infectious disease are noticeably more prevalent among unhappy (melancholy) people than among those who are vigorous and enthusiastic (sanguine). Delayed recovery and prolonged convalescence have also been mentioned as complications of emotional disturbance superimposed on infection. This is supported by experimental evidence showing that psychiatric patients exhibit a depressed humoral response to certain antigens. It seems certain, then, that some types of emotional

disorders can decrease host resistance to infection.

As in the case of infectious disease, the tendency for cancer to be more common among emotionally disturbed individuals was noticed centuries ago and has been reiterated among medical writers of every era. The tumor most often mentioned is carcinoma of the breast in women, although bronchogenic carcinoma in the male has been shown to be correlated with similar psychic problems.

Additional Reading

Balner, H. Perspectives of immunosuppression. Transplant. Proc. III:949, 1971
Bellanti, J. A. and Schlagle, R. J. The diagnosis of immunologic deficiency diseases. Pediat. Clin. N. Amer. 18:49, 1971
Douglas, S. D. Analytic review: disorders of phagocyte function. Blood 35:851, 1970
Friedman, S. B. et al. Differential susceptibility to a viral agent in mice housed alone or in groups. Psychosom. Med XXXII:285, 1970
Jooste, S. V. Immunological effects of heterologous antilymphocyte sera. Lymphology 3:79, 1970
Kirkpatrick, C. H. et al. Chronic mucocutaneous candidiasis model-building in cellular immunity. Ann. Int. Med. 74:955, 1971
Lehrer, R. I. The role of phagocyte function in resistance to infection. California Med. 114:17, 1971
Mirsky, H. S. and Cuttner, J. Fungal infections in acute leukemia. Cancer 30:348, 1972
Solomon, G. F. et al. Secondary immune response to tetanus toxoid in psychiatric patients. J. Psychiat. Res. 7:201, 1970

ALLERGY

LEARNING OBJECTIVE

To be able to define allergy and outline the immunologic mechanisms, pathogenesis, clinical picture and complications of the following basic types:

    a) anaphylaxis
    b) immune-complex injury
    c) atopy
    d) cytotoxicity
    e) infection allergy
    f) contact allergy
    g) graft rejection
    h) graft-versus-host response

4-10. ALLERGIC DISEASE
ALLERGIES OF HUMORAL IMMUNITY 1) ANAPHYLAXIS 2) ATOPY 3) IMMUNE-COMPLEX INJURY 4) CYTOTOXICITY **ALLERGIES OF CELLULAR IMMUNITY** 1) INFECTION TYPE 2) CONTACT TYPE 3) GRAFT REJECTION 4) GRAFT-VERSUS-HOST REACTION

1. Allergy as a Kind of Immunologic Disease

Allergy (defined in Illustration 4-9) is the second of our 4 major categories of immunologic disease. The definition presented in Illustration 4-9 was not the original meaning of the term, but corresponds approximately to its past usage. When the concept of allergy was first proposed by von Pirquet, very little was known of the mechanism of immunity. His intention was that the word denote an altered response upon the second exposure to an environmental stress, a definition entirely in keeping with the level of knowledge of that time. Throughout intervening years, the term became inexact owing to its casual use in referring to a variety of poorly understood conditions. In a rather general way, it can be said to have been confined to those diseases

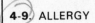

4-9. ALLERGY
1) AN IMMUNOLOGIC RESPONSE 2) TO AN *EXOGENOUS* ANTIGEN 3) THAT IS INAPPROPRIATE OR DAMAGING AND 4) NOT SHOWN BY ALL MEMBERS OF A SPECIES

characterized by a harmful immunologic response, although its use in popular parlance has sometimes been far afield. As a result of its original meaning and this long period of ambiguity, almost everyone has a working idea of allergy, but no definition can be said to be generally accepted. Some authors *do* and some *do not* consider the term synonymous with *hypersensitivity*, whereas some have even advocated its abandonment. For purposes of this discussion the definition presented in Illustration 4-9 will be used. The term, hypersensitivity, on the other hand, should either be abandoned (which is highly unlikely) or at least avoided as a synonym.

It has been recognized for some time that allergies can be based on either the humoral or cellular immunologic response and occur in a limited number of clinical patterns. If we extend the usual limits of cellular response allergy just slightly to include the graft rejection and graft-versus-host phenomenon, the complete roster of allergic disease becomes that presented in Illustration 4-10. We will now consider each type of allergy in brief outline, beginning with allergies of humoral immunity.

2. Allergies of Humoral Immunity

Humoral response allergies are those in which immunoglobulin systems are known to be operative. Illustration 4-11 lists the known associations between immunoglobulin classes and allergic disease. Allergies of the humoral

KNOW *allergins - allergy provoking antigen*

4-11. IMMUNOGLOBULINS AND ALLERGIC DISEASE

IgG

probably mediates most kinds of immune-complex injury, complexes can be soluble at certain Ag-Ab ratios

IgA

no known active participation in allergy

IgM

role in allergy is indefinite, complexes are large and usually insoluble, probably precluding its mediating immune-complex injury

IgD

nothing is known of its participation in allergy

IgE

mediates anaphylaxis, atopy and asthma *cytophilic*

---

to attach themselves to fixed tissue cells and are not found in any abundance in the serum. Although a very small amount of the same types of immunoglobulins with similar specificities are present in the serum and can be detected serologically, these circulating antibodies do not participate in the reaction and its vigor is not always proportional to their concentration. Anaphylaxis can be transferred passively, but the ability to react to the antigen is delayed 8 to 18 hours, during which time antibodies fix to participating cells. In combination with antigens these cell-bound antibodies cause the release of histamine and other vasoactive substances from mast cells and other reservoirs in the area of the antigen-antibody complex. This results in sudden vasodilatation and bronchiolar constriction, the effect being the onset of shock and bronchospasm as well as the possibility for edematous obstruction of the upper respiratory tract. In the usual human anaphylactic reaction, vascular collapse may predominate, although a wide variety of responses has been reported. In experimental guinea pig anaphylaxis, bronchial spasm is most prominent and the usual cause of death. Human asthma resembles guinea pig anaphylaxis, but is rarely severe enough to be fatal.

PASSIVE TRANSFER?

Atopic reactions, like anaphylaxis, are humoral allergies in which the antibodies mediating the response are fixed to cell surfaces. Although some antibodies with identical specificity are circulating and can be demonstrated serologically these, as in anaphylaxis, are not operative in the reaction. The term atopy generally implies a constitutional tendency

response fall very neatly into 4 principal clinical patterns as listed in Illustration 4-12. The first 2 produce no necrosis while the latter 2 are associated with some degree of tissue damage. We will consider these 4 patterns in 2 groups.

usually begins as feeling of uneasiness, nausea

Anaphylaxis and Atopy (Humoral Allergy without Necrosis)

Very conspicious and familiar types of humoral allergy are those which can be grouped as anaphylaxis and atopy. Many authors consider these as 1 group, for reasons which will be discussed. *loss of peripheral vas.*

Anaphylaxis is a shock-inducing and potentially fatal allergy in man. In the guinea pig, it results in hypotension and severe bronchial spasm and is also potentially fatal. In anaphylaxis, the antibodies which mediate the response are thought to be fixed to the smooth muscle cells of arterioles and bronchioles. They are said to be strongly cytophilic, i.e. they tend

4-12. ALLERGIES OF HUMORAL IMMUNITY

NO NECROSIS	1) anaphylaxis — *danger of dying from shock*
	2) atopy — *multiple reactions, including*
NECROSIS	3) immune-complex injury
	4) cytotoxicity

toward multiple similar allergies, including anaphylaxis. Thus, *the patient exhibiting atopic sensitivity to one allergen is liable to react to many others.* In fact, although poorly defined, there are genetic, environmental, and even psychologic factors operative in atopic disease.

The principal difference between anaphylaxis and atopy is in the sites of localization of the cell-fixed (cytophilic) antibodies and in the potential for a suddenly fatal outcome. There is no clear-cut line of division between certain types of atopy and anaphylaxis. If the reaction is life-threatening and involves shock and respiratory distress, it is usually considered the latter. Insofar as can now be determined, atopic reactions and anaphylactic reactions are mediated by IgE. Another designation for atopy-producing antibodies is "reagins," the term "reagin reaction" being roughly equivalent to atopy. They are also called "skin sensitizing antibodies," sometimes abbreviated SSA. All of these denote an immunologublin system with antibody fixed to the immediately subepithelial tissue of skin and mucosal surface.

The familiar hay fever, urticaria, superficial erythema and other common reactions to pollens, foods and drugs which occur in relation to some body surface are atopic reactions and may be diseases resulting from exaggerated reactivity of the IgE system.

Immune-Complex Injury and Cytotoxicity (Humoral Allergy with Necrosis)

Immune-complex and cytotoxic reactions are humoral allergies based on a mechanism very different from the preceding 2. They are particularly significant in that they are the only humoral reactions that result in necrosis. All antibodies participating in both reactions are circulating. Reactions can be elicited immediately after passive transfer of serum, since no time is needed to allow immunoglobulins to fix to tissue. Since there are important differences between the immune-complex and cytotoxic reactions we will consider each as a separate phenomenon.

Immune-complex injury is a fairly recent concept. The term is preferable to Arthus reaction since it is broad enough to include the many newly discovered examples of this kind of allergy. Immune-complex injury begins with the formation of an antigen-antibody complex

within a blood vessel and depends upon the participation of neutrophils for its completion. Its pathogenesis is outlined in Illustration 4-13. Examples of immune-complex injury are the hyperacute rejection of human renal allografts and the glomerulonephritis of systemic lupus erythematosus and serum sickness.

The cytotoxic reaction is a humoral response to allergy which has certain features in common with the immune-complex reaction, but differs slightly in its results. As in the immune-complex reaction the participating antibodies are circulating. However, in the cytotoxic reaction the antigen is always part of a surface of an intact cell such as a foreign blood cell, an altered native blood cell, a bacterial cell or another intact but alien structure. Reaction in the bloodstream results in the fixing of complement and the lysis of the cell. Again, as in the immune-complex reaction the fixing of comple-

---

4-13. PATHOGENESIS OF IMMUNE-COMPLEX INJURY

1) ANTIGEN REACTS WITH CIRCULATING ANTIBODY FORMING SOLUBLE COMPLEX

2) COMPLEX BECOMES ATTACHED OR LODGED IN SOME VASCULAR STRUCTURE

   AND FIXES COMPLEMENT

3) COMPLEX-COMPLEMENT AGGREGATE ATTRACTS NEUTROPHILS

4) NEUTROPHIL ENZYMES DIGEST AND DESTROY VESSEL WALL LOCALLY

5) PLATELETS ADHERE, CONGLUTINATE AND THROMBUS FORMS

6) SMALL VESSELS MAY BURST: PUNCTATE HEMORRHAGE RESULTS

4-14. ALLERGIES OF CELLULAR IMMU-NITY

INFECTION TYPE: Infection or the injection of extracts of a microorganism results in immunization. Later exposure causes destruction of tissue in which organism is found

CONTACT TYPE: Small molecule forms complex with normal tissue protein. Complex provokes immunologic response. Tissue is destroyed

GRAFT REJECTION: Graft of foreign tissue results in sensitization. Graft is invaded and destroyed

GRAFT-VERSUS-HOST REACTION: Transplanted mature lymphoid cells attack an immunologically incompetent host

Neutrophil participation essential to completion of immune-complex injury

ment is a necessary step: however, the participation of neutrophils is not required. This type of allergy is responsible for thrombocytopenia and for the massive hemolysis seen in erythroblastosis fetalis and the rejection of incompatible transfused erythrocytes.

3. Allergies of Cellular Immunity

Just as in humoral immunity, when the cellular immune response to an exogenous antigen is inappropriate and results in tissue damage the condition can be thought of as allergy. The allergies of cellular immunity are not as easily classified as those of humoral immunity, because comparatively little is known of the cellular response itself. At least for the present, it is convenient to consider cellular-response allergies under the subcategories listed in Illustration 4-14. Also included in 4-14 are comparative features of these 4 allergies.

Infection Type of Cellular Allergy

The first of the 4 patterns of cellular allergy we will consider is the so-called "infection" allergy. The infection type of cellular allergy results from actual invasion by microorganism or by the injection of killed cells or their extract. Sensitized lymphocytes encounter the infective antigen and in the resulting lesion the organism is destroyed or sequestered but, much to our occasional distress, it seems that native tissue to which antigens of the organism are adhering is also destroyed. This destruction of host tissue may be protective and may have evolved as a means of eliminating organisms that would otherwise go unnoticed. Whatever the reason, necrosis can be very extensive and may, for example, account for much of the damage to lung parenchyma in tuberculosis. The time-honored example of an infection type of allergy induced by exposure to a bacterial extract is the tuberclin skin test. In an immunized individual the intradermal injection of the purified protein dereviative (PPD) of the tubercle bacillus will cause formation, after 42 to 78 hours, of a raised, red, indurated lesion in which many lymphoid cells are seen. A significant amount of necrosis does not usually develop in the test lesion, because a very small amount of soluble antigen is used.

necrosis can be extensive - account for

Contact Allergy

In the contact type of cellular allergy, immunologic sensitivity is generated toward a complex between a native tissue protein and a foreign small molecule (Illustration 4-15). Neither substance is antigenic alone; the native protein is tolerated and the foreign molecule is too small. However, when joined, the resulting complex is a foreign-appearing, antigenic macromolecule which provokes a vigorous cellular response. A small molecule which acts in this way when exposed to tissue is said to be a hapten, i.e. one half of an antigen.

The best example of a contact allergy is the familiar *poison ivy*. Since the plant is of the genous Rhus, the condition is often called Rhus dermatitis. Here, the plant toxin acts as the hapten causing a reaction against native protein of the normal epithelium. In the usual case, the toxin does not penetrate into deeper tissue and, since the epithelium regenerates completely, no

complex itself antigen drains in lymph nodes

4-15. PATHOGENESIS OF CONTACT AL-
LERGY

---

1) SMALL MOLECULE (HAPTEN) FORMS
COMPLEX WITH NATIVE TISSUE
PROTEIN. COMPLEX IS ANTIGENIC

2) COMPLEX DRAINS INTO REGIONAL
NODE AND ELICITS CELLULAR IM-
MUNOLOGIC RESPONSE

3) SENSITIZED LYMPHOCYTES ARE
BROADCAST AND ENCOUNTER
COMPLEX AT SITE OF HAPTEN CON-
TACT

4) EPITHELIUM CONTAINING COMPLEX
IS DESTROYED

4-16. REJECTION OF A GRAFT

GRAFT

antigen | sensitized
        | lymphocytes

PERIPHERAL
LYMPHOID
TISSUE

afferent | efferent
(affector) | (effector)

---

strict localization to area contacted by hapten

scar results. Many reactions to salves and
cosmetics are based on the same mechanism
and are manifested as contact dermatitis,
contact stomatitis or surface inflammation
elsewhere in the body.

Graft Rejection as Transplantation Allergy

Know The graft rejection reaction is the cellular
response to transplanted alien tissue (Illustration 4-16). There is reason to believe that it
represents the allergic counterpart of a normal
immunologic facility which protects us against
tumor development and growth. In speaking of
tissues used as grafts, it is convenient to classify
them with regards to their genetic similarity to
the recipient, since this will give some insight
into the severity of the rejection response to be
expected. Tissues with identical or very similar
genetic constitutions will be well accepted,
whereas, if grossly dissimilar, they will provoke
a severe reaction. Using this type of classification, grafted tissue is designated as one of the 4
classes listed in Illustration 4-17.

The rejection of transplanted tissue is ultimately dependent upon a cellular immunologic
reaction. Humoral immunity is not involved
(except in the highly abnormal hyperacute
phenomenon) and, indeed, antibodies coating

4-17. CLASSIFICATION OF GRAFTS AND
GRAFTED TISSUE

GRAFT CLASSIFICATION
   AUTOGRAFT: same individual

   HOMOGRAFT: same species

   HETEROGRAFT: different species

TISSUE CLASSIFICATION (OF GRAFT)
   ISOGENEIC: same genetic constitution

   SYNGENEIC: very similar genetic constitution: inbred animals

Know ALLOGENEIC: different genetic constitution: same species

   XENOGENEIC: different species

[handwritten margin notes: "humoral only involved in hyperacute rejection", "about 14 days to reject graft"]

antigenetic determinants of the graft may actually protect it from attack by the cellular immune system. The initial graft of a foreign tissue fragment will appear, at first, to be accepted; only later, after healing has progressed, will the actual rejection occur. The second graft of this same tissue is rejected much more readily, however, since it is transplanted to an already sensitized animal. The ready rejection of the second graft is frequently referred to as the "second-set" response. The second-set response cannot be transferred with serum, supporting the hypothesis of a cellular immunologic basis for graft rejection.

[handwritten margin note: "counterpart of anamnesis of humoral reaction"]

Graft-versus-Host Reaction as a Rare Cellular Allergy

The graft-versus-host type of allergy is an immunologic reaction in which transplanted, mature lymphoid cells attack a tolerant host organism. It is not conventionally considered an allergy, but is included here because it is based on immunity and results in tissue damage. Pathogenesis of the graft-versus-host reaction is presented in Illustration 4-18. At present, the graft-versus-host reaction is most important as a laboratory disease model. No clear-cut examples of spontaneous disease can be attributed to this mechanism: however, it has been mentioned as an explanation for certain kinds of autoimmune phenomena. A disease exactly corresponding to the laboratory model has been accidentally generated in congenitally immunodeficient children as the result of attempts to transplant competent lymphoid cells of maternal origin.

Additional Reading

Bickley, H. C. A concept of allergy with reference to oral disease. J. Periodont. 41:302, 1970

Brent, L. Tolerance and enhancement in organ transplantation. Transplant. Proc. IV:363, 1972

Congdon, C. C. Bone marrow transplantation. Science 171:1116, 1971

Dausset, J. Polymorphism of HL-A system. Transplant. Proc. III:1139, 1971

Frank, M. M. The relationship of complement to allergic disease. Ann. Allerg. 27:490, 1969

Henson, P. M. Pathologic mechanisms in neutrophil-mediated injury. Am. J. Path. 68:593, 1972

Ishizaka, K. and Ishizaka, T. The significance of immunoglobulin E in reaginic hypersensitivity. Ann. Allergy 28:189, 1970

Kruger, G. R. F. et al. Graft-versus-host disease. Am. J. Path. 63:179. 1971

McDevitt, H. O. Relationship between histiocompatibility antigens and the immune response. Transplant. Proc. III:1321, 1971

Russell, P. S. and Winn, H. J. Transplantation (3 parts). N. Engl. J. Med. 282:786, 848, 898, 1970

Singal, D. P. Tissue typing and organ transplantation. Canad. J. Surg. 15:295, 1972

Winn, H. Humoral antibody in allograft reactions. Transplant. Proc. II:83, 1970

4-18. THE GRAFT-VERSUS-HOST REACTION

1) MATURE, IMMUNOCOMPETENT *[handwritten: KNOW]* CELLS ARE TRANSFERRED TO IMMUNOLOGICALLY INCOMPETENT HOST

2) HOST CANNOT REJECT FOREIGN CELLS BUT CELLS ATTEMPT TO REJECT HOST

3) MULTIPLE, DISSEMINATED LESIONS TYPICAL OF VARIOUS AUTOIMMUNE DISEASES RESULT

   experimental disease called "runt disease" or homologous disease

   human counterpart has resulted from attempts to unconstitute a congenitally deficient child with maternal cells

[handwritten margin note: "animal remains small & doesn't grow — homologous cells cause it"]

[handwritten note at bottom: "ex. knock out immunologic response + then inject spleen cells from another subj"]

AUTOIMMUNITY

LEARNING OBJECTIVE

To be able to define autoimmunity and discuss causes of the breakdown of self tolerance, briefly considering the immunologic mechanisms involved and some prominent clinical examples of each of the following types:

  a) immune-complex autoimmune injury
  b) autologous antitissue antibody injury
  c) homologous antitissue antibody injury (as exemplified in erythroblastosis fetalis)
  d) cellular autoimmune injury (including the possible involvement of infectious agents)

Autoimmunity (immunity directed against one's self) remains a controversial subject but, despite its being incompletely understood, it is now a well accepted mechanism of disease. We have seen in the previous learning objective that allergy is based on an inappropriate immunologic response to an antigen that orginates outside the body; we must now establish that autoimmunity is a comparable response, except that the antigen is of endogenous origin (Illustration 4-19). Autoimmunity differs from allergy only in that the antigen originates within the body (in most cases) and not in its environment. Indeed, allergy and autoimmunity are closely interrelated and often difficult to separate.

KNOW

4-19. AUTOIMMUNITY

1) AN IMMUNOLOGIC RESPONSE

2) TO AN *ENDOGENOUS* ANTIGEN THAT. IS *ONLY difference FROM Allergy*

3) INAPPROPRIATE OR DAMAGING AND

4) NOT SHOWN BY ALL MEMBERS OF A SPECIES

4-20. TYPES OF AUTOIMMUNE PHENOMENA

1) BASED ON HUMORAL IMMUNITY

KNOW

  autologous immune-complex injury *STARTS & IN body*
  autologous anti-tissue antibody
  homologous anti-tissue antibody (erythroblastosis fetalis)

2) BASED ON CELLULAR IMMUNITY*

  anti-tissue sensitized lymphocytes ("forbidden" clone)
  involvement of "slow", latent or inapparent infection with virus, mycoplasma or other intracellular pathogen

---

* in many cases of cellular auto-immune phenomena, immune-complex injury will occur secondary to the appearance of tissue debris

---

Like other types of immunologic disease, autoimmunity can be divided into examples based on the humoral immunologic system and those based on the cellular immunologic system (Illustration 4-20).

1. Humoral Autoimmunity

Certain autoimmune phenomena can be clearly shown to be based on malfunction of the humoral immunologic system. These humoral autoimmune mechanisms are of 3 types: 1) autologous immune-complex injury; 2) autologous anti-tissue antibody injury; 3) homologous anti-tissue antibody injury (as exemplified by erythroblastosis fetalis).

Autoimmunity Based on Immune-Complex Injury

Material released from disrupted cells is undoubtedly antigenic and probably incites a humoral immunologic response that aids in its

out of place

elimination. In Chapter 1 we classified such material as *ectopic non-self.* Because of the constant breakdown of cells throughout a person's lifetime, it is felt that a low level of autoantibodies directed against ectopic non-self is constantly circulating in the blood stream. This is normal when held to its usual low concentration, but may cause trouble if provoked to extreme concentrations by the sudden appearance of a massive amount of tissue debris. Under these circumstances a large number of immune complexes are formed which may, in turn, lead to the subsequent development of immune-complex tissue injury. As with other examples of immune-complex injury, IgG appears to be the offending immunoglobulin, because IgG complexes are soluble and fix complement. These complexes lodge in the walls of blood vessels and in vascular structures such as the renal glomerulus and result in tissue damage. Two examples of such immune-complex injury are listed and described in Illustration 4-21.

Autoimmunity Based on the Anti-Tissue Antibody

The second variety of humoral autoimmunity results from an antibody being generated within the body that reacts not with ectopic antigens but with *normal* body material

Idiopathic ? → thrombocytopenia

4-21. AUTOIMMUNE IMMUNE-COM-PLEX INJURY

1) NEPHRITIS OF SLE   *KNOW*
   primary damage releases an abundance of tissue debris: complexes form which lodge in glomerular filter, fix complement and cause glomerulonephritis

2) POST-MYOCARDIAL INFARCTION SYNDROME
   complexes formed with necrotic debris from infarct cause a variety of damage

---

4-22. POSSIBLE REASONS FOR LOSS OF SELF TOLERANCE

1) ACTUAL CHANGE IN THE ANTIGENIC NATURE OF THE TISSUE
   hapten complex
   somatic mutation

2) DEFICIENCY OF IMMUNOLOGIC PROTECTIVE MECHANISM

3) CROSS REACTIVITY BETWEEN A DETERMINANT OF AN EXOGENOUS ANTIGEN AND ONE OF NORMAL TISSUE

4) APPEARANCE OF ABNORMAL IMMUNOCYTES
   mutation
   proliferation of "forbidden" clone

5) RELEASE OF A NORMALLY SEQUESTERED ANTIGEN   *occur in hypothalamus*

Good-Pasteur's syndrome - disease from body's production

in a *normal* location; we will refer to these as anti-tissue antibodies. The formation of anti-tissue antibodies suggests that the body's tolerance for its own tissue has somehow been violated. Self (even though it remains in its normal position) is construed as non-self. It is postulated that the cause for this would be one or more of the factors listed in Illustration 4-22. Examples of diseases produced by anti-tissue antibodies are listed in Illustration 4-23. A thorough discussion of each of these 3 examples is beyond the scope of this objective: however, there is strong evidence in each case that the disease is actually produced by an autologous anti-tissue antibody.

autologous anti-tissue antibodies against certain component of glomerular basement membrane - cross react → glomerular nephritis → hemorrhage + renal failure FATAL

Autoimmunity Based on the Homologous Anti-Tissue Antibody

The third category of autoimmune disease produced by humoral immunity is that in which the antibody is obtained passively. Most examples of such disease center around hemolytic disorders of the newborn and, in partic-

preparation of antibodies anti-Rh antibodies known as Rho-gam

4-23. DISEASES PRODUCED BY ANTI-TISSUE ANTIBODIES

1) GOODPASTURE'S SYNDROME

2) IDIOPATHIC THROMBOCYTOPENIC PURPURA

3) ACQUIRED HEMOLYTIC ANEMIA

ular, the syndrome of *erythroblastosis fetalis* (Illustration 4-24). Erythroblastosis fetalis is a disease resulting from incompatibility between a mother and fetus based on the Rh blood group antigen. The Rh antigen was discovered when it was noted that blood from a Rhesus monkey when injected into a rabbit, caused its serum to agglutinate the red blood cells of 85 per cent of humans. This 85 per cent of the population is said to be Rh-positive and are known to carry the Rh antigen on the surface of their erythrocytes, just as the Rhesus monkey does. It was later found that the antigen was inherited as an autosomal dominant trait and that there were no naturally occurring antibodies toward the Rh antigen in the serum of individuals not manifesting Rh on their blood cells. In order to be sensitized against the Rh antigen a person must be immunized against it. This usually occurs either as the result of an incompatible blood transfusion or a pregnancy in which the fetus is Rh-positive and the mother Rh-negative. Development of erythroblastosis fetalis requires the 3 factors listed in Illustration 4-24. When the mother's IgG is transferred to the fetus some anti-Rh is included. These anti-Rh antibodies destroy fetal blood cells, causing a severe hemolytic disorder. Since the mother cannot be effectively desensitized the only practical means of preventing erythroblastosis is to *prevent maternal sensitization.* Fetal blood cells are usually transferred to the mother's blood stream during delivery as part of the birth trauma. Thus, sensitization occurs at the end of 1 pregnancy and the mother is sensitized for the next. To prevent fetal cells from sensitizing the mother, it is now routine practice to inject a preparation of

difference from ABO system

Cannot be de-sensitized

human anti-Rh antibodies within a week of delivery of an Rh-incompatible child. These antibodies coat the Rh antigens on the transferred cells and prevent the mother's mounting an immunologic reaction against them. The use of this preparation at the end of each pregnancy has proven effective in the prevention of erythroblastosis fetalis.

2. Cellular Autoimmunity

The mechanism of cellular autoimmunity is similar to that described for the humoral immunologic system. Anti-tissue sensitized lymphocytes are generated for many of the same reasons listed in Illustration 4-22. In addition, however, many authorities believe that infection with an unusual pathogen may somehow be involved in many autoimmune phenomena based on the cellular immunologic system.

It has recently been discovered that certain intracellular parasites can live inobtrusively within cells. They do not kill the host cell

4-24. ERYTHROBLASTOSIS FETALIS

1) SYNDROME CAUSED BY MASSIVE DESTRUCTION OF FETAL BLOOD CELLS *IN UTERO*
   anemia
   jaundice
   hydrops fetalis — *generalized edema in fetus*

2) DESTRUCTION CAUSED BY ANTI-Rh COMPONENT OF NATURALLY TRANSFERRED IgG

3) REQUIREMENTS
   KNOW
   Rh negative mother
   Rh positive fetus
   mother sensitized to Rh (incompatible blood transfusion or previous pregnancy)

---

4) MATERNAL SENSITIZATION MUST BE PREVENTED TO PREVENT DISEASE
   postpartum use of human anti-Rh

primary tissue damage of SLE is from cellular immunity (gives rise to most of debris)

SLE seen in woman of child bearing age.

4-25. CELLULAR AUTOIMMUNITY

1) POSTVIRAL ENCEPHALOMYELITIS *nervous system damaged following viral infection*

2) PRIMARY TISSUE DAMAGE IN SYSTEMIC LUPUS ERYTHEMATOSUS *after this* renal damage is caused by immune-complex injury *cellular immune attack*

3) SCLERODERMA (PROGRESSIVE SYSTEMIC SCLEROSIS)

4) OTHERS *ALL collagen or connective tissue disease*

---

immediately (if ever), and apparently cause such a subtle alteration of its surface that their presence only gradually comes to the attention of the cellular immunologic system. A list of such pathogens would include certain viruses, L-form bacteria, mycoplasma and perhaps even some intracellular parasitic protozoa. Examples of diseases known to be caused by pathogens of this type are scrapie in sheep, certain kinds of pneumonia and perhaps even rhematoid arthritis in man. Their role in autoimmunity may be such that they change the antigenic characteristics of the parasitized cell just enough to render it liable to attack by the cellular immune system (either chronically or in periodic episodes). In effect, only parasitized cells are eliminated but the infection is so low-grade that it appears as if normal somatic cells are being destroyed without provocation.

Whatever the true cause there seem to be a number of diseases based on cellular autoimmunity (Illustration 4-25). We will simply mention these here as examples, since the more common will be encountered again as diseases of specific organ systems.

Additional Reading

Karpatkin, S. Autoimmune thrombocytopenic purpura. Am. J. Med. Sci. 261:127, 1971

Levine, P. Prevention and treatment of erythroblastosis fetalis. Ann. N.Y. Acad. Sci. 169:234, 1970

Russell, W. O. Fifth annual ASCP research symposium: Viruses and Autoimmune disease. Am. J. Clin. Path. 56:259, 1971

Shean, M. A. The clinical spectrum of Sjogren's syndrome. California Med. 117:63, 1972

Stein, S. The early appearance of the post-myocardial infarction syndrome. Angiology 20:262, 1969

Tuffanelli, D. L. Lupus erythematosus. Arch. Dermatol. 106:553, 1972

Tuffanelli, D. L. and La Perriere, R. Connective tissue diseases. Pediat. Clin. N. Amer. 18:925, 1971

Tuismorio, F. P. et al. Autoimmunity in thermal injury: Occurrence of rheumatoid factors, antinuclear antibodies and antiepithelial antibodies. Clin. Exp. Immunol. 8:701, 1971

Weir, D. M. and Elson, C. J. Antitissue antibodies and immunological tolerance to self. Arth. Rheum. 12:254, 1969

White, C. A. et al. Rh_O (D) immune globulin to prevent Rh hemoloyte disease. Am. Family Phys. 3: 85, 1971

KNOW

debris - primarily nuclear, occasional neutrophils stuffed c nuclear-basophilic that has picked up nuclear material during incubation = LE cell

LE preparation - blood test of LE cells incubate blood at 37°

IMMUNOPROLIFERATIVE DISEASE

Seen in other diseases - all related to SLE

LEARNING OBJECTIVE

To be able to define immunoproliferative disease and discuss briefly the following:

   a) monoclonal gammopathies, including the significance of paraproteinemia

   b) proliferative disease of cells mediating cellular immunologic phenomena

---

Somatic cells that undergo mitotic division as part of their normal function frequently give rise to tumors, whereas cells which do not proliferate, such as the mature neuron or myocardial fiber, do so only rarely. Most lymphoid cells are thought to be capable of mitosis, at least at some stage in their differentiation. In fact, as we have seen, proliferation is an essential part of the primary and secondary immunologic responses. As would be expected, lymphoid neoplasia (proliferative disease) is not rare.

stable cells give rise to tumors rarely.

Proliferative disease of lymphoid tissue has been termed lymphoproliferative or immunoproliferative disease. The latter, being more general, is favored for this discussion. Immunoproliferative disease affects the humoral and cellular immunologic systems, but so little is

some pathogens don't kill host immediately (viruses + other intracellular parasites) never - just cause subtle change - cause gradual one

unprovoked proliferation of lymphoid cells sometimes accompanied by synthesis of functionless immunoglobulin

known of either that it is difficult to even distinguish between the 2 much less characterize human diseases which represent them.

1. Proliferative Disease of the Humoral Immunologic System

Proliferative disease of tissues mediating the humoral immunologic response occurs in a bewildering spectrum ranging from benign plasmacytosis and plasmacytoma through Waldenstrom's macroglobulinemia and multiple myloma to true plasma cell leukemia (Illustration 4-26). The last 3 of these are frequently associated with the appearance in blood of an abnormal immunoglobulin (paraprotein or myeloma protein) and this protein is most often, but not always, homogeneous. The light chain component is frequently found in the urine (Bence-Jones proteinuria) and is of great diagnostic value.

The homogeneity of paraproteins is strong evidence in favor of the Clonal Selection theories of immunologic specificity, since it suggests that the neoplastic plasmacytoid tissue has arisen from a single clone. Recognizing this, Waldenstrom has suggested the term *monoclonal gammopathy* as more appropriate for immunoglobulin-producing neoplastic disease. It is also of great interest that most immunoglobulins produced in monoclonal gammopathies are recognizable as one of the principal isotypes, IgG, M or A, and that their occurrence in these diseases roughly parallels their proportions in normal blood. Paraproteins may have immunologic specificity and in certain rare diseases occur only as the heavy chain component rather than the entire molecule. An infectious disease of the horse resembles human immunoproliferative disease of the humoral type and has been proposed as a laboratory model.

2. Proliferative Disease of the Cellular Immunologic System

Immunoproliferative disease affecting the cellular immune system is more poorly understood than that of the humoral system. It is entirely possible that Hodgkin's disease in its many varieties is the spontaneous human representative of this class, but this is only speculation.

Additional Reading

Pruzanski, W. et al. Leukemia form of immunocytic dyscrasia. Am. J. Med. 47:60, 1969

Fishkin, B. G. et al. IgD multiple myeloma: A report of five cases. Am. J. Clin. Path. 53:209, 1970

4-26. IMMUNOPROLIFERATIVE DISEASE

1) OF CELLS MEDIATING *HUMORAL* IMMUNITY

  benign plasmacytosis and plasmacytoma

  monoclonal gammopathies*

  Waldenstrom's macroglobulinemia
  multiple myeloma
  certain forms of lymphoma

2) OF CELLS MEDIATING *CELLULAR* IMMUNITY

  Hodgkin's disease
  certain forms of lymphoma

---

* term denotes single-clone neoplasm with production of large amounts of essentially functionless immunoglobulin (or fragment), the immunoglobulin is referred to as paraprotein and the blood picture as a dysproteinemia

part 2

modes of injury

chapter 5
PHYSICAL AND CHEMICAL INJURY

MECHANICAL INJURY (TRAUMA)

LEARNING OBJECTIVE

To be able to discuss the 6 traumatic lesions presented, in terms of the principles of mechanical injury

No mode of injury is more relevant to contemporary culture than trauma. Indeed, considering war, transportation accidents and crime, trauma is perhaps the most important form of injury in the world.

Agents of trauma are those that transfer a damaging excess of kinetic energy to tissues. Trauma has always been common because of mankind's propensity to violence. Even in pre-history it must have been readily apparent that the swinging club or speeding projectile could be charged with an enormous amount of kinetic energy and conveniently directed into contact with the tissues of one's prey or adversary. Many of the traumatic lesions listed in illustration 5-1 require no explanation and so we will single out only 2 for description.

1. Contusion

A blow with a blunt instrument that does not penetrate the surface of the body is called a *contusion* or bruise. As in other forms of mechanical injury, the shock represented by the sudden absorption of large amounts of energy is the damaging effect. Tissues are crushed, dislocated or disrupted resulting in death or sublethal disease.

Hemorrhage into the skin resulting from the crushing of superficial vessels is usually a prominent effect of contusion. As blood pigment is processed by macrophages, the color of

---

5-1. TRAUMA (MECHANICAL INJURY)

examples

1) LACERATION — tearing

2) ABRASION

3) INCISION

4) PUNCTURE

5) CONTUSION

6) PROJECTILE WOUND

---

the skin changes from red to blue to greenish-yellow. Discoloration of this type is called *ecchymosis*.

2. Projectile Wound

A projectile, penetrating the body surface, injures in 2 ways. As velocity is decreased the energy represented is transferred to tissues as a sudden wave of shock. But there is also the additional hazard of its penetrating and directly disrupting vital structures such as the central nervous system, cardiovascular system or gastrointestinal tract.

Additional Reading

De Muth, W. E. Bullet velocity as applied to military rifle wounding capacity. J. Trauma 9:27, 1969

Gaston, S. R. Accidental death and disability: the neglected disease of modern society (a progress report). J. Trauma 11:195, 1971

Know reln. of hemorrhage (ecchymosis) w/ contusion

79

Hi! Moon

THERMAL INJURY

LEARNING OBJECTIVE

To be able to outline the principles of thermal injury and discuss burn injury in detail mentioning:

a) terminology used in specifying and describing a burn

b) complications of serious burn injury

The human organism tolerates only slight variations in the thermal quality of its surroundings. An environment that is too hot prevents the body from radiating excess heat and causes an elevation of body core temperature. Extremely high temperatures disrupt delicate metabolic processes and denature critical protein components of cells.

An environment that is too cold precludes the maintenance of proper temperatures, slowing metabolic processes and ultimately disrupting their interaction. Extremes of cold, of course, will freeze body water and growing intracellular crystals will burst cell membranes resulting in fatal damage. These principles are outlined in Illustration 5-2.

body rids itself of heat, how?

5-2. THERMAL INJURY

1) EXTREMELY LOW TEMPERATURE
   hypothermia
   frostbite

2) EXTREMELY HIGH TEMPERATURE
   hyperthermia
   burn injury

5-3. BURN INJURY

1) EXTENT OF SURFACE AFFECTED
   in per cent of total skin area

2) DEPTH OF INJURY *describe*
   partial thickness (first and second degree)
   full thickness (third degree)

---

1. Burn Injury

Of all types of thermal injury, the burn is perhaps most common and significant. The seriousness of a burn depends upon the 2 factors listed in Illustration 5-3. The *extent* of burn injury is usually referred to as the percentage of total body area affected whereas its *depth* is expressed in terms of the thickness of the skin involved. The former is self-explanatory: however, the latter requires some elaboration.

The skin consists of 2 layers, epidermis and dermis. The epidermis forms a thin covering over the tough, fibrous dermis, but also extends into the dermis as sweat glands and hair follicles. Since these are derived from epithelial cells, they are referred to as epithelial appendages; the epithelial covering itself can be regenerated from cells that make up these structures.

If a burn injury destroys only the epithelial covering but does not extend into the dermis, it is called a *partial thickness burn.* Since sweat glands and hair follicles escape damage, the epithelial covering is regenerated from their cells and a graft is not required. If a burn destroys both the epidermis and the dermis, it is called a *full thickness burn.* In the case of the full thickness burn, no regenerative source remains for epithelial surface tissue and the surface must be restored by grafting such tissue from unaffected areas of the body.

2. Complications of Burn Injury

A list of common complications of burn injury is provided in Illustration 5-4. Colonization of the burn area by opportunistic pathogens, septicemia and shock is the most common sequence of events leading to death in the severely burned patient. Some of the principal pathogens involved are organisms relatively

5-4. COMPLICATIONS OF BURN INJURY
1) PAIN
2) SHOCK
3) INFECTION AND SEPTICEMIA   leading to septicemic shock

4) CURLING'S ULCER
    hemorrhage
    perforation

5) NEPHROSIS

harmless to healthy subjects. These include *Pseudomonas aeruginosa, Staphylococcus aureus* and other such organisms which can be relied upon to contaminate the burned area.

Further complicating this picture is a constellation of factors that seemingly result from the high output of adrenocortical steroids provoked by the severe stress imposed by this kind of injury. As might be expected, high circulating levels of such hormones suppress the immunologic defenses of the body and render the patient even more vulnerable to infection and septicemia. IgA and IgG immunoglobulins fall to dangerously low levels within 48 hours after a serious burn and are restored gradually through a period of 7 to 14 days. Cellular immunity becomes severely depressed somewhat later in the postburn period and may remain so for up to 2 months.

An additional complication resulting from high steroid levels is the occurrence of Curling's ulcers (stress-induced ulcers of the stomach), which can progress to hemorrhage or even perforation.

Additional Reading

Haynes, B. W. Current problems in burns. Arch. Surg. 103:454, 1971

Lowbury, E. J. L. Infection associated with burns. Postgrad. Med. J. 48:338, 1972

Munster, A. M. Alterations of the host defense mechanism in burns. Surg. Clin. N. Amer. 50:1217, 1970

Silva, Y. J. Thomas Blizard Curling—the man and the ulcer. Surgery 69:646, 1971

IONIZING RADIATION

LEARNING OBJECTIVE

To be able to define ionizing radiation and discuss each of the following:
   a) Meaning of the term "ionizing" and examples of radiant energy that penetrates and ionizes
   b) theories of radiation tissue damage
   c) the law of Bergonie and Tribondeau
   d) classification of human tissues with regard to susceptibility to ionizing radiation
   e) difference between local and whole-body irradiation
   f) difference between acute and delayed effects of whole-body irradiation

Injury through ionizing radiation results when high intensity photons are directed at living tissue. It is important to recognize that, although this kind of injury does not cause pain, a damaging dose of energy is just as surely transmitted to irradiated tissue as if it were struck by a projectile. Radiant energy is encountered in 2 forms as indicated in Illustration 5-5. Particulate emissions do not penetrate intact skin but are considered ionizing. Electromagnetic emissions take the form of photons (units that share characteristics of wave and particulate forms); they do penetrate intact skin, cause widespread ionization of water and are the form of radiant energy most likely to be encountered as an agent of injury. The discussion that follows applies, for the most part, to electromagnetic radiation of X and gamma energy levels.

1. Radiation Tissue Damage

Currently held theories of the means by which ionizing radiation damages tissue hold that most injury is produced indirectly. The photon in transit through the cell interacts with a molecule of solvent water, splitting it into highly reactive ions known as free radicals. These ions react immediately with critical components of the cells, the effect being to crosslink macromolecules, changing their tertiary structures in such a way that they can no

```
┌──────────────────────────────────────┐
│ 5-5. FORMS OF RADIANT ENERGY         │
├──────────────────────────────────────┤
│                                      │
│ 1) PARTICULATE OR CORPUSCULAR        │
│      Alpha                           │
│        nucleus of the helium atom    │
│      Beta                            │
│        electron                      │
│                                      │
│ 2) ELECTROMAGNETIC                   │
│      X-ray                           │
│      λ = approx. 10⁻⁷ cm* generated  │
│        by orbital shift of electrons │
│      Gamma                           │
│      λ = approx. 10⁻⁹ cm* generated  │
│        by disintegration of unstable nu-│
│        clei                          │
│                                      │
│      – – – – – – –                   │
│                                      │
│                                      │
│ * λ shorter than 10⁻⁵ cm are considered│
│ ionizing                             │
└──────────────────────────────────────┘
```

5-5. FORMS OF RADIANT ENERGY

1) PARTICULATE OR CORPUSCULAR
   Alpha
     nucleus of the helium atom
   Beta
     electron

2) ELECTROMAGNETIC
   X-ray
   λ = approx. 10^{-7} cm* generated by orbital shift of electrons
   Gamma
   λ = approx. 10^{-9} cm* generated by disintegration of unstable nuclei

   – – – – – – –

* λ shorter than 10^{-5} cm are considered ionizing

longer function adequately in metabolism. Any degree of injury is possible, from subtle interference with a critical molecule to the absolute destruction of a cell by overwhelming disturbance of its vital functions. It can also be seen that the damaging quantity of radiation is not that to which a tissue has been exposed, but rather that which has been absorbed. The most useful unit, considering the need to express absorbed dose, is the rad. See Illustration 5-6 for further explanation of this energy unit.

2. Classification of Human Tissue by Radiation Sensitivity

Radiation appears to be most lethal to dividing cells. This was pointed out in a paper by Bergonie and Tribondeau in 1906 and has since become known as the "Law of Bergonie and Tribondeau." It is actually less of a law than a consistent observation. In fact, it has proven so consistent that it would seem that tissues of the human body can be arranged into 3 groups on the basis of their response to ionizing radiation. These are listed and defined in Illustration 5-7. Because of its unusual significance in understanding the pathologic effects of radiation, the student should master this scheme of classification.

3. Local and Whole-Body Irradiation

In assessing or predicting the effects of radiation one must be sure to differentiate between local and whole-body modes of administration. Local irradiation (such as that used in the radiotherapy of cancer) affects only the tissues in the path of the beam; very high doses can therefore be used with relative safety. In whole-body irradiation the entire body is exposed at once and all susceptible tissues are similarly affected; a much lower dose is permissable.

The acute effects of whole-body irradiation are based on the destruction of the 3 most radiosensitive tissues, bone marrow, lymphoid tissue, and gastrointestinal epithelium. As might be expected, acute radiation sickness resulting from whole-body irradiation is characterized by early lymphopenia and bloody diarrhea followed by anemia and granulocytopenia. A somewhat delayed effect of whole-body irradiation that is not apparent is the appearance of chromosome abnormalities. The significance of this phenomenon is not fully understood although some of these chromosomal changes persist for years.

Long-delayed effects of whole body irradiation are noticed only when a population of

```
┌──────────────────────────────────────┐
│ 5-6. RADIATION INJURY                │
├──────────────────────────────────────┤
│                                      │
│ 1) RADIOLYSIS OF TISSUE WATER        │
│    FORMS FREE RADICALS (ION PAIRS)   │
│                                      │
│ 2) SECONDARY REACTIONS OF FREE       │
│    RADICALS DESTROY FUNCTION OF      │
│    CRITICAL MACROMOLECULES           │
│                                      │
│ 3) DOSE USUALLY EXPRESSED IN "rad"   │
│    UNITS                             │
│        (100 ergs per gram of tissue, ab-│
│        sorbed)                       │
└──────────────────────────────────────┘
```

5-6. RADIATION INJURY

1) RADIOLYSIS OF TISSUE WATER FORMS FREE RADICALS (ION PAIRS)

2) SECONDARY REACTIONS OF FREE RADICALS DESTROY FUNCTION OF CRITICAL MACROMOLECULES

3) DOSE USUALLY EXPRESSED IN "rad" UNITS
   (100 ergs per gram of tissue, absorbed)

5-7. CLASSIFICATION OF HUMAN TISSUES BY RADIOSENSITIVITY

LAW OF BERGONIE AND TRIBONDEAU (paraphrased)

Mitotic cells are more susceptible to radiation damage than nonmitotic cells

— — — — —

1) RADIOSENSITIVE (2500r or less)
   lymphoid tissue
   hematopoietic marrow
   g.i. epithelium

2) RADIORESPONSIVE (2500 to 5000r)
   connective tissue, bone
   epithelium
   endothelium

3) RADIORESISTANT (5000r or more)
   —brain
   muscle
   kidney

— — — — — —

A single dose of whole-body radiation of 500r has a direct lethal potential

Additional Reading

Haber, A. H. and Rothstein, B. E. Radiosensitivity and cell division: "Law of Bergonie and Tribondeau." Science 163:1338, 1969

Hempleman, L. H. Risk of thyroid neoplasms after irradiation in childhood. Science 160:159, 1968

Miller, R. W. Delayed radiation effects in atomic bomb survivors. Science 166:569, 1969

Polland, E. C. The Biological action of ionizing radiation. Am. Scientist 57:206, 1969

Symposium: The Medical Consequences of Thermonuclear War. N. Engl. J. Med. 266:1126, 1962

5-8. IMMEDIATE AND DELAYED MANIFESTATIONS OF WB IRRADIATION

1) A SINGLE DOSE OF WHOLE-BODY RADIATION OF 500r HAS A DIRECT LETHAL POTENTIAL

2) MANIFESTATIONS (sublethal)
   immediate (syndrome of radiation sickness)
   lymphopenia
   bloody diarrhea
   delayed
   anemia, agranulocytosis
   susceptibility to infection
   chromosomal abnormalities
   long-delayed
   increased incidence of leukemia
   shortening of life
   genetic damage

irradiated individuals is observed. Such effects include the increased incidence of leukemia and other cancers and a shortening of the mean lifespan of the population. An additional effect is radiation-induced mutations which become manifest, not in the irradiated individual, but in subsequent generations. It is axiomatic that practically all such mutations having effects large enough to be detected are harmful and result in genes that do not function properly in transcription. Tragically, these genes will contribute to health problems of subsequent generations for as long as can be foreseen.

HEAVY METAL INTOXICATION

LEARNING OBJECTIVE

To be able to compare and contrast acute and chronic intoxication with mercury and lead, mentioning the following:

a) toxic forms of both
b) morphologic and functional changes associated with intoxication
c) importance as ecologic or industrial hazard

Heavy metal poisoning is often produced by lead (Pb), mercury (Hg), arsenic (As), Thallium (T1), cadmium (Cd), iron (Fe), gold (Au) and copper (Cu). The clinical picture varies depending upon the heavy metal involved and whether exposure is acute or chronic. Patients surviving serious intoxication due to lead, mercury, thallium or arsenic may be left with permanent injury to the brain and kidneys. As examples of heavy metal poisoning, we will discuss the 2 most prominent, those due to lead and mercury.

1. Lead Poisoning *most in children*

The vast majority of clinically overt cases of lead poisoning occur in children 12 to 36 months of age. These children usually reside in ancient, urban slum housing in which old, flaking, lead-pigment paints are found on interior surfaces. In practically every case, the additional behavioral idiosyncrasy of pica is seen. (Pica is defined in Illustration 5-9). Lead poisoning or *plumbism* occurs after prolonged, repeated ingestion of flaking paint. Accumulation of lead over a period of weeks to years results in a toxic body burden.

5-9. PICA

Craving for unnatural articles of food; a depraved appetite

Dorland (22nd Ed.)

5-10. LEAD   POISONING   (PLUMBISM)

---

1) MOST CASES OCCUR IN CHILDREN 1–3 YEARS OF AGE
   lead pigment paint
   pica

2) ADDITIONAL SOURCES INCLUDE
   lead glazed pottery
   illicit whiskey
   automobile exhaust

3) ACUTE TOXICITY
   encephalopathy with possible permanent brain damage

The most serious manifestation of plumbism is acute encephalopathy, with permanent brain damage resulting in 40 per cent of survivors. Sequellae include convulsive disorders, learning defects, impulsive antisocial behavior and profound mental retardation.

On occasion, acute plumbism is traced to the consumption of acidic foods and beverages (fruit juice, tomato juice, etc.) served in lead-glazed ceramic containers. Another common cause of plumbism is improperly distilled illicit whiskey. An increasingly significant source of lead absorption may be traced to atmospheric contamination by the combustion of leaded gasolines. In recent years inhalation of airborne lead is thought to be causing its accumulation to levels of incipient toxicity in some inhabitants of larger cities (Illustration 5-10).

2. Mercury Poisoning

Mercury is encountered in many forms, each of which exhibits a somewhat different toxicity (Illustration 5-11). It occurs naturally in fish, birds and some animals, but in recent years natural levels are being raised by industrial pollution. It is estimated that only half of the 5 to 6 million pounds of mercury produced each year in the United States is recycled. Despite this rather impressive rate at which mercury is being released the health hazard of environ-

Heavy metals - primary damage to bra[in]

5-11. MERCURY POISONING

1) MANY DIFFERENT FORMS ARE ENCOUNTERED

Hg^{++} (highly toxic: once a common instrument of suicide)

elemental mercury (relatively non-toxic unless inhaled as vapor)

Various organic mercurials (mercury has unusual propensity toward forming organic complexes)

2) SYNDROMES

suicide with $HgCl_2$

chronic poisoning with organic or metallic mercury (pink disease)

acute poisoning with organic or metallic mercury

3) SIGNIFICANCE IN FOOD CHAIN

mental mercury appears to be limited, for the time being, to persons using fish as the dominant component of their diet. Normal concentrations of mercury in the aquatic food-chain, when combined with that released in industrial wastes can result in severely toxic concentrations in people using fish as a dietary staple. This was vividly demonstrated in an incident occurring in Minamata, Japan, where inhabitants, existing primarily on fish from a local bay, were poisoned in great numbers by the effluent from a factory.

Metallic mercury is relatively harmless when ingested or even injected directly into tissues. However, the vapor of metallic mercury is highly toxic when inhaled. Since metallic mercury divides into tiny globules which vaporize readily this form of mercury can constitute a hazard in areas where it is in routine use. These include hospitals, dental operatories and industrial installations.

Clinical manifestations of mercury poisoning vary with the dose and form of the agent. Mercuric chloride is violently poisonous and acute doses were quite commonly used for suicide. More familiar today is the clinical picture of subacute or chronic exposure to metallic mercury vapor or organic mercurials. The syndrome produced by the latter is known as *acrodynia* or pink disease (Illustration 5-11). Pink disease is historically important as the disease of the "Mad Hatter," because it was often seen in gilders and hatters who apparently employed mercurial compounds on a regular basis.

Additional Reading

Chisolm. J. J. Poisoning due to heavy metals. Ped. Clin. N. Amer. 17:591, 1970

Gronka, P. et al. Mercury vapor exposure in dental offices. J. Am. Dent. Assn. 81:923, 1970

Guinee, V. F. Lead poisoning in New York City. Trans. N.Y. Acad. Sci. 33:539, 1971

Klein, M. et al. Earthenware containers as a source of fatal lead poisoning. N. Engl. J. Med 283:669, 1970

Milne, J. et al. Acute mercurial pneumonitis. Brit. J. Indus. Med. 27:334, 1970

Peakall, D. B. and Lovett, R. J. Mercury: its occurrence and effects in the ecosystem. BioScience 22:20, 1972

Reddick, L. P. Plumbism exists today. South. Med. J. 64:446, 1971

Schroeder, H. A sensible look at air pollution by metals. Arch. Environmental Health 21:798, 1970

Smith, R. A. Current concepts: sialorrhea. N. Engl. J. Med. 283:917, 1970

Elemental mercury / Metallic / "Quick Silver" — non-toxic as long as liquid

CARBON MONOXIDE POISONING

LEARNING OBJECTIVE

To be able to describe the effects of acute and chronic carbon monoxide poisoning mentioning the following:

a) its importance as environmental or industrial hazard

b) pathogenesis of CO injury

c) acute and chronic poisoning syndromes and their sequellae

Asphyxiants are toxic agents that interfere with the exchange or transport of respiratory gasses. As our single example of an asphyxiant,

Mercuric - highly toxic; used in rat poisoning c̄ Cl $HgCl_2$

5-12. CARBON MONOXIDE (CO) POISONING

1) COLORLESS, TASTELESS, ODORLESS
   1 per cent fatal in 10 to 20 min
   auto exhaust = 7 per cent
   natural gas = 16 per cent

2) INJURES BY PREVENTING OXYGEN TRANSPORT
   COHb is more stable than OHb
   brain is most sensitive to O_2 deprivation

3) SYNDROMES
   ACUTE POISONING
   confusion
   coma
   death
   CHRONIC POISONING
   apathy, headache
   personality disturbances

4) POSSIBILITY OF PERMANENT BRAIN DAMAGE

we will consider the ubiquitous and lethal carbon monoxide (CO).

Exposure to carbon monoxide commonly results from its presence in automobile exhaust, cigarette smoke and airborne industrial wastes (Illustration 5-12). Significant intoxication may mimic organic disease of mental disorder. In higher concentrations it may result in coma or death. Survivors of serious carbon monoxide poisoning are often affected with permanent brain damage secondary to the cerebral anoxia experienced in this kind of poisoning.

Carbon monoxide is a colorless, tasteless, odorless gas. A leaky automobile exhaust system is the usual source of CO in cases of severe poisoning. Other important sources include faulty nonelectric heating appliances, obstructed chimneys and the smoking of cigarettes. The concentration of CO reaching the alveoli in the average smoker is about 400 ppm, a level well above the allowable maximum atmospheric concentration recommended by the American Conference of Governmental Industrial Hygienists (50 ppm).

CO is not a direct tissue poison; it injures by depriving the tissues of oxygen. Combining with hemoglobin to form carboxyhemoglobin (COHb), it prevents normal transportation of oxygen by red blood cells. COHb is far more stable than oxygenated hemoglobin, dissociating 250 times more slowly. The effect of acute longterm exposure to dangerous concentrations of CO is to render the patient functionally "anemic." In another sense, CO poisoning is comparable to massive hemorrhage in that it deprives the body of functioning red cells. Since the brain is the organ most sensitive to oxygen deficit, most manifestations of CO poisoning are referrable to the central nervous system. It is not uncommon for patients to be discharged following apparent recovery from an acute dose of carbon monoxide only to return within a few days suffering relapse. Signs of acute poisoning include delirium, confusion, disorientation and death. Chronic exposure to low atmospheric concentrations may become manifest as anorexia, nausea, apathy, fatigue, headache, dizziness, insomnia, personality disturbances or memory defects. Chronic exposure may also aggravate existing organic disease and constitute a danger to the child *in utero*.

Additional Reading

Gilbert, D. L. Oxygen and life. Anesthesiology 37:100, 1972

Lawther, P. J. and Commins, B. T. Cigarette smoking and exposure to carbon monoxide. Ann. N.Y. Acad. Sci. 174:135, 1970

Moore, M. E. The case of the disappearing headache. N. Engl. J. Med. 278:1216, 1968

Rose, E. G. and Rose M. Carbon monoxide: a challenge to the physician. Clin. Med. 78:12, 1971

name a common source
?
auto exhaust

SELF-INFLICTED INJURY

LEARNING OBJECTIVE

To be able to discuss the social, psychiatric and physical syndromes associated with each of the following 3 examples of self-inflicted injury:

a) smoking
b) alcoholism
c) drug abuse

One of the most serious of all sources of injury is the kind that a person inflicts upon himself. In the last analysis all of these are disorders of behavior, some being far more important than others.

1. Smoking

Recognized authorities now claim that the use of tobacco is the single greatest public health hazard in the United States today. The smoking of cigarettes, in particular, decreases life expectancy and predisposes an individual to cardiovascular, gastrointestinal and pulmonary disease.

Although the potential dangers of tobacco were well known 100 years ago, it was not until the 1930's that the use of cigarettes came under systematic investigation as a cause of illness and death. Since that time the relationship has been confirmed by thousands of scientific reports. Yet, despite overwhelming evidence discouraging the use of cigarettes, more people smoke today than ever before and the number is still rising.

Even the causes of cigarette smoking remain obscure (Illustration 5-13). Genetic factors, cultural factors, personality factors and a dependency phenomenon have been implicated. Whatever the reason, cigarette smoking is universally recognized as a habit easy to acquire but difficult to break. In this regard it is sobering to reflect on the fact that, given today's social climate, of those who smoke more than a single cigarette during adolescence some 70 per cent will continue smoking for the next 40 years.

Deleterious effects of cigarette smoking on various organ systems will be taken up in a number of subsequent subjects.

5-13. SMOKING

1) USE OF TOBACCO IS THE GREATEST PUBLIC HEALTH HAZARD IN THE U.S. TODAY (PARTICULARLY CIGA-RETTES)
   - shortens life
   - predisposes to cardiovascular, g.i. and pulmonary disease

2) CAUSES REMAIN OBSCURE
   - genetic factors
   - culture
   - personality
   - dependency phenomena

---

2. Alcoholism

Alcoholism, like the use of cigarettes, is an example of self-inflicted injury affecting both the quality and duration of the lives of millions of people throughout the world. In the case of alcohol abuse, however, there appears to be a sharper line of division between the person who indulges occasionally and the person suffering from a clearcut addictive disorder.

As in other addictive conditions the 2 criteria used as definitive are *tolerance* and *physical dependence*. Individuals who consistently consume more ethanol than can be safely processed by detoxication facilities of the body must be considered addicts.

Derangements of liver functions are particularly prominent and will be covered in detail in Chapter 19. As in the case of smoking, the causes of alcohol abuse are numerous and obscure. They undoubtedly include genetic, physiologic and endocrine factors, as well as influences derived from culture (Illustration 5-14)

3. Drug Abuse

Any substance that causes a change in affect (feelings), thought, behavior or perception is a drug that can be abused. Five major groups of these agents are listed in Illustration 5-15. Alcoholism, of course, remains the primary

5-14. ALCOHOLISM

1) ADDICTIVE DISORDER WHEN THERE IS CONSISTENT CONSUMPTION OF MORE ALCOHOL THAN CAN BE PROCESSED BY DETOXICATION ENZYMES

   most important drug addiciton problem in U.S.

2) CAUSES OBSCURE

   genetic, physiologic and cultural

3) DERANGEMENT OF LIVER FUNCTION IS PARTICULARLY PROMINENT

5-15. MAJOR   GROUPS   OF   ABUSED DRUGS

1) NARCOTICS   *most misused*

   opium

   morphine

   heroin (90 per cent of abuse)

   codeine

2) SEDATIVE-HYPNOTICS   *wrong answer*

   barbiturates

3) MINOR TRANQUILIZERS

   meprobamate

   Librium®

   Vallium®

4) STIMULANTS

   amphetamines

5) HALLUCINOGENIC AGENTS

   marijuana

   LSD

   mescaline

   psilocybin

---

national drug addiction problem with nearly 5 per cent of all Americans addicted to its use. A number of other very familiar drugs such as marijuana, LSD and amphetamines are widely misused, but not addictive. The agents producing the most serious health problems are the narcotics.

Because intravenous administration of illicit narcotics produces a complex organic syndrome, the remainder of our discussion will be devoted to this kind of drug abuse.

Recent reports estimate that there are 100,000 or more heroin addicts in the United States. Most are found in urban communities and are in the age group between 20 and 40. Adverse effects of the chronic intravenous administration of illicitly procured drugs are listed in Illustration 5-16.

Again, as in the preceding 2 examples, the causes of drug abuse are many and obscure. Undoubtedly, cultural and psychologic factors predominate. Most people first take drugs out of curiosity or in response to peer pressure.

5-16. COMPLICATIONS OF THE INTRAVENOUS ABUSE OF NARCOTICS

1) "ACUTE REACTION" OR "OVERDOSE"

   sudden death due to direct toxic effect of drug or poisonous contaminant (nicotine, quinine, strychnine, cyanide): accounts for 80 per cent of fatalities.

2) INFECTIOUS DISEASE

   hepatitis

   tetanus

   septicemia

   bacterial endocarditis

   malaria (from common use of equipment)

   abscess

3) DISSEMINATED   VASCULITIS   OR GRANULOMATOUS DISEASE CAUSED BY CONTAMINANT

Continued use and eventual addiction, however, depends upon need. A recent review concludes that the ultimate reason proved to be the need to control one's affect, that is, either to escape from feelings or discover them.

Additional Reading

Becker, C. E. Medical complications of heroin addiction. California Med. 115:42, 1971

Gossett, J. F. Extent and prevalence of illicit drug use as reported by 56,745 students. J. Am. Med. Assn. 216:1464, 1971

Halpern, M. Fatalities from narcotic addiction in New York City. Human Path. 3:13, 1972

Mendelson, J. H. Biologic concomitants of alcoholism. N. Engl. J. Med. 283:24, 1970

Ochsner, A. The health menace of Tobacco. Am. Scientist 59:246, 1971

Peterson, G. C. and Wilson, M. R. A perspective on drug abuse. Mayo Clinic Proc. 46:468, 1971

Rubin, E. Alcoholism, alcohol and drugs. Science 172:1097, 1971

Russell, M. A. H. Cigarette smoking: natural history of a dependence disorder. Brit. J. Med. Psychol. 44:1, 1971

U.S. Government Printing Office Federal Sourcebook. Answers to the most frequently asked questions about drugs. Washington, D.C. Division of Public Documents, 1970

chapter 6
NEOPLASIA

BENIGN AND MALIGNANT NEOPLASMS

LEARNING OBJECTIVE

To be able to discuss the meaning of the terms neoplasia and neoplastic disease, comparing the clinical and morphologic differences between a benign and malignant tumor, considering the following:

a) rate of growth
b) pattern of growth
c) propensity for distant speed
d) means of injuring host
e) radiation sensitivity
f) gross architecture
g) microscopic architecture

Neoplasia is a morbid process that begins as a new and uncontrolled growth of abnormal tissue. This growth always arises by transformation of normal body cells, never serves any useful purpose and is frequently fatal to its host. A growth of this kind is called a neoplasm or tumor. Strictly speaking, the term, tumor, can refer to any swelling or enlargement; but after many years of use in the context of neoplastic disease it has come to be almost a synonym for the word, neoplasm. As customary, we will use the terms interchangeably in this discussion.

Tumors are grouped into 2 large categories, benign and malignant; the former are usually harmless, whereas the latter are potentially lethal. Actually, the behavior of tumors describes a continuous spectrum from the completely innocuous, through those that are aggressive and difficult to control, to a group that can be reliably predicted to be fatal if untreated. No sharp line of division exists anywhere in this spectrum and tumors of all kinds continue to be seen in all parts of the world. Yet despite this potential for uncertain behavior, most tumors can be assigned fairly confidently to one category or another. This is because many years of experience have shown that certain morphologic and behavior qualities are associated with benign tumors and others with malignant tumors. Illustration 6-1 lists some of the features commonly used in the evaluation and prediction of tumor behavior.

Just as infectious disease results from a parasite's injuring its host, so neoplastic disease becomes apparent only when a tumor causes damage sufficient to lead to its being detected. A tumor such as a small benign neoplasm of the stomach wall may persist unnoticed throughout most of a person's lifetime and could hardly be said to be the source of neoplastic disease. Other benign tumors occasionally cause disease by obstruction, compression, or interference with metabolism. But, by far, most neoplastic disease is the result of malignant tumors.

Benign tumor:
smooth mus. - leiomyoma
rhabdomyoma - skeletal mus.

Hypersecretion b7 breasts
parathyroid calcify

rodent - malignant autogrows

6-1. COMPARATIVE FEATURES OF BENIGN AND MALIGNANT TUMORS

	BENIGN TUMORS	MALIGNANT TUMORS
Mode of growth	usually grow by expansion, displacing surrounding normal tissue	invade, destroy and assimilate surrounding normal tissue
Metastasis (formation of distant growing colonies	do not metastasize but remain at site of formation unless transplanted	most will metastasize: distant colonies form and grow
Rate of growth	grow slowly: may stop or regress	grow rapidly never (or very rarely) stop or regress
Architecture	encapsulated: have complex stroma and adequate blood supply	not encapsulated: usually have poorly developed stroma: may become necrotic at center
Danger to host	most are without lethal significance	always ultimately lethal: must be removed or destroyed *in situ*
Injury to host	usually negligible but may become very large and compress or obstruct vital tissue	can kill host directly by destruction of vital tissue
Radiation sensitivity	radiation sensitivity near that of normal parent cell: rarely treated with radiation	radiation sensitivity increased in rough proportion to degree of malignancy: frequently treated w/radiation
Behavior in tissue culture	cells are cohesive and inhibited by mutual contact	cells do not cohere, are frequently not inhibited by mutual contact
Resemblance to tissue of origin	cells and architecture resemble tissue of origin	cells atypical and pleomorphic: disorganized bizarre architecture
Mitotic figures	mitotic figures rare and normal	mitotic figures may be numerous and abnormal in polarity and configuration
Shape of nucleus	shape of nucleus is normal and regular: shows usual stain affinity	shape of nucleus is irregular: nucleus is frequently hyperchromatic
Size of nucleus	size of nucleus is normal: nucleus/cytoplasm ratio is near normal	nucleus is frequently large: nucleus/cytoplasm ratio increased
Nucleolus	nucleolus not conspicuous	nucleolus hyperchromatic and larger than normal

DAMAGING EFFECTS OF THE MALIGNANT TUMOR

LEARNING OBJECTIVE

To be able to discuss malignant tumors with regard to means of inflicting injury, mentioning the following:
   a) local damaging effects
   b) metastasis (definition, routes, preferential sites)
   c) systemic effects (DIC, synthesis of hormones, associated autoimmune phenomena, tumor cachexia)

The malignant tumor is dangerous because, quite in contrast to the benign tumor, it grows out of control, invading and destroying normal tissue, spreading throughout the body and, on occasion, producing widespread systemic effects that are unpredictable and often perplexing. We will examine 3 aspects of disease produced by the malignant tumor: 1) local damaging effects, 2) metastasis, and 3) systemic effects.

1. Local Damaging Effects

Examples of local damaging effects of the malignant tumor are presented in tabular form in Illustration 6-2. Malignant tumors commonly obstruct the intestine, airway or urinary outflow tract causing stasis and infection. They destroy vital tissue such as brain and adrenal, they perforate hollow viscera causing peritonitis or erode blood vessels resulting in massive or chronic hemorrhage.

Disseminated malignant tumor cells frequently cause pathologic fractures as well as adhesions of thoracic and abdominal viscera. Malignant tumors of the skin can serve as a portal of entry for infection, whereas those of marrow will displace critically needed myeloid tissue, resulting in thrombocytopenia and anemia.

2. Metastasis

The malignant tumor is also dangerous because it does not remain confined. In addition to direct extension into adjacent tissue it spreads by the formation of distant colonies

---

6-2. LOCAL DAMAGING EFFECTS OF THE MALIGNANT TUMOR

1) INVASION AND DESTRUCTION OF NORMAL CONTIGUOUS TISSUE

2) OBSTRUCTION
   intestine
   airway
   urinary tract
   biliary tract

3) PERFORATION OF HOLLOW VISCERA

4) EROSION OF BLOODVESSEL WALLS
   acute and chronic hemorrhage

5) PATHOLOGIC FRACTURES

6) ADHESIONS

7) PORTAL OF ENTRY FOR INFECTION

8) MYELOPHTHISIC EFFECTS

---

that duplicate all of the destructive effects of the primary neoplasm. This latter phenomenon is called *metastasis*. Metastasis undoubtedly requires the spread of cells but the simple dissemination of tumor cells is far from being its only requirement. Circulating tumor cells are common in malignancy but do not, alone, constitute metastasis. True metastatic tumor always has the 2 distinguishing qualities listed in Illustration 6-3.

Although by no means an absolute rule, it is common for malignant epithelial tumors to metastasize via lymphatics whereas mesenchymal malignancies usually spread through the blood stream. A third kind of metastasis is seen in body cavities where cells shed from a primary tumor may scatter over serous surfaces, fix to another structure within the same cavity and grow out into a metastatic nodule. This is termed *metastasis by implantation.*

For reasons yet unexplained certain malignant tumors metastasize with greater frequency

6-3. METASTASIS (TWO COMPONENTS)

6-3. METASTASIS (TWO COMPONENTS)

1) DISSEMINATION OF TUMOR CELLS FROM PRIMARY SITE

2) GROWTH OF SECONDARY (META-STATIC) TUMOR AT DISTANT SITE

– – – – – – – – – –

both must occur before metastasis becomes clinically detectable

6-4. EXAMPLES OF THE SYSTEMIC EFFECTS OF MALIGNANT TUMORS

1) DISSEMINATED INTRAVASCULAR COAGULATION (DIC)

2) DISRUPTION OF METABOLISM BY THE UNCONTROLLED SECRETION OF HORMONES
    functional tumors:
        tumors (benign and malignant) of glandular epithelium that produce all or part of the product of the parent gland
    paraendocrine syndromes:
        malignant tumors of nonglandular epithelium that produce endocrine substances

3) MESENCHYMAL AUTOIMMUNE SYNDROMES

4) ANEMIA

5) TUMOR CACHEXIA

to some locations than others. This phenomenon of site preference undoubtly has something to do with the growth requirements of the tumor: however, other factors are thought to be equally important. Perhaps the most clear-cut examples of preferential metastatic sites can be seen in the pronounced tendency of cancer of the prostate to metastasize to the bone and cancer of the colon to metastasize to the liver. The liver is a particularly fertile site for metastatic tumor growth. It has been estimated that approximately 50 per cent of all cases of cancer death show liver metastasis. Equally as striking is the apparent resistance of other sites to the growth of metastatic tumor; skeletal muscle and spleen, for example, are far less frequently involved.

3. Systemic Effects of Malignant Tumors

In addition to direct extension and metastasis, the malignant tumor may endanger its host with a variety of systemic effects. Some examples are listed in Illustration 6-4 and described below:

1) A large number of circulating tumor cells may activate the intrinsic coagulation mechanism causing disseminated intravascular coagulation (DIC). This often occurs as a terminal incident in cancer of the pancreas or stomach: however, it can be seen in association with other tumors as well.

2) Tumors of glandular tissue may synthesize the product of the parent gland in an uncontrolled manner causing severe metabolic disturbance. This is seen with both benign and malignant neoplasms. A tumor secreting all or part of the normal product of its parent tissue is called a functional tumor. However, in no instance is such a tumor beneficial despite the misleading terminology.

3) Another kind of functional tumor is seen in the propensity of malignant epithelial tumors to secrete a variety of both peptide and steroid hormones. Certain varieties of lung cancer secrete ACTH or a parathyroid hormone-like agent. Cancers of the breast often elaborate a sterol that overrides the calcium homeostatic mechanism and causes sustained hypercalcemia.

4) Mesenchymal autoimmune syndromes are often associated with malignant tumors. The one most often seen is dermatomyositis, an autoimmune inflammatory dis-

ease of skin and muscle. Approximately 50 per cent of patients over 40 presenting with dermatomyositis will have an associated malignancy.

5) Most malignant tumors produce a kind of wasting disease as part of their terminal ravages. This is known as tumor *cachexia*; it is probably the result of the tumor's competing with the patient's body for metabolites in critically short supply. The patient actually wastes away as if starving.

Additional Reading

Armstrong, D. Infectious complications of neoplastic disease. Med. Clin. N. Amer. 55:729, 1971

Baserga, R. and Kisieleski, W. E. Autobiographies of cells. Sci. Amer. Aug, 1963

Beacham, W. D. et al. Uterine and/or ovarian tumors weighing 25 pounds or more. Am. J. Obstet. Gynec. 109:1153, 1971

Day, E. A. Tumor sterols. Metabolism 18:646, 1969

Paul, J. The cancer cell *in vitro*: a review. Cancer Res. 22:431, 1962

Rous, P. The challenge to man of the neoplastic cell. Science 157:24, 1967

Scherbel, A. L. et al. Association of certain connective tissue syndromes and malignant disease. Postgrad. Med. 35:619, 1964

Schottenfeld, D. Medical syndromes associated with malignant tumors. Cancer 20:35, 1970

Special Issue. Current concepts of cancer. Postgrad. Med. 48:1, 1970

Taylor, S. G. Common medical problems in disseminated cancer. Geriatrics Oct., 1970

Theologides, A. Pathogenesis of cachexia in cancer. Cancer 29:484, 1972

CLASSIFICATION AND NOMENCLATURE OF NEOPLASMS

LEARNING OBJECTIVE

To be able to assign a systematic or non-systematic name (where applicable) to any benign or malignant tumor of epithelial, mesenchymal, embryonal or compound origin

The scheme of naming tumors is systematic to a degree but, owing to the wide variety of sources and cell types, it is neither consistent nor comprehensive. In addition to many recently coined non-systematic terms, some older terms and eponyms have managed to persist and are often used along with or in place of the preferred nomenclature.

To be able to talk about tumors in a clinical context, one must resign oneself to learning both the systematic terminology and the many non-systematic synonyms. If any part of this task could be said to be complicated it would be the latter. Regular tumor nomenclature is extremely simple and requires the observation of only a few basic rules:

1) The suffix -oma refers to a neoplasm.
2) Benign neoplasms are named by adding the prefix appropriate for the tissue of origin. A benign tumor of fibrous tissue, for example, is a *fibroma*, that of cartilage, a *chondroma*, whereas a benign

---

6-5. SYSTEMATIC TUMOR NOMENCLATURE

PARENT TISSUE	BENIGN	MALIGNANT
SIMPLE TUMORS		
epithelium (glandular)	adenoma	adenocarcinoma
epithelium (surface)	papilloma	carcinoma
mesenchymal tissue	tissue prefix + oma (fibroma)	tissue prefix + sarcoma (fibrosarcoma)
COMPLEX TUMORS		
totipotential cell	teratoma	teratocarcinoma
embryonic rest		embryonal tumor
mature tissue	mixed tumor	malignant mixed tumor

tumor of any gland is called an *adenoma.*

3) A malignant tumor of epithelial origin is called a *carcinoma.* Those originating in glandular epithelium are called *adenocarcinomas,* whereas those arising from surface epithelium are named according to the type of surface from which they take origin. In the latter catagory, 2 very prominent examples would be the *squamous cell carcinoma* and the *transitional cell carcinoma* originating in stratified squamous and urinary epithelium respectively.

4) Malignant tumors of mesenchymal origin are called *sarcomas.* A tumor of this type is named by simply adding the prefix appropriate for the tissue of origin. A malignant tumor of fibrous tissue is a *fibrosarcoma,* that of cartilage a *chondrosarcoma,* etc.

In addition to the above there are tumors that appear to consist of more than one tissue. When these arise from mature tissues they are called *mixed tumors* and when they take origin from cells of multiple potential they are called *teratomas.* In a mixed tumor, usually only 1 of the cell types is neoplastic, the other being an overgrowth of normal tissue elicited by the neoplasm. In a teratoma, the entire collection of tissue is part of the tumor process and 1 or more component tissues may even become malignant. Another kind of tumor that usually exhibits mixed composition is the *embryonal tumor.* Embryonal tumors arise from nests of cells that have failed to complete their differentiation into adult tissue. Embryonal tumors usually occur in very early childhood and almost all are malignant.

One pitfall of naming a neoplastic disease according to the cell that forms the tumor is that the student tends to lose sight of the fact that the cancer patient is afflicted with more than just a rampant cell. Bear in mind, then, that cancer consists of not only the malignant cell but also the patient's failure to cope with it.

CLINICAL DESCRIPTION OF NEOPLASTIC LESIONS

LEARNING OBJECTIVE

To be able to define each of the terms that will be presented as useful in the clinical description of neoplastic lesions

As in other areas of pathology, one is obliged to be familiar with not only the principles of neoplasia but also the language. The need for accurate language is acute in all branches of clinical practice since an accurate description of a tumor *in situ* must be communicated to the pathologist if he is expected to come to a reliable diagnosis.

Generally speaking, benign tumors grow by symmetrical expansion if located within a tissue mass or by outward expansion if located at a surface. Since the clinical description of tumors will more often be directed toward those observable at a surface we will emphasize characteristics of this kind of growth.

Benign tumors projecting from a surface of the body are said to be demonstrating an *exophytic* pattern of growth, whereas malignant tumors, extending into normal subjacent tissue, are said to be growing in an *endophytic* manner (Illustration 6-6). Actually, malignant tumors exhibit a variety of surface configurations. Some grow outward as well as inward, most ulcerate, whereas others, particularly those seen on mucosal surfaces, may become manifest as areas of hyperkeratosis or a red lesion.

Exophytic neoplasms assume a variety of characteristic shapes (Illustration 6-7). The student should memorize these and make them part of his working vocabulary. Although endophytic (malignant) neoplasms are capable of great variety, they too exhibit certain characteristic patterns of growth. Examples of these are listed and briefly described in Illustration 6-8.

6-6. EXOPHYTIC AND ENDOPHYTIC TUMOR GROWTH

EXOPHYTIC

ENDOPHYTIC

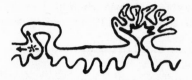

6-8. TERMS USED TO DESCRIBE ENDO-PHYTIC NEOPLASMS

1) INFILTRATING: evidence of the local spread of cells

2) INVASIVE: obviously growing into contiguous normal tissue

3) SCIRRHOUS: invasion with strong desmoplastic (connective tissue-eliciting response)

4) ANNULAR CONSTRICTION: "napkin ring" constriction of gut wall

6-7. TERMS USED TO DESCRIBE EXOPHYTIC NEOPLASMS

1) POLYPOID: forming an outward projection

2) PEDUNCULATED: on a stalk

3) VILLOUS: thin, finger-shaped projections

4) PAPILLARY: nipple-shaped projections

5) SESSILE: raised above the surface but with a broad base of attachment

EXAMPLES OF PROMINENT HUMAN NEOPLASMS

LEARNING OBJECTIVE

To be able to describe each of the 10 tumors presented, assigning a systematic name where possible

In general, human neoplasms are best studied as specific diseases of an organ or system. Since we need examples at this point to show the application of principles under discussion, we will present and briefly describe each of the 10 neoplasms listed in Illustration 6-9. In most cases, these will be encountered again in later subjects.

1. Wart (Verruca Vulgaris)

The common wart or verruca vulgaris is a benign papillary neoplasm occurring commonly on the fingers, palms and forearms. Histologically, the wart consists of an area of acanthosis (thickening of the prickle-cell layer of the

6-9. NON-SYSTEMATIC TERMS FOR PROMINENT HUMAN NEOPLASMS

1) WART

2) FIBROID

3) MELANOMA

4) HEPATOMA

5) PHEOCHROMOCYTOMA

6) CHORIOCARCINOMA

7) WILM'S TUMOR

8) BOWEN'S TUMOR

9) LYMPHOMA

10) CARCINOID TUMOR

epidermis) and a greatly thickened keratotic layer (hyperkeratosis). Viral particles have been detected in these lesions by electronmicroscopy, supporting their viral etiology. They are almost always benign and often disappear spontaneously.

Using systematic nomenclature, the wart would be classified as a squamous papilloma or fibroepithelial papilloma.

2. Fibroid

The fibroid is a benign tumor of the smooth muscle of the uterine wall. It occurs at either surface of the uterus or within the wall itself. It exhibits strong estrogen dependency and undergoes a degree of regression after menopause.

Using systamatic nomenclature, the fibroid is termed a uterine leiomyoma.

3. Melanoma

The melanoma is a neoplasm arising from melanin-producing (or dopa-positive) cells. When properly delimited this term can be used interchangeably with "nevus," although the latter includes other examples of congenital skin blemishes. Some authorities consider the melanoma (nevus) a developmental error, others a neoplasm. On occasion, the term melanoma is used in reference to a malignant tumor of dopa-positive or melanin-producing cells: however, such a lesion is more appropriately called a melanocarcinoma.

The origin of neval cells is a matter of controversy. Some authorities consider them altered epidermal basal cells, others propose their origin as neurogenic. The nevus occurs in a number of histologic types, the most common being a lesion in which neval cells are found both at the dermo-epidermal junction and within the dermis (compound nevus).

Most melanocarcinomas arise from a junctional nest of neval cells or from the junctional component of a compound nevus. The melanocarcinoma of the skin can be one of the most aggressive of malignant tumors depending upon its location and histologic type.

4. Hepatoma

The hepatoma is a malignant tumor primary to the liver. Most arise from hepatic cells, but a small percentage take origin in the epithelium of bile ducts. The incidence of hepatoma differs strikingly among areas of the world. In the United States and Europe such tumors are seen in less than 1 per cent of all autopsies and then usually as a complication of cirrhosis. In most cases in which the predisposing cirrhosis was not of alcoholic etiology, the patient with carcinoma of the liver will manifest the antigen of the hepatitis virus in his serum. To many, this suggests a strong causative association between this virus and the tumor.

5. Pheochromocytoma

The pheochromocytoma is a tumor of the adrenal medulla. Most are benign (94 per cent) and secrete epinephrine, norepinephrine or both. There seems to be no appropriate systematic term for this tumor.

6. Choriocarcinoma

Choriocarcinoma is a malignant tumor of the trophoblastic cells of the placenta. Most cases are seen following an abnormal pregnancy. The tumor is unusually aggressive and, before the advent of modern chemotherapeutic methods, was most often fatal.

Because this tumor is unique in that it takes origin from placental tissue, it does not fit within the regular system of tumor nomenclature.

7. Wilms' Tumor

Wilms' tumor is an embryonal tumor of the kidney. Because of its origin from pluripotential mesodermal cells it most often exhibits at least 2 kinds of neoplastic tissue, a highly cellular connective tissue surrounding numerous epithelial tubular structures. Wilms' tumor accounts for about 20 per cent of all childhood malignancies, with most cases occurring before the 7th year of life.

8. Bowen's tumor *is MAL. just HASN't INVADED*

Bowen's tumor is carcinoma *in situ* of the skin, usually occurring on the trunk, buttocks and extremities. Lesions exhibit marked dyskeratosis (interruption in the orderly process of epithelial cell maturation) with acanthosis and hyperkeratosis. Large anaplastic, keratin-producing cells are found within all layers of the epidermis and may exhibit numerous, and even abnormal, mitotic activity.

9. Lymphoma *ALWAYS MALIGNANT*

The lymphoma is a neoplasm of peripheral lymphoid tissue. Since all neoplasms primary to peripheral lymphoid tissue are malignant, the lymphoma is actually a form of sarcoma. Because of the histologic variety exhibited by these tumors and the complex subclassification required, no attempt is made to include them in the standard system of nomenclature.

10. Carcinoid Tumors

The carcinoid tumor is a neoplasm of the argentaffin cells found at the base of the epithelial crypts of the gut. They occur throughout the gastrointestinal tract as well as, less commonly, within the epithelium of the upper respiratory tract. Most are found within the appendix and rarely give rise to any clinical manifestations. Extra-appendiceal carcinoid tumors that metastasize widely often secrete serotonin giving rise to the "carcinoid syndrome," which consists of diarrhea, flushing of the skin and deformity of valves on the right side of the heart.

ELEMENTS OF MALIGNANT DISEASE

LEARNING OBJECTIVE

To be able to discuss the following 2 qualities of malignant disease:

 a) the malignant cell
 b) the permissive personal constitution of the host

The results of elegant experiments with laboratory animals suggest that at least 2 stages of transition must be completed before a detectable neoplasm emerges from normal tissue. These 2 stages are called *induction* and *promotion*; the clear dichotomy between these 2 stages accurately reflects the dual-component nature of malignant disease.

Induction is the event that creates the malignant cell; promotion is a quality of its environment that encourages its growing out into a clinically detectable tumor. Induction is presumably a single event, comparatively sudden and irreversible. Promotion, quite in contrast, is a persistent influence that acts over a variable but more extended period of time to finally set the changed cell free of body regulation.

Application of the 2-stage hypothesis to the development of spontaneous human tumors is still very speculative; however, it does impose some order in a multitude of factors that are known to be causative malignant disease. It suggests that such factors should be considered, first of all, as consisting of 2 major groups, those concerned with creation of the *malignant cell* and those contributing to the *permissive constitution* of the host (Illustration 6-10).

6-10. ELEMENTS OF MALIGNANT DISEASE

1) THE MALIGNANT CELL
changed genome

each division produces two cells with full mitotic capability

predatory behavior

2) PERMISSIVE CONSTITUTION OF THE HOST
neoplastic transformation of somatic cells may occur frequently (daily?) but without support from the host a tumor does not develop

In this learning objective, we will compare and contrast these 2 groups of factors. Subsequent learning objectives will be devoted to a more detailed discussion of each.

1. The Malignant Cell

Tumors occur only in many-celled organisms. This is because a tumor begins with the failure of 1 cell to respond to the controlling influences of the body community; this unruly cell is said to be neoplastic. A neoplastic cell, particularly one that is clearly malignant, is a changed cell. It acquires certain dangerous characteristics that set it apart from normal cells of its parent tissue. It does not (or cannot) heed the body's direction to stop and specialize. Further, it is apparent that, whatever the nature of this change, it is passed from 1 generation of tumor cells to the next, since the progeny of these cells are all comparably neoplastic. Axiomatic in any description of malignancy, then, is *that the malignant cell has undergone genetic change.*

Of critical concern to the oncologist (one who specializes in the study of tumors) is the question of whether neoplastic transformation is irreversible. Does the fact that the cancer cell and its offspring behave in such an antisocial manner mean that the genome has been unalterably disrupted? Has a cancer cell been provided with new information for delinquency that cannot be exorcised? Some investigators think not. The ability of normal cells to equal or better cancer cells in activities considered characteristically malignant suggests that neoplastic transformation need not be based on irreversible change, but may represent a heritable disturbance in these cells' regulatory machinery. For example, because some tumors grow so fast, it is frequently thought that cancer cells proliferate more rapidly than normal cells. Yet, despite this first impression, one sees on closer scrutiny that the rapid growth of a malignant tumor is not attributable to rapid mitosis but rather to the fact that each daughter cell from each mitotic division retains its full ability to divide. This is distinctly different than the reproductive behavior of all normal adult somatic cells, even those specializing in mitosis. The most rapidly dividing of all normal cells always gives rise to 1 daughter cell with full mitotic capability and 1 that goes on to more specialized function. As a consequence, normal adult tissue never grows in geometric increments, whereas a malignant tumor frequently does so.

Another quality usually considered characteristic of the cancer cell is invasiveness. Malignant cells burrow deeply into adjacent normal tissue, in many cases destroying it and assimilating the digested material as nutrient. But even this is not a unique characteristic of malignancy; consider that invasiveness is the very specialization of the normal trophoblast. It rapidly invades the tough uterine wall where it acts as an interface between maternal and fetal blood for the exchange of food material and waste. Although it does this at least as well as a malignant cell, it stops short of invading any deeper than necessary. It is the equal of the cancer cell in a quality usually attributed to malignancy, but still responds to control.

Metastasis, the formation and growth of distant colonies, is another criterion of malignancy. Cancer cells, particularly in the terminal stages of neoplastic disease, frequently spread throughout the body forming colonies in the brain, lung, liver, bone or virtually any organ (with the usual exception of spleen and skeletal muscle). Again, we can point out normal cells that exhibit very comparable behavior. Lymphocytes circulate throughout other tissue as part of their normal function. They can be found almost anywhere and easily form growing colonies (follicles) whenever the need arises.

It would seem, then, that cancer cells have not acquired any really novel abilities; rather *they express information that normal cells have, but hold in check.* Being insensitive to coordinating signals they set out behaving like free-living predators. They may have lost some element of their own intrinsic control system or they may be responding to direction by foreign nucleic acid, but there is no reason to give up hope that some day it will be possible to rehabilitate the malignant cell.

2. Permissive Constitution of the Host

It is tempting to think of a tumor in the same way one would think of a more common infectious disease. If we can catch a cold, is it not reasonable that we might also fall victim to neoplastic disease when we encounter an agent in our environment that causes the formation of a malignant cell?

Although valid to a limited extent this concept neglects the second major factor in both infectious and neoplastic disease, that of the permissive personal constitution of the host. Induction creates the transformed cell, promotion encourages its expression as a tumor; 1 will not lead to overt neoplastic disease without the other. The malignant cell may be the actual biologic basis of the tumor, but a permissive (promotional) host constitution must also prevail or the malignant cell is suppressed (and perhaps even destroyed) before it is able to grow out into a clinically detectable neoplasm. Indeed, there is reason to believe that malignant cells arise periodically within all normal individuals, but, in the overwhelming majority of such instances, these cells are held in check until destroyed by immunologic defenses. Good evidence for this is adduced from the high frequency of multiple or additional primary tumors in the cancer patient.

The permissive host constitution is an exceedingly complex concept. Whereas agents that generate the malignant cell are usually impressed on a person from his environment (exogenous), those that go into the makeup of the permissive personal constitution arise from within the body (endogenous). The former, although diverse, are usually identifiable as

single agents. The latter, like all physiologic functions, are highly interdependent and difficult to consider singly or in isolation. In the next 2 learning objectives we will examine the agents of malignant transformation and the components of the permissive constitution of the host, respectively. Bear in mind, however, that although we will discuss each factor in both groups individually, in actual fact all are inextricably mixed within the patient and his environment.

Additional Reading

Berg, J. W. et al. The prevalence of latent cancers in cancer patients. Arch. Path. 91:183, 1971

Braun, A. On the origin of the cancer cells. Am. Scientist 58:307, 1970

Kauffman, S. Differentiation of malignant to benign cells. J. Theor. Biol. 31:421, 1971

Pierce, B. and Johnson, L. D. Differentiation and cancer *in vitro* 7:140, 1971

Temin, H. M. RNA-directed DNA synthesis. Sci. Amer. 226:25, 1972

Thoma, G. W. Incidence and significance of multiple primary malignant tumors. Am. J. Med. Sci. 247:427, 1964

EXOGENOUS FACTORS— AGENTS THAT GENERATE THE MALIGNANT CELL

LEARNING OBJECTIVE

To be able to discuss each of the 5 kinds of exogenous factors (carcinogens) presented with respect to its potential for the induction of malignancy

Neoplasia is almost certainly a collection of very different diseases, all of which converge at the single endpoint of uncontrolled cell proliferation. The validity of this interpretation is inferred from the variety of widely different factors that contribute to the cause of tumors. We have seen that the 2 requirements for neoplastic disease are: 1) the malignant cell and

2) the permissive constitution of the host. We must now study the first of these groups of factors in some detail. Bearing in mind their usual role as agents of induction, let us examine the series of exogenous cancer-causing agents (carcinogens) listed in Illustration 6-11.

1. Mechanical and Thermal Injury

It is clear that, under some circumstances, longstanding mechanical irritation is associated with cancer. This cannot be held true of most types of acute trauma, since repeated examinations of groups of wounded war veterans has disclosed no difference in the incidence of tumors between these and other groups of comparable age. The carcinogenic effect of chronic irritation requires a period of several years and even then will not predictably cause a tumor. Yet, despite all reservations, it is undeniable that a broken-down, jagged tooth is occasionally found opposite a malignancy of the tongue (Illustration 6-12). Perhaps this kind of irritation acts only as a promoting agent for dormant tumor cells initiated by a true carcinogen. Whatever the relationship, the clinical association has been verified by repeated observations.

Thermal injury, on the other hand, is far more dangerous as a cause of neoplasia. A number of well authenticated cases has been described in which a malignancy of the skin has developed at the site of a burn or scald injury.

6-12. MECHANICAL AND THERMAL INJURY

1) MECHANICAL INJURY
    chronic, longstanding (not acute) trauma has questionable association with malignancy
    may act as promoting agent
 	
 2) THERMAL INJURY
    many cases of epithelial malignancy in skin covering burn or scald injury

Also, to invoke a bizarre but interesting example, carcinoma of the abdominal skin is virtually non-existent except in those natives of Kashmir who make a practice of holding an appliance (kangri) containing glowing charcoal to their bodies as a means of keeping warm. The tumor caused by this practice is known as the kangri cancer and, although often cited as an example of thermal carcinogenesis, it may be provoked in part by hydrocarbons in the fumes.

2. Ionizing Radiation

There is now overwhelming evidence that radiant energy can act as a carcinogen. This is particularly true of electromagnetic radiation in the shorter wave lengths such as x-ray and gamma-rays, but even ultraviolet light and alpha particles are associated with cancer under certain circumstances. High energy radiation such as x-rays and gamma rays are generally more dangerous as carcinogens, because they penetrate deeply and do not require long exposure. Their mode of action on the cell is not understood, but must involve damage due principally to water ionization and free radical formation.

Several examples of radiation carcinogenesis can be drawn from the dynamic and, for some, tragic history of radiobiology. For instance, only 5 years after the discovery of x-rays, the first radiation-induced skin cancer was reported; thereafter, many of the early workers in

---

6-11. EXOGENOUS FACTORS IN MALIGNANCY (CARCINOGENS)
Agents that generate the malignant cell   1) MECHANICAL AND THERMAL INJURY   2) IONIZING RADIATION   3) ENVIRONMENT AND HABIT   4) CHEMICALS   5) ONCOGENIC VIRUS

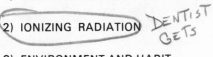

6-13. IONIZING RADIATION (AS A CAR-
        CINOGEN)

1) LOCAL IRRADIATION
       skin cancer in early radiobiologists

2) OCCUPATIONAL HAZARDS
       watch dial painters
       uranium miners
       radiologists

3) THERAPEUTIC IRRADIATION
       irradiation of infants for "thymic
       enlargement"

4) THERMONUCLEAR WAR
       increased incidence of leukemia
       in survivors at Hiroshima and
       Nagasaki

blasts that were exposed within 5,000 meters of the hypocenter at Hiroshima and Nagasaki showed a much higher incidence of leukemia, reaching a peak some 5 to 7 years after exposure.

Although the mechanism of radiation carcinogenesis is not understood, it is clear that it requires a long latent period. Also, a greater dose can be roughly correlated with a higher cancer incidence within the exposed population. Beyond these rudimentary facts little is known.

3. Environment and Habit

Predominant forms of cancer vary among nations as well as among occupational and socio-economic groups within a single nation. This kind of variability in cancer incidence is undoubtedly based, to some extent, on genetic differences. But, in the case of many tumors, it has proven to be more strongly related to the carcinogenic quality of environment and habit.

In the United States, bronchogenic squamous cell carcinoma is the most common visceral

radiology succumbed to cutaneous cancer and leukemia. The names of hundreds of these scientific martyrs are inscribed on a monument in Hamburg, Germany. Even Mme. Curie may have died from overexposure to radiation.

Radiation carcinogenesis has also proved a serious occupational hazard. Dial painters in a watch factory in Massachusetts at one time used their lips and tongue to point brushes used in applying luminous paint. The inevitable result was the absorption of minute amounts of radium which is readily incorporated into bone and excreted very slowly. It required only a very short exposure to lead to the later occurrence of osteogenic sarcoma and carcinoma of sinus epithelium.

Other examples of radiation and cancer include the alarming discovery that the incidence of pulmonary carcinoma is much higher in uranium miners, whereas that of leukemia was at one time greater among radiologists.

Finally, the use of radiation to both cure and destroy has resulted in cancer. Infants irradiated at birth for presumed thymic enlargement were later found to have developed cancer of the thyroid and a higher incidence of other tumors whereas survivors of the atomic bomb

6-14. ENVIRONMENT AND HABIT IN
        CARCINOGENESIS

1) SOCIO-ECONOMIC DIFFERENCES
       carcinoma of breast: higher
       carcinoma of cervix: lower

2) GEOGRAPHIC DIFFERENCES
       U.S.: lung
       Japan: stomach
       Taiwan: nasopharynx

3) OCCUPATIONAL DIFFERENCES
       aniline dye and synthetic rubber
       workers
       asbestos workers, carpenters,
       uranium miners
       workers exposed to oil, arsenic,
       sunlight

4) USE OF TOBACCO

malignancy of males. In Japan, cancer of the stomach and, in Taiwan, cancer of the nasopharynx make up about half of all cancer in males. Migration from 1 country to another results in the migrant group's assuming the cancer risk of the adopted country, usually within 2 generations, evidence that the pattern of the ancestral country was the result of its environment rather than the genetic composition of its people.

Cancer of the stomach and cervix show a 3 to 4 times higher rate of occurrence in unskilled workers and their wives whereas cancer of the breast, leukemia and multiple myeloma are more common among those of higher economic classes. Interestingly, carcinoma of both the stomach and cervix are showing a marked decline in the United States.

A number of examples of cancer patterns associated with occupational groups can be mentioned. Workers in the aniline dye or early synthetic rubber industries experienced an alarming incidence of carcinoma of the urinary bladder caused by routine exposure to beta-naphthylamine and related chemicals. Asbestos workers, carpenters and uranium miners are known to have a higher incidence of carcinoma of the lung, whereas skin cancers are found with increased frequency in workers exposed to oil, arsenic or sunlight. *CAUSE CANCER*

Without any doubt the use of tobacco is the single most prominent example of a habit-related cancer pattern. *Tobacco in one form or another is responsible for more human cancer (and cancer deaths) than any other known agent.* In fact, in assessing the whole problem the only conclusion possible is that we are experiencing a bona-fide epidemic of a tobacco-related syndrome of diseases, a prominent component of which is cancer of the lung. It has been estimated that over 90 per cent of the current incidence of lung cancer in the United States would vanish, if all smoking of cigarettes was discontinued.

4. Chemicals

Any summary of the status of chemical carcinogenesis must begin with an acknowledgement of the initial report of this phenomenon by Sir Percival Pott, a London surgeon who 2 centuries ago described the occurrence of scrotal cancer in English chimneysweeps. Pott called this occupational disease the "soot wart" and his book in 1775 incited the first general awareness of chemical carcinogenesis. Experimental confirmation of Pott's findings languished until the work of Yamagiwa and Ichikawa in 1915 showed that skin cancer could be induced at will in rabbits by the simple application of coal tar to the surface of the ear.

Since that time, the number and variety of recognized carcinogens have increased alarmingly. Chemical carcinogens now comprise a diverse group of non-viral, non-radioactive substances ranging from the originally cited polycyclic hydrocarbons to aliphatic structures, metals (arsenic) and even metabolites of living cells (Illustration 6-15). Also, it is now clearly understood that we are confronted not only with the specific cancer-causing activity of single compounds but also with a complex interplay among such agents.

5. Oncogenic Virus

Our final example of a class of exogenous agents capable of producing tumors is the virus. Although it can be demonstrated that the virus can cause a variety of benign and malignant tumors in lower animals, its association with human neoplasms (except for the common wart and the laryngeal papilloma) is still quite vague. Identification and isolation of a virus responsible for a major human malignancy would be a truly significant achievement in medicine.

6-15. CHEMICAL CARCINOGENESIS

---

1) POTT'S DISEASE (1775)

2) YAMAGIWA AND ICHIKAWA (1915)

3) CURRENTLY KNOWN CHEMICAL CARCINOGENS INCLUDE
   polycyclic hydrocarbons
   aliphatic hydrocarbons
   metals
   metabolites of living cells

6-16. THE ONCOGENIC VIRUS

1) VIRAL MALIGNANCY IS WELL DOCU-MENTED PHENOMENON AMONG LOWER ANIMALS

2) SUSPECTED TO APPLY TO CERTAIN HUMAN NEOPLASMS: HOWEVER, ONLY WELL DOCUMENTED VIRAL TUMOR OF MAN IS COMMON WART
(and laryngeal papillomatosis)

Many, especially those associated with younger-aged groups, are suspected to be of viral etiology: however, absolute proof is still lacking.

The whole picture of viral infection, including viral oncogenesis, will be presented in a systematic way in the following chapter.

Additional Reading

Allen, D. W. and Cole, P. Viruses and human cancer. N. Engl. J. Med. 286:70, 1972

Cook, P. J. and Burkitt, D. P. Cancer in Africa. Brit. Med. Bull. 27:14, 1971

Ho, H. C. Incidence of nasopharyngeal cancer in Hong Kong. Bull, Cancer 9:5, 1971

McMahon, B. Epidemiologic aspects of cancer. *In* Cancer: A Manual for Practitioners. American Cancer Society, 1968

Miller, J. A. Carcinogenesis by chemicals: An overview. Cancer Res. 30:559, 1970

Warren, S. Radiation carcinogenesis. Bull. N.Y. Acad. Med. 46:131, 1970

Wynder, E. L. et al. The epidemiology of lung cancer. J. Am. Med. Assn. 213:2221, 1970

ENDOGENOUS FACTORS—COMPONENTS OF THE PERMISSIVE CONSTITUTION

LEARNING OBJECTIVE

To be able to discuss each of the 5 kinds of endogenous factors presented with regard to its significance as a component of the permissive host constitution in malignant neoplasia

---

Having considered exogenous factors in the previous learning objective, we must now turn to a more detailed discussion of those that arise within the individual. As declared earlier, these are to be considered components of the permissive constitution. With reference to the 2-stage evolution of the tumor, these would be more nearly akin to agents of promotion than induction. Although difficult to specify as single factors, we will consider the 5 examples listed in Illustration 6-17.

1. Age

The influence of an individual's age on his liability to contract a malignant disease seems to be 2-fold (Illustration 6-18). In the first of these, we see that advancing age is generally associated with a greater frequency of malignant disease. An overwhelming body of evi-

---

6-17. ENDOGENOUS FACTORS IN MALIGNANCY

(Components of the permissive constitution)

1) AGE

2) SEX

3) HEREDITY

4) HORMONAL IMBALANCE

5) IMPAIRED IMMUNOLOGIC DEFENSES

6-18. AGE AS A FACTOR IN MALIGNANCY
1) MOST MAJOR MALIGNANCIES OCCUR WITH GREATER FREQUENCY IN ADVANCED AGE

2) CERTAIN TUMORS SHOW A PROPENSITY TO OCCUR WITHIN A PARTICULAR AGE RANGE AT SOME TIME DURING THE EARLIER YEARS
    embryonal tumors in infancy
    sarcomas in adolescence and early adulthood

6-19. SEX AS A FACTOR IN MALIGNANT DISEASE INCIDENCE

1) STRUCTURAL RESTRICTIONS
    uterus
    prostate

2) NO STRUCTURAL RESTRICTIONS*
    breast
    stomach
    others

3) SEX INCIDENCE BASED ON
    genetic differences
    hormonal differences
    differences in gender role

* most major malignancies without structural restrictions occur with greater frequency in the male

dence persuades us to accept the psalmist's estimate of 3-score and 10 years as the average human life span. Clearly, something slowly happens to an individual over this amount of time that undermines his grip on life. Whatever the nature of the aging process, it seems certain that it predisposes the human body to cancer. Indeed, it has been estimated that 85 per cent of all cases of cancer occurs beyond the age of 60. Biologic aging has been discussed in Chapter 3 and will not be considered in detail here. However, with respect to its significance in neoplasm, it would seem that in order to develop a tumor all one has to do is to live long enough.

Another relationship between age and tumor incidence is seen the phenomenon of the age specificity of certain tumors. We have seen that embryonal tumors occur at a very early age, sarcomas show a pronounced propensity for adolescence and early adulthood, whereas carcinomas favor the older patient. Leukemia is a malignant tumor of early childhood, osteogenic sarcoma a tumor of adolescence and early adulthood, whereas other tumors exhibit comparable age-related peaks of occurrence.

2. Sex

Some tumors show a clear-cut predilection for 1 or the other sex (Illustration 6-19). In certain cases, of course, this is absolutely obligate. Testicular or prostatic tumors could not possibly occur in the normal female, nor would tumors of female generative structures be expected in a normal male.

But, even with regard to those tumors where there are no structural restrictions, a striking difference in sex-related incidence can often be seen. For example, although the male possesses breast tissue analogous to that of the female, cancer of the breast is almost exclusively a disease of women. Only about 1 per cent of reported cases occur in men, a situation undoubtedly related to the well established estrogen dependence of this tumor.

Cancer of the stomach, on the other hand, occurs far more often in men, as does transitional cell carcinoma, bronchogenic squamous cell carcinoma *and most other major malignancies.* In the case of some tumors, the reason for a clear-cut sex related propensity is undoubtedly based on genetic differences between male and female. In others, increased incidence in the male probably reflects gender role differences that lead to greater exposure to carcinogens (Illustration 6-20).

6-20. INCIDENCE OF MAJOR CANCERS BY SITE AND SEX (per cent total)		
(American Cancer Society)		
	female per cent	male per cent
SKIN	13	23
ORAL	2	3
BREAST	23	1
LUNG	3	18
COLON AND RECTUM	13	11
OTHER DIGESTIVE	8	10
UTERUS	15	—
PROSTATE	—	10
URINARY	3	7
LEUKEMIA AND LYMPHOMA	6	7
ALL OTHER	15	11

6-21. HEREDITY AND CANCER

1) THE TENDENCY TO CONTRACT A TUMOR CAN BE INHERITED
some cancers are inherited as single-gene defects
cancer is more common among individuals with cytogenetic defects
known mutagenic agents also cause cancer

2) THE MALIGNANT CELL IS GENETICALLY ALTERED

6-22. SINGLE-GENE TUMORS OR PREDISPOSING CONDITIONS*

1) AUTOSOMAL DOMINANT
familial polyposis of the colon
retinoblastoma
cancer families

2) AUTOSOMAL RECESSIVE
xeroderma pigmentosum
Chediak-Higashi syndrome
ataxia-telangiectasia

– – – – –

* selected examples of such conditions

3. Heredity

The fact that a cancer cell is a changed cell and that this change is passed on to its progeny suggests that cancer is a disease that somehow involves the genome. This is further supported by the 3 additional observations regarding the nature and the course in human cancer listed in Illustration 6-21. We will now consider each of these observations in more detail.

Although most human cancers are not inherited as single-gene defects, some tumors and conditions predisposing the tumors clearly are. In fact a few (listed in illustrated 6-22) are actually passed from generation to generation in a simple Mendelian pattern. Some other cancers, including malignant melanoma, adenocarcinoma of the colon and adenocarcinoma of the endometrium (but not squamous cell carcinoma of the cervix), show a very pronounced tendency toward familial grouping, whereas many others, including carcinoma of the breast, tend to occur with a slightly greater frequency among consanguinous groups.

Individuals with certain cytogenetic defects appear to be far more prone to contracting cancer than those with a normal chromosome complement. This is particularly apparent in Down's Syndrome (mongolism, trisomy 21) where the incidence of leukemia is 11 times normal. A somewhat higher than normal risk of leukemia is also seen in Klinefelter's Syndrome and in others based on chromosomal abnormalities. Genetic disease will be covered in greater detail in Chapter 9.

Finally, mutagenic agents such as ionizing radiation, some chemicals and some viruses also produce cancer in man or experimental animals. Concordance between the ability of these agents to produce chromosomal breakage and induce neoplasia suggests that the former is somehow involved in the latter.

4. Hormonal Imbalance

Hormonal alteration, like radiation, can both cause and cure cancer. Its practical use in cancer therapy is one of the great triumphs of medical research, but its potential for causing cancer has only recently become generally accepted. The hormones most suspect in cancer are the estrogens. Although it is true that neither these nor any other hormone has been shown to be carcinogenic in man, most oncologists feel that this is due only to the fact that the appropriate experiment is outside the limits of ethical investigation (Illustration 6-23). Estrogens have been shown to cause cancer of the breast and other organs in laboratory animals and 2 cases have been reported of male transsexuals who almost certainly developed breast cancer as a result of high doses of

---

6-24. IMMUNITY AND CANCER

1) ALL NEOPLASTIC CELLS HAVE ALTERED GENETIC STRUCTURE (GENOME): HENCE RESEMBLE ALLOGENEIC GRAFTS

2) IF TUMOR-SPECIFIC ANTIGENS ARE RECOGNIZED TUMOR MAY BE REJECTED

3) INCREASED INCIDENCE OF MALIGNANCY WITH AGE IS ASSOCIATED WITH DECLINING IMMUNOCOMPETENCE

4) CONTINUED, LONGSTANDING IMMUNOLOGIC STIMULATION IS SUSPECTED TO BE ASSOCIATED WITH THE OCCURRENCE OF MALIGNANCY

---

estrogens. Also, and quite portentious for the further indiscriminate use of drugs, the treatment of pregnant women with estradiol has resulted in the unusual incidence of carcinoma of the vagina, not in the women treated, but in the female children born of such pregnancies after they reached the age of 20.

5. Impaired Immunologic Defenses

There is strong evidence that the cellular immune system is one of our most indispensible means of defense against a malignant tumor. In a recent study it was shown that both survival and freedom from recurrence following surgery for malignancy can be correlated directly with the patient's ability to mount a vigorous, immunologic reaction of the cellular type.

Also, it has been known for some time that patients being treated with immunosuppressive agents to enhance acceptance of a grafted organ such as a kidney are more prone to the development of malignant tumors. Deficiency of the cellular immune response constitutes a strong predisposition to cancer (Illustration 6-24).

6-23. HORMONES AND CANCER

1) HORMONES MOST SUSPECT ARE THE ESTROGENS
   breast
   vagina (in offspring)

2) ANDROGENS ARE NEEDED FOR CARCINOMA OF THE PROSTATE

Despite the unusual significance of cellular immunity in cancer protection, one must not overlook other possible defenses. There is a growing appreciation of the possibility of a mechanism of cancer defense based on the genetic apparatus of the somatic cell itself. The picture is far from complete however, the future promises exciting and unexpected discoveries in cancer research.

Additional Reading

Dumars, K. W. Cancer, chromosomes and congenital abnormalities. Cancer 20:1006, 1967

Editorial: Sibling cancers—statistics and biology. N. Engl. J. Med. 279:159, 1968

Herbst, A. L. Adenocarcinoma of the vagina. N. Engl. J. Med. 284:878, 1971

Huggins, C. Endocrine-induced regression of cancers. Science 156:1050, 1967

Humphrey, L. J. Current status of cancer vaccine. Am. J. Surg. 120:329, 1970

Klein, E. Tumor-specific transplantation antigens. Ann. N.Y. Acad. Sci. 164:344, 1969

Knudson, A. G. Genetics and cancer. Postgrad. Med. 48:6, 1970

Lynch, H. T. and Krush, A. J. Cancer genetics. South. Med. J. 64:(Suppl. 1), 1971

Miller, R. W. Fifty-two forms of childhood cancer: United States mortality experience, 1960-1966. J. Pediat. 75:685, 1969

Symposium: Immunological Aspects of Cancer. Collection of Reprints from the British Medical Journal, 1970

chapter 7
VIRAL, CHLAMYDIAL, AND RICKETTSIAL INFECTION

PRINCIPLES OF INFECTIOUS DISEASE

LEARNING OBJECTIVE

To be able to discuss each of the following subjects in terms of its broad application to infectious disease

- a) the hierarchy of human pathogens based on complexity
- b) symbiosis, commensalism, parasitism
- c) reservoir (zoonosis, inanimate reservoirs and single-host human pathogens)
- d) carrier (human)
- e) vehicle, fomite, vector
- f) inoculum, portal of entry
- g) endemic, epidemic, pandemic
- h) intrauterine infection

The human body can be successfully parasitized by organisms ranging in complexity from simple viruses to complex animals. This hierarchy of human parasites is shown in Illustration 7-1. At its lowest (least complex) end are the viruses, chlamydiae and rickettsiae, all 3 of which are *obligate intracellular parasites*.* Midway we find bacteria, the mycotic organisms (yeasts and fungi) and protozoa; these occur as both intracellular and extracellular parasites. Finally, at the most complex terminus of our spectrum, we find the metazoan parasites, all of which occupy an extracellular position, some even being classified as ectoparasites and actually living on or near the surface of the body.

In the parasitic relationship (Illustration 7-2), 1 organism lives at the expense of another. All infectious disease is due to this kind of

* One variety of rickettsia has been grown in vitro, outside of cells.

relationship between a human being and a pathogenic organism. The successful pathogen does not kill its host, so most examples of fatal infections can be presumed natural mistakes.

1. The Spread of Infection

The transmission of infection from host to host is essential to the biologic success of a pathogen. Good pathogens can be expected to have developed efficient means of communicability. The entire population of a single pathogen existing at any one time will be distributed among a group of infected individuals, either animal or human or both. This infected group is said to be the "reservoir" of the infection. In those diseases where a pathogen is passed from one human being to another, the only reservoir is human. Some pathogens, however, can multiply in 2 or more hosts, thus animals, insects or, in rare cases, all 3 can act as reservoirs for human infection (Illustration 7-3). Some pathogens also employ inanimate reservoirs.

Agents of transmission can be either animate or inanimate. Living agents of disease transmission are called *vectors*, whereas passive, non-living carriers of infection are classified as either food or *fomite* (a fomite is any non-living substance other than food that serves to harbor and transmit infectious organisms).

Vectors of infection are usually either insects or animals. When a human being functions as an agent for the transmission of infection, he is called a *carrier*. Some infections, such as venereal diseases, must be transmitted by direct contact with the infectious organism. The agent of syphilis, for example, is extremely delicate and cannot withstand desiccation. It would be impossible for such a pathogen to persist in nature were it not for the unusual opportunity for transmission presented by human coitus.

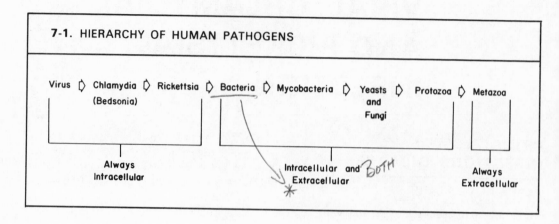

7-1. HIERARCHY OF HUMAN PATHOGENS

Virus ▷ Chlamydia ▷ Rickettsia ▷ Bacteria ▷ Mycobacteria ▷ Yeasts ▷ Protozoa ▷ Metazoa
       (Bedsonia)   and
                                                              Fungi

Always   Intracellular and *BOTH*   Always
Intracellular   Extracellular   Extracellular

7-2. KINDS OF SYMBIOSIS (DORLAND, 22ND EDITION)

SYMBIOSIS:
The living together or close association of two dissimilar organisms

1) MUTUALISM: the association is beneficial to both

1st ques.

2) COMMENSALISM: the association is beneficial to one without injury to the other

3) PARASITISM: the association is beneficial to one but detrimental to the other

---

7-3. RESERVOIRS OF INFECTIOUS DISEASE

1) ANIMAL RESERVOIRS

FALSE ANS.
zoonoses: infectious diseases transmitted between vertebrate animals and man
includes hundreds of diseases caused by all kinds of pathogens
extremely difficult to eradicate or control

2) INANIMATE RESERVOIRS
principally soil and dust

3) SINGLE-HOST HUMAN DISEASES
whole reservoir in human population (smallpox, measles, polio, etc.)
could be eradicated by eliminating all susceptible hosts

7-4. SPREAD OF INFECTION

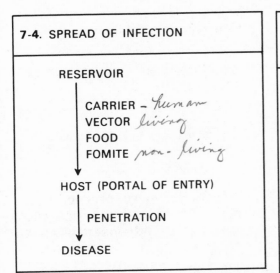

RESERVOIR

CARRIER – *human*
VECTOR *living*
FOOD
FOMITE *non-living*

↓

HOST (PORTAL OF ENTRY)

PENETRATION

↓

DISEASE

7-5. RELATIONSHIP OF INFECTIOUS DISEASE TO HOST POPULATION

1) **ENDEMIC**
   disease is prevalent within a given community where it exhibits a low but constant incidence   *Not*

2) **EPIDEMIC**
   incidence increases, disease spreads affecting an ever-increasing number of people

3) **PANDEMIC**
   incidence increases further, all susceptible hosts are affected

Important details regarding the spread of disease are recapitulated in Illustration 7-4.

2. Dynamics of Infection

Epidemiology (among other things) is the study of the behavior of a disease within a population of susceptible individuals. Most infectious diseases are simply *endemic*; that is, they persist within such a population from year to year without much variation in incidence or attack rate. Occasionally, conditions will favor the occurrence of an enormous increase in the incidence of a single disease within a limited area. Such an occurrence is called an *epidemic*. If the epidemic spreads unchecked throughout the entire population of the world, it is called a *pandemic*. Pandemics, fortunately, are unusual, the last one occurring as a wave of influenza in 1914 to 1918 that infected the population of every known area of the world with the single exception of the island of Tristan da Cunah (Illustration 7-5). The relationship between a disease and a population of susceptible individuals is a dynamic one. When a disease exhibits endemicity, it means that factors favoring its spread and containment are in balance. Disturbance of this balance may have either favorable or unfavorable results; it may lead to suppression of the disease or to its increasing incidence. A program of mass prophylactic inoculation, for example, has all but eliminated poliomyelitis, whereas in contrast, the mutation of an influenza virus periodically leads to new epidemics.

7-6. MAJOR EPIDEMIC DISEASES

VIRAL
influenza, yellow fever, poliomyelitis, encephalitis

RICKETTSIAL
typhus

BACTERIAL
plaque, cholera, syphilis, typhoid fever

PROTOZOAN
malaria

For a number of very complex reasons, certain diseases are more liable to burst forth in epidemics than others (Illustration 7-6). The reasons are not uniform and may depend, in 1 case, on a change in the organism, in another, on a change in the host and in a third, on a change in the reservoir or vector. The student should study the diseases listed in Illustration 7-6 and be prepared to recognize them as major epidemic diseases of current or historic importance.

Which of following are viral disease?
exclude Typhoid & malaria

NOT ON TEST

*used throughout Text

3. Virulence

The quality of being able to produce disease is referred to as *pathogenicity* whereas the degree of pathogenicity exhibited by an organism is referred to as its *virulence*. Thus, pathogens may be more or less virulent, but all share the quality of pathogenicity.

Virulence is a measure of an organism's ability to penetrate the body, destroy tissue and sustain attack by defense mechanisms. An overwhelmingly virulent organism such as the bacillus of plague, for example, has little trouble thriving despite every effort by the host to purge it from the body. We will discuss both the modes of infection and the elements of host resistance in greater detail as we consider each disease.

4. Intrauterine Infection

Although the fetus would seem liable to any infection contracted by the mother, only a limited number of human pathogens seem to be able to cross placental membranes and establish a significant infection in fetal tissues. The 5 organisms most commonly observed to do this are listed in Illustration 7-7. The effects of such an infection on the developing child will depend upon a number of factors, among which are the nature of the infection and the time of its onset relative to the progress of the pregnancy. Each of the 5 agents listed has a somewhat different potential. The agent of syphilis, for example, cannot cross placental membranes until the fifth month, after which the untreated fetal infection follows a predictable course. The rubella virus, by far the most common intrauterine infectious agent, seems to be able to establish an infection at any time during the pregnancy and causes a variety of untoward effects ranging from miscarriage to a chronic infection syndrome in the offspring.

Since the intrauterine environment should be devoid of significant immunologic challenge, a child delivered at term in a normal pregnancy will have only those antibodies of the IgG class given him by his mother. In the case of an intrauterine infection, however, the developing child has been forced to respond to immunologic challenge *in utero*. In doing so, he will have generated a significant amount of IgM antibodies and these will be detectable in the

---

7-7. INTRAUTERINE INFECTION

1) **MOST COMMON INTRAUTERINE INFECTIONS ARE:**
   rubella
   syphilis
   cytomegalic inclusion disease
   toxoplasmosis
   listeriosis

2) **EFFECTS ON CHILD DEPEND UPON THE NATURE OF THE INFECTION AND THE TIME OF ITS ONSET RELATIVE TO PROGRESS OF THE PREGNANCY**
   abortion or stillbirth
   congenital defects
   chronic infection syndrome

3) **PRESENCE OF IgM IN CORD SERUM MEANS CHILD HAS SUSTAINED INTRAUTERINE INFECTION**

---

cord serum at the time of birth. The presence of IgM in cord serum, therefore, is strong evidence that a child has sustained an intrauterine infection.

Additional Reading

Cooper, L. Z. German measles. Sci. Amer. 215:30, 1966

Foege, W. H., et al. Current status of global smallpox eradication. Am. J. Epidemiol. 93:223, 1971

Hardy, J. B. Viruses and the fetus. Postgrad, Med. Jan., 1968

Hilleman, M. R. Toward control of viral infections in man. Science 164:506, 1969

Krugmen, S. Present status of measles and rubella immunization in the U.S.: A medical progress report. J. Pediat. 78:1, 1971

Muul, I. Mammalian ecology and epidemiology of zoonoses. Science 170:1275, 1970

Sabin, A. B. Control of infectious diseases. J. Infectious Dis. 121:91, 1970

THE TRUE VIRUS

LEARNING OBJECTIVE

To be able to list the specifications of the true virus and compare its mode of life with that of higher organisms

The true virus is the smallest and most simple of human pathogens (Illustration 7-8). Aside from its size the virus exhibits several characteristics that serve to distinguish it from kinds of other pathogens. These have been summarized as follows:

1) Viral genetic material consists of either DNA or RNA *but not both*.
2) The virus has a relatively simple structure in which a protein shell surrounds the centrally located nucleic acid.
3) The virus functions only within living cells, occupying either the nucleus or cytoplasm or both; it exhibits no metabolic activity when extracellular.
4) The virus does not possess genetic information for the synthesis of a system for energy metabolism.
5) A virus does not divide in the manner of cells (binary fission).

6) The nucleic acid of the invading virus takes over control of the infected cell causing it to synthesize new viral particles.
7) The invading virus makes use of the ribosomes of the infected host cell for all synthetic activity.
8) The 2 major components of the complete virus (nucleic acid and protein) are produced separately and assembled in the cell shortly before release.
9) During the process of release, some viruses acquire an outer envelope containing lipid and other materials derived, at least in part, from the infected cell.
10) The complete viral particle is known as the *virion*, and consists of a nuclei acid core (either DNA or RNA) surrounded by an antigenitically specific capsule of protein.

These qualities define the "true" virus. Viruses infect higher animals, insects, plants and even bacteria (bacteriophages).

Additional Reading

Evans, E. A. Viruses and evolution. Persp. Biol. Med. III:213, 1960

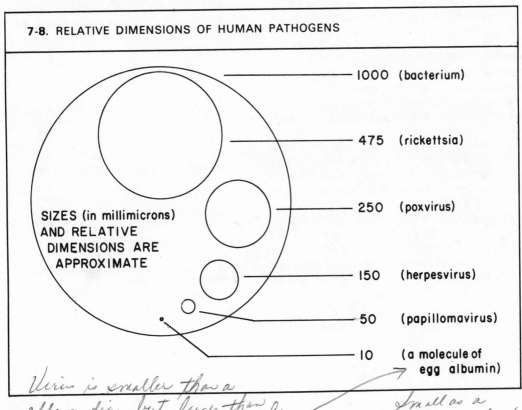

7-8. RELATIVE DIMENSIONS OF HUMAN PATHOGENS

SIZES (in millimicrons) AND RELATIVE DIMENSIONS ARE APPROXIMATE

1000 (bacterium)
475 (rickettsia)
250 (poxvirus)
150 (herpesvirus)
50 (papillomavirus)
10 (a molecule of egg albumin)

Virus is smaller than a chlamydia but larger than a

Small as a protein molecule.

INTERACTION BETWEEN A VIRUS AND ITS HOST CELL

LEARNING OBJECTIVE

To be able to discuss the essential features of the necrotizing or cytocidal viral infection describing each of the following stages:
   a) fixation
   b) penetration
   c) uncoating and release
   d) synthesis and re-assembly of new virions
   e) bursting of the infected cell and release of virions

1. The Cytocidal (Cytolytic or Necrotizing) Viral Infection

As long ago as 1923 it was proposed that viruses were not microbes in the usual sense, but rebellious genes that had somehow escaped the controlling influence of a parent cell. In this concept, the virus would have evolved by retrograde development from higher organisms. As could be predicted, such an utterly speculative idea caused an outburst of heated discussion and promptly fell into disfavor; today there are reasons for second thought. It is known, for example, that viruses and the genetic material of their host cell have significant nucleotide sequences in common, suggesting that virus has either developed from the host cell genome or has acquired the sequences as a means of adapting to the cell it must parasitize. Many authorities favor the former interpretation, that the virus has indeed devolved from higher forms of life. But, whatever its origin, it must be conceded that the virus is a biologic success. To have been so successful, the virus must have arrived at certain modes of relationship with its host which, while allowing the host to go on living, still permit adequate replication and spread of the virus. On the basis of todays appreciation of the subject, it would seem that the type of relationship usually assumed between a virus and its host cell is the kind known as the *cytocidal* (cytolytic or necrotizing) infection (Illustration 7-9).

In carrying out the cytocidal infection, the virus, an obligate intracellular parasite, must first contrive to penetrate to the interior of the cell it will parasitize. This is accomplished by interaction with a specific receptor protein at the cell's surface. Having fixed to the cell surface, the virus, in some way, induces the cell to engulf and ingest it through endocytosis. Once inside, the virus sheds its protein coat, escapes from the vacuole and the viral nucleic acid assumes direction of the cell's synthetic activity, causing it to produce new viral components. Finally, the newly synthetized virus is assembled and the cell (which has now been reduced to little more than a limp bag of virus) bursts, releasing new virions for distribution throughout the body.

2. Viral Infection and Viral Disease

Infection and disease are not synonymous terms: the former describes the relationship of the parasite to the host whereas the latter encompasses all changes observed in the host as a result of this relationship. Infection may be totally asymptomatic, but disease is usually manifest (Illustration 7-10). Every viral infection will not necessarily result in overt disease; some, we will see, cause a form of disease that remains occult for years or for a person's entire lifetime.

Having examined the sequence of steps that lead to the typical viral infection, we must now turn our attention to the classification of viral disease, allowing that in some cases the infectious process will differ importantly from that described. The classification of viral disease to be used in this discussion is outlined in Illustration 7-11.

Additional Reading

Lwoff, A. Interaction among virus, Cell and Organism. Science 152:1216, 1966

7-9. THE CYTOCIDAL (CYTOLYTIC OR NECROTIZING) VIRAL INFECTION

PENETRATION AND UNCOATING   SYNTHESIS, REASSEMBLY AND RELEASE

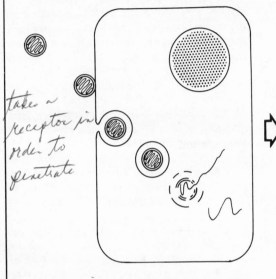 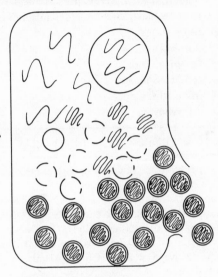

takes a receptor in order to penetrate

1) Virus is adsorbed to cell probably by interaction with specific receptor

★ 2) Enters cell through endocytosis   *way it gets to ctr. of cell*

3) Released from vacuole and uncoated

1) Viral nucleic acid pre-empts cell synthetic activity allowing only viral components to be made

2) Protein and nucleic acid are reassembled

3) Cell bursts and new virions are released

NOT

7-10. VIRAL INFECTION AND VIRAL DISEASE

1) VIRAL INFECTION
process through which the virus assumes and maintains a parasitic relationship with a susceptible host cell

2) VIRAL DISEASE
syndrome manifested by host (organism) as a result of sustaining a viral infection

7-11. CLASSIFICATION OF VIRAL DISEASE

1) ACUTE (TYPICAL) VIRAL DISEASE
based on cytocidal (cytolytic or necrotizing) infection
typified by ectromelia model

2) ATYPICAL VIRAL DISEASE
inapparent
chronic
latent
slow
oncogenic

ACUTE (TYPICAL) VIRAL DISEASE

LEARNING OBJECTIVE

To be able to differentiate viral disease from viral infection and describe the pathogenesis of the acute (typical) viral disease mentioning the following stages:

a) inoculation
b) incubation
c) acute illness
d) exanthem
e) recovery

Acute viral disease is the type that almost everyone will recognize. It is so common and so familiar that each of us probably experiences at least one such episode per year and perhaps many more. Acute viral disease is based on the cytopathic (cytocidal or necrotizing) infectious process shown in Illustration 7-9. The steps in this type of infection must be kept firmly in mind, as we now look at how it leads to acute viral disease.

The pathogensis of acute viral disease has been most critically studied using the mousepox virus (ectromelia) system and the steps to be described apply largely to that disease. Since mousepox strongly resembles similar human infections, it is most probable that the steps to be described (Illustration 7-12) are very com-

---

7-12. PATHOGENESIS OF TYPICAL VIRAL DISEASE

(as exemplified by ectromelia model)

1) INOCULATION   *mousepox virus*

2) INCUBATION — *primary viremia (feel bad)*

3) ACUTE ILLNESS — *secondary viremia*

4) EXANTHEM

5) RECOVERY

---

parable to those in human diseases that result in skin rashes (exanthems) such as smallpox, measles, varicella, rubella and others.

1. Inoculation

In the first step of the developing viral disease, a cytopathic infection is established at the portal of entry of the virus. In experimental mousepox, this is accomplished by simply injecting the virus.

2. Incubation   *DEFINE*

The incubation period is the time elapsing between inoculation and the appearance of the acute disease syndrome. Events included in this period are:

1) *Primary viremia*. The cytopathic infection at the portal of entry proceeds to the stage of virus release. At approximately the same time, all infected cells suddenly burst, liberating newly synthesized virus into the blood stream and surrounding tissue. This gives rise to the *primary viremia*. At this point the patient feels slightly ill and (if he is not a mouse) may complain of "coming down with something."

2) *Clearance of Primary Viremia*. The primary viremia is quickly cleared from the blood stream by macrophages of the lymphoreticular system, particularly those of the liver and spleen. There follows a phase in which the virus undergoes a second cycle of replication within these cells. Having undergone 1 previous cycle of replication within this same host at the portal of entry, the virus is better adapted and will enjoy easier passage in this second cycle. Also, assuming that this is the first exposure of an otherwise healthy and immunologically competent patient, there will be no pre-existing immunologic defenses against this virus.

3. Acute Illness

Again, in a synchronous manner, the infected cells burst and release a second (and much larger) wave of virus into the blood stream. This is known as *secondary viremia*. At this point the patient becomes acutely ill and exhibits all of the familiar signs and symptoms of the "syndrome of being sick."

4. Exanthem

Now widely distributed in great numbers, the virus begins to concentrate at its preferred tissue location (tropism). In mousepox as well as exanthematous human diseases, this preferred site will be the epithelial cells of the skin and mucous membranes. With localization of the virus at the preferred site, the secondary viremia subsides, the exanthem breaks out and the patient experiences a remission of the acute illness.

Clearance of 2nd ary viremia + appearance of exanthem both mark end of acute illness

5. Recovery

Having been intimately exposed to the lymphoreticular system, the virus has elicited very strong immunologic reponses of both the humoral and cellular types. Antibodies will be instrumental in completing the clearance of the secondary viremia. Sensitized lymphocytes are released from peripheral lymphoid tissue and, finding their way to infected epithelial cells, destroy both the virus and the cells that contain them. In the more superficial infections, the exanthem is confined totally to epithelial cells which regenerate and no scar results. If cells of the dermis are involved (usually through secondary bacterial infection), dermal tissue is destroyed and a scar results. A second component of recovery is the synthesis of interferon by cells in the area of viral infection. The mode of action of interferon will be covered in detail later.

Finally, we must bear in mind that the details of the sequence described above apply only to the pathogenesis of exanthematous viral disease. Many human diseases of viral etiology such as influenza and mumps may not produce a significant viremia or exanthem as an essential part of the disease. The common wart (verruca vulgaris) is perhaps most representative of a localized human viral infection.

Additional Reading

Blanden, R. V. Mechanisms of recovery from a generalized viral infection: mousepox. J. Exp. Med. 132:1035, 1970

Which of following false:
4. Virus definitely been prove cause of osteo - Cancer.

GENERAL CHARACTERISTICS OF ACUTE (TYPICAL) VIRAL DISEASE

LEARNING OBJECTIVE

To be able to discuss each of the 5 general characteristics of acute (typical) viral disease presented, mentioning its relevance in the diagnosis, clinical picture and treatment of the disease. Also, to be able to list several prominent human diseases of viral origin using both scientific and common terminology for each

Regardless of the exact specifications of the infecting virus, acute diseases of viral etiology share certain general qualities. The following are a collection of these and are useful in differentiating between viral disease and that caused by other kinds of pathogens:

1. Most Are Acute

different

Most systemic viral infections are acute and self-limiting. There are several conspicuous examples of *chronic* viral disease (cytomegalic

---

7-13. GENERAL CHARACTERISTICS OF ACUTE (TYPICAL) VIRAL DISEASE

1) ACUTE COURSE. SELF LIMITING

2) TROPISM DETERMINES LOCALIZATION OF DEFINITIVE INFECTION

3) SYNCHRONY AND REPETITION OF STAGES

4) MANY CONFER LONGSTANDING IMMUNITY
   (resistant)

5) REFRACTORY TO TREATMENT

6) INCLUSION BODIES *infect either cytoplasm or nucleus or both*

7) SPECIFICITY OF SYNDROME

false — ans. all involve lymphocytosis

composed of viral material & debris from desintegration host

inclusion disease, congenital rubella syndrome), but, by far, the acute forms are more common and familiar.

2. Tropism

Viruses exhibit a genetically determined specificity for a particular cell type within the host. This specificity is referred to as the *tropism* of the virus. Thus, viruses, depending upon their cellular preference, can be thought of as dermotropic, neurotropic, hepatotropic, pneumotropic, or other. This tropism is not absolute, but represents the preferred site of localization of the virus within the host. It will determine where the definitive and most serious infection occurs.

3. Synchrony and Repetition

It is typical of cytopathic, systemic viral infections that the course of the disease is predictably repetitive and synchronous in all infected hosts. Two patients exposed to smallpox virus will pass through the successive stages of the disease at approximately the same time. A third patient infected by one of these will repeat the stages.

4. Many Confer Longstanding Immunity

Also characteristic of some viral infections of the type that result in systemic illness is longstanding immunity to second infection. Those of us who experienced measles in childhood, for example, will, in most cases, be free of any second attack. This immunity is thought to result from the widespread exposure of the virus to the lymphoreticular system during viremia or, in certain cases, to the retention of a small amount of virus in the body.

5. Difficulty in Treatment

Viral infections tend to be unaffected by all but the most sophisticated and specific therapeutic strategy. Recovery from viral infection is almost totally dependent on an adequate and appropriate response by the host. This response is, in some way, based on the cellular immunologic system and on the synthesis of interferon. Patients with cellular immunologic deficiency

have far more difficulty containing and terminating viral infection than those with normal cellular immune system. This is vividly demonstrated in the response of the patient with cellular immunologic deficiency to the normally innocuous procedure of vaccination. Instead of developing a small localized lesion, he may succumb to a disease produced by generalized dissemination of the vaccinia virus.

6. Inclusion Bodies

Infecting viruses occupy either the cytoplasm or the nucleus of the host cell (in some cases, both). The infected cell, when stained and examined under the microscope, exhibits deposits of an abnormal material known as *inclusion bodies*. Inclusion bodies are thought to be composed of viral material and debris from the disintegrating host cell; in many cases, the location and appearance of the inclusion body is diagnostic of the infecting virus. The so-called negri body of rabies is the usually cited example of a very pathognomonic inclusion body.

7. Specificity of Disease Syndromes

Although the cytolytic infection is common to most acute viral diseases, differences in the details of the relationships between virus and host result in the production of a specific clinical syndrome for each disease that is usually clearly recognizable. It would be far beyond the scope of this discussion to describe each important human viral disease in detail. Rather than this, a selected group of human viral diseases is presented in tabular form in Illustration 7-14. The student is advised to commit these diseases to memory and be prepared to recognize them as being of viral etiology. He should also memorize as much of the accessory information as he feels will be useful in his professional career.

N.O.T.

7-14. EXAMPLES OF HUMAN DISEASES CAUSED BY TRUE VIRUS

Major Virus Group*[1]	Approx. size	Core	Disease or Specific Infection	Common Terminology
Poxvirus	mμ 200 to 350	DNA	Variola	Smallpox
			Vaccinia	Vaccination
Myoxvirus[2]	80 to 300	RNA	Influenza	Flu
			Rubeola	Measles
			Epidemic parotitis	Mumps
			Rubella	German measles
Rhabdovirus	225[3]	RNA	Rabies	Hydrophobia
Herpesvirus	100	DNA	Herpes simplex	Coldsore
				Chickenpox
			Varicella-zoster	Shingles
			CID[4]	
			Epstein-Barr[5]	Infectious mononucleosis
Papovavirus	40 to 50	DNA	Verruca vulgaris	Wart
Au(1) or HAA[6]	18 to 20	?	Serum hepatitis	Transfusion hepatitis
			Infectious hepatitis	
Arbovirus	15 to 20	RNA	Yellow fever	Yellow fever
			Equine encephalitis	
Picornavirus	18 to 30	RNA	Polio	Infantile paralysis
			Echovirus	Aseptic meningitis
			Coxsackievirus	Herpangina
			Rhinovirus[7]	Common cold

caused by herpes virus

* This is not a complete list of major virus groups; only those with prominent human pathogens are included.

[1] The classification of virus is still in flux. Major groups are here distinguished by commonly accepted or recently proposed terminology and arranged in rough order of decreasing size and chemical complexity.

[2] The term, myxovirus, as used here includes the closely related paramyxoviruses and the rubella virus. The latter has been shown recently to be actually unrelated to myxovirus; however, it is included here since no new major group has been established to accomodate it.

[3] The rhabdovirus is actually bullet-shaped with dimensions of 60 by 225 mμ.

[4] Cytomegalic Inclusion Disease.

[5] Epstein-Barr virus has been found in association with the benign, self-limiting disease, infectious mononucleosis and the malignant Burkitt's lymphoma. It is thought causative of the former but its association with the latter is still undefined.

[6] This virus or, more accurately, virus antigen is generally known as Australia antigen or hepatitis-associated antigen. It is more clearly associated with serum hepatitis than infectious hepatitis.

[7] Rhinovirus is a common but not exclusive cause of the common cold. Other virus such as influenza, parainfluenza, adenovirus and coronavirus can give rise to similar disease.

ATYPICAL VIRAL DISEASE

LEARNING OBJECTIVE

To be able to describe each of the following types of a typical viral disease in some detail:

    a) inapparent
    b) chronic
    c) latent
    d) slow
    e) oncogenic

A number of viral infections produce disease syndromes which differ radically from that described above. We will assemble these under the single heading of *atypical viral disease*. In this category we will consider those kinds of viral diseases listed in Illustration 7-15.

N.V.T.

1. Inapparent Viral Disease

Not all viral infections lead to overt, clinically apparent disease; in fact there is reason to believe that we actually experience a far greater number of infections than we recognize. Some of these are not even cytopathic and will be discussed below, others are caused by weakly cytopathic viruses and progress to mild systemic disease that is so lacking in signs and symptoms that it remains occult. This phenomenon has come to light through experience with vaccines employing live, attenuated virus which causes the recipient to experience a complete disease even though he never becomes aware of it.

Viruses producing inapparent disease are said to be *avirulent*. An apparent disease produced by an avirulent strain of virus frequently results in lifelong immunity against a closely related virulent (wild) counterpart. This is the principle underlying the use of live, attenuated viral vaccine.

Not

2. Chronic Viral Disease

There are at least 2 principal components of acute viral disease that give rise to the clinical picture of illness, the cytocidal effect of the virus and the necrotizing effect of the host's cellular immune response. Some viral infections are not particularly cytocidal and the virus, left

---

7-15. ATYPICAL VIRAL DISEASE

1) INAPPARENT

    subclinical disease: seen in infections with "wild" virus such as CID or vaccine virus such as measles

2) CHRONIC

    example is chronic rubella syndrome

3) LATENT

    example is herpes labialis

4) SLOW   *multiple sclerosis*

    conventional agents, unconventional agents   *causes death*

5) ONCOGENIC

    best studied human virus with *suspected* oncogenic effect is E-B virus

---

to its own devices, would loiter in the host cells, causing an indolent disease and substandard cellular functions. There is reason to believe that this kind of infection is counteracted by immunologic destruction of infected cells.

Rubella is such a weakly cytopathic virus. In the usual adult case of German measles the virus is probably finally eliminated from the body by immunologic destruction of cells harboring it (in combination with interferon synthesis to prevent spread to neighboring cells). The results are a mild acute disease, complete recovery and strong immunity against recurrence. In maternal rubella, where the virus manages to infect the fetus, however, the story is completely different. Very early fetal infection may result in miscarriage or stillbirth, whereas late infection causes birth defects and the *congenital rubella syndrome*. In the former situation, the fetus, being immunologically incompetent is simply overwhelmed; in the latter, it develops what appears to be a degree of immunologic tolerance for the virus which then persists in its tissues causing poor development *in utero* or a lingering, chronic infection in infancy.

A similar picture of chronic viral disease is seen in the case of *cytomegalic inclusion disease*. Mild or inapparent maternal infection gives rise to tolerance on the part of the developing child and a lingering infection in infancy and childhood. Although these 2 viruses are the most seriously offensive in this regard, others have also been mentioned as being able to cause birth defects and chronic neonatal infections.

3. Latent Viral Disease

Latent viral disease is the syndrome in which the virus lives for a period of many years within the hosts' body, bursting forth on occasion to give rise to clinically overt disease. Latent viral disease is based on the *temperate infection*. In this kind of infection, the virus enters the cell but, rather than causing the usual cytopathic effect, assumes a kind of static relationship. In this state, the virus does not cause active disease because it does not injure its host. Also, it is apparently not detectable by tissue surveillance mechanisms; hence the infected cells are not immunologically rejected.

Given certain kinds of provocation the infection is activated and a full-blown necrotizing (but usually localized) disease breaks out.

Latent viral disease is usually preceded by a single episode of acute infection that occurs when the virus first comes in contact with the host. This so-called *primary infection* may be obvious or inapparent.

In man, the most common example of latent viral disease is the familiar "cold sore" or "fever blister" caused by latent infection with the herpes simplex. Primary herpetic infection usually occurs in childhood as an acute, febrile disease with the exanthem of gingivostomatitis. It is often confused with some other illness or resolves and is quickly forgotten. Thereafter, a person may experience the periodic appearance of clusters of small vesicular eruptions occurring around the mouth. This is triggered by a variety of stimuli ranging from menstruation to the common cold (hence the term cold sore).

Another, rather common, latent human viral disease is *herpes zoster* infection in which the acute episode gives rise to the familiar varicella (chickenpox) while the recurrent secondary disease is seen as a painful, localized eruption, *shingles*.

4. Slow Viral Disease

A type of atypical viral disease that may some day prove extremely important is the so-called "slow" viral disease. In the slow viral infection, the agent enters the cell, but propagates so lethargically and caused such delayed destruction that the association between exposure and the eventually ensuing disease may become obscure. In effect, a slow viral disease is one that manifests an enormously long incubation period (up to 3 years or more), and then a protracted course that almost invariably culminates in death. Agents causing slow viral disease seem to be of 2 fundamentally different types, *conventional viruses* and *unconventional viruses*. The former are thought to cause a number of rare demyelinating diseases of the central nervous system, perhaps including multiple sclerosis, whereas the latter are responsible for 4 quite distinct and unusual diseases of man and lower animals. We will take this occasion to look more closely at the latter.

The diseases known to be caused by *unconventional* slow viruses are kuru and Creutzfeld-Jakob (C-J) disease in the human and scrapie and transmissable mink encephalopathy (TME) in lower animals. Morphologic and clinical signs of these 4 conditions are very similar and the physical and biologic properties of their causative agents appear to be identical. These agents are described as "unconventional," because they fail to exhibit many of the criteria established for the true virus. Recent research suggests that they are comparable to the "viroid," self-replicating, infectious RNA molecules that produce certain plant diseases. They have no protein coat and are of unusually low molecular weight. To date, they have resisted all attempts at isolation and characterization; they have never been observed with electron microscopy, nor has any evidence of their antigenicity been demonstrated. Some investigators have even proposed that these agents are actually replicating protein molecules or membrane fragments.

Perhaps the most interesting of the 4 is the disease, kuru. This disease has been found only

slow human viral disease

in the Fore people and their neighbors in New Guinea, where its incidence is reported as extremely high. According to recently acquired data, 2,500 people (of a total population of only 35,000) have died from this disease since it was first studied in 1957. Its alarming prevalence is thought to be due to a practice of ritual cannibalism through which the Fore honored their dead. With the cessation of this practice, the incidence of kuru has declined dramatically.

Both kuru and C-J disease can be transmitted to subhuman primates. The effect on brain tissue strongly resembles that seen in common degenerative diseases of the central nervous system such as amyotrophic lateral sclerosis, Parkinson's disease, Pick's disease, Alzheimer's disease and others. Although none of these diseases has been proven infectious, their resemblance to kuru suggests that slow viral infection may be more widely distributed in animal populations than previously thought. As a result, practically all degenerative diseases of unknown etiology (but especially those involving the central nervous system), are now at least suspected of being caused by slow infection with unconventional viral agents.

Not.

5. Viral Oncogenesis

Viral oncogenesis is the final variety of atypical viral disease that we will be considering. It is based on the *proliferative* viral infection in which the virus enters the cell but, rather than destroying it, stimulates its uncontrolled proliferation. There is no observable cytopathic effect and because waves of newly-synthesized virions are not released the infection tends to remain localized. This last quality is not absolute, however, and systemic virus has been detected in oncogenic infections.

If purpose can be attributed to a virus, it is reasonable that the "intention" of viral infection is to produce billions of new, complete virions. This is the usual and, in every respect, natural object of viral disease. Should the virus fail to induce the host cell to produce protein coat as well as nucleic acid, the virus is said to be defective. Lacking a protein coat, virus would not be released or, even if it was, could not manage to infect another cell. The defective virus must remain within the host cell and settle

---

7-16. VIRAL ONCOGENESIS

1) TUMOR VIRUSES OF LOWER ANIMALS ARE WELL DEFINED

2) ASSOCIATION BETWEEN VIRUS AND HUMAN TUMORS SUSPECTED IN (examples):
    Burkitt's lymphoma (E.B. virus), lymphocytic leukemia, osteogenic sarcoma, carcinoma of the cervix

3) ISOLATION OF VIRUS IS FIRST STEP TOWARD PREPARING VACCINE

---

for an aborted cycle of reproduction. Some authors believe that it is these defective viruses that produce neoplasia and that oncogenesis is a kind of corrupt cytopathic infection. Others feel that it is a well-developed viral adaptation.

We have seen that viruses are separable into two chemical categories, those that contain RNA as genetic material and those that contain DNA. Both of these can cause tumors, but one curious and important difference has been noticed; DNA viruses cannot be recovered from the tumors they produce whereas RNA viruses can. Existing evidence points to the fact that, although DNA viruses are not recoverable from tumors, they nonetheless persist within the cells of the tumor. They have apparently entered into the nuclear material of the infected cell and are acting as a kind of newly acquired gene. The cell is said to be transformed by the infecting virus; its normally latent faculty for replication has been activated and the cell reproduces out of control.

Acting in a somewhat similar way, RNA viruses apparently assume the role of messenger RNA within the infected cell. It is possible that they cause the synthesis of an agent that redepresses the normal but latent cell replication system resulting again in uncontrolled proliferation. It is also possible that RNA viruses function through some kind of reverse transcription mechanism.

Animal Tumor Viruses

in lower animals

The clearest examples of viral oncogenesis are seen in tumors of lower animals. Pure examples of tumor-producing viruses have been isolated and will repeatedly cause tumors when inoculated into susceptible hosts. These viruses will transform a cell either *in vivo* or *in vitro* and a great deal of insight has been gained from such laboratory experiments.

Human Tumor Viruses

With a seemingly unequivocal association established between viruses and tumors of experimental animals it would be reasonable that human tumors might now be confidently attributed to viral oncogenesis; this has certainly not been the case. Although a great deal of provocative evidence has been put forth, it remains that the only clearly demonstrated example of a tumor caused by virus in man is the common wart. At this writing an extensive long-term program is going forward at the National Institutes of Health intended to demonstrate the role of the virus in the etiology of such important human neoplasms as leukemia. The purpose of this program is far more than the gathering of information. It is well known that most viral leukemias in mice are preventable by vaccine. Assuming that some forms of human leukemia are caused by a virus and vaccine-preventable we will have conquered one of our most tragic diseases.

Burkitt's Lymphoma

No discussions of human tumor viruses would be complete without some mention of Burkitt's lymphoma. In fact, it is the peculiar epidemiology of this disease combined with the observance of virus-like particles in electron micrographs of human leukemic cells that warrants the determined expenditure of time and effort to uncover a human leukemia virus. In 1958, Dennis Burkitt, a British physician in Africa, reported the occurrence of a lymphoma in children that seemed to be concentrated in a relatively restricted area of high humidity and low altitude. The distribution of this neoplasm coincided with that of mosquito density and

---

7-17. EPSTEIN-BARR VIRUS

1) HERPES-LIKE VIRUS PRESENT IN CELLS OF BURKITT's LYMPHOMA
   also present in 50 per cent of healthy children in area of lymphoma endemic

2) PRESENT IN SERUM OF SMALL PERCENTAGE OF HEALTY AMERICAN CHILDREN

3) PRESENT IN SERUM OF ALL HETEROPHILE-POSITIVE CASES OF INFECTIOUS MONONUCLEOSIS

---

suggested that an insect vector might be in some way associated with its occurrence. Adding to this conviction, Epstein and his collaborators succeeded in finding virus-like particles in Burkitt tumor cells. This virus resembled herpesvirus morphologically, but was found to be antigenically distinct. It has been called the Epstein-Barr (EB) virus, a term that is becoming generally accepted. They found that the serum of all Burkitt's tumor patients contained this virus but, confusingly, so did the serum of about 50 per cent of all healthy African children. In fact, when the serum of American children was examined, it was found that many of these also contained this same antigen. Then, quite by accident, it was discovered that the identical virus antigen was present in the serum of all heterophile-positive patients suffering from *infectious mononucleosis*. It now appears that this 1 virus may be causing a lymphocytic neoplasm, a cytopathic infection and a symptomless latency in different classes of individuals. The implications are astounding but not inconsistent with inexperience in viral tumors of laboratory animals.

E. B. virus
Ans.
Lymphoma

Additional Reading

Cooper, L. Z. Rubella: A preventable cause of birth defects. Birth Defects: Original Article Series IV:23, 1968

Chitwood, L. A. Herpesvirus infections. Postgrad. Med. 48:213, 1970

Henle, G. and Henle, W. EB virus in the etiology of infectious mononucleosis. Hospital Pract. July, 1970

Katz, S. and Griffith, J. F. Slow virus infections. Hospital Pract., Mar., 1971

Kinard, R. Cancer viruses in primates. Science 169:828, 1970

Paraf, A. Relationship between immune reactions to viruses. Ann. N.Y. Acad. Sci. 181:223, 1971

Weller, T. H. Cytomegaloviruses: Ubiquitous agents with protean clinical manifestations. N. Engl. J. Med. 285:203, 267 (two parts), 1971

Which of following couldn't stop spread of viral infection
A. intercellular SOMETHING

DEFENSE AGAINST VIRAL INFECTION

LEARNING OBJECTIVE

To be able to discuss human defense against viral infection, mentioning each mechanism within the following 4 general categories:

    a) **extracellular defenses (the deciduous body surface, secretory immunoglobulin, surface reactivity, circulating immunoglobulin, cellular immunity)**

    b) **intracellular defense (genetically determined resistance and interferon)**

    c) **prophylaxis (passive immunity, active immunity, pretreatment with interferon)**

    d) **viral chemotherapy**

    e) **effects of viral infection on host defenses**

The obvious fact that we are not all critically threatened by viral disease all of the time suggests that the normal body possesses effective means of defense against viral pathogens. These defenses are roughly separable into the 2 categories listed in Illustration 7-18. We will look briefly at elements of each of these categories of defenses in turn.

1. Extracellular Defenses

The most effective defenses against viral infections will be those that prevent the virus from reaching or penetrating a susceptible cell. These include the following:

7-18. DEFENSE AGAINST VIRAL INFECTION

1) **EXTRACELLULAR DEFENSES**
    deciduous body surfaces
    secretory immunoglobulin
    surface reactivity
    circulating immunoglobulin
    cellular immunity

2) **INTRACELLULAR DEFENSES**
    genetically determined resistance
    interferon

The Deciduous Body Surface

Sloughing of the cornified layer of skin, shedding of superficial cells of mucus membranes and gastrointestinal epithelium, the flow of mucous toward the mouth in the respiratory system and urine toward the exterior in the urinary tract and the constant lavage of the surface of the eye with tears sets up a complete mechanical barrier that normally prevents a virus or other pathogens from remaining in contact with a surface long enough to penetrate.

Secretory Immunoglobulins

In those individuals where prior experience with a virus has resulted in local immunity, specific antibodies of the IgA class will be secreted onto mucous membranes and other normally moist surfaces. Since surfaces such as these are most often used as the portal of entry for a virus, secretary IgA provides effective protection against the communication of viral disease. In fact, it has been shown that resistance to influenza A virus, a pathogen that remains localized in the respiratory tract, is mediated primarily by antibodies present in local secretions, whereas antibody serum is relatively ineffective.

Surface Reactivity

There is no doubt that the catarrhal reaction of a nasopharynx and respiratory tract is

[handwritten margin note top: infected cell synthesizes protein (interferon) → message to unaffected cell]

instrumental in washing away noxious material. It may also serve to prevent or minimize viral pentrations once an irritation is set up.

Circulating Immunoglobulins

The effect of passive immunization against viral disease suggests that circulating immuno-globulins play some role in preventing or at least attenuating acute, systemic viral disease. Its principal effect may be in the neutralization of viremia. In this way, the process of the disease is interrupted at an incipient stage, usually before that of systemic illness.

Cellular Immunity

The role of cellular immunity in protection against viral disease may be principally one of destroying infected cells. We have already seen that viruses may cause the appearance of a new antigen at the surface of the host cell. Since the cellular immune system is responsible for tissue surveillance, it is reasonable that cells altered in this way would be detected and destroyed.

2. Intracellular Defense against Viral Infection

Once a virus has reached a susceptible cell it must attach to its surface, be ingested by endocytosis, break out of the vacuole, shed its protein coat and take over the cell's synthetic machinery. These are the necessary steps preliminary to successful viral infection. The key strategy of cellular defense viral infection is interruption of this sequence; 2 factors seem most imporant:

Genetically Determined Resistance

It is well known that viruses are extremely fastidious regarding species and cell types. For example, certain viruses that readily invade guinea pig cells in vitro will fail to penetrate human cells under these same conditions. The absolute resistance provided by genetic constitution is not understood, but may someday provide us with a means of preventing virus infections.

Interferon

The second principle cellular defense against viral attack is interferon. The story behind the discovery and development of interferon is somewhat complex, but, in view of its potential importance in controlling viral infection, it warrants our attention. It has been recognized for some time that infection with 1 virus may exclude infection with another, even if the second is unrelated to the first. This is known as the phenomenon of *viral interference.* Some time later it was found that interference was mediated by a protein of low molecular weight, subsequently termed "interferon." Interferon is now known to be not 1 but a number of proteins that are synthesized by cells as a means of protection against the spread of viral infection. Interferon, itself, has no direct antiviral activity; cell protection is achieved by its preventing the translation of viral (but not cellular) RNA. This is accomplished as diagrammed in Illustration 7-19.

The synthesis of interferon, curiously, is provoked by many different kinds of agents, most of which are not even related to viral infection. Endotoxin, for example, ellicits cellular production of this material. Presumably most kinds of cells are able to synthesize interferon when properly stimulated. Pretreatment with interferon is needed to protect cells against viral infection and recovery from an established infection seems to be based, in no small part, on the quickness with which an organism can begin synthesizing interferon to head off the spread of virus from cell to cell. Interferon exhibits a rather strict species specificity and, except for isolated examples, material produced in 1 animal is usually ineffective in another.

3. Prophylaxis of Viral Infection

Three means of achieving prophylactic protection against viral infection are listed in Illustration 7-20. The first 2 are employed routinely, but the last is still in early stages of development.

Passive Immunization

While useful in the immediate treatment of patients exposed to a virulent virus, passive immunization confers only temporary immunity at best. Except for certain special applications, it is not considered adequately reliable nor its protection adequately durable.

[handwritten margin note: VACCINE]

[handwritten note at bottom: What stops spread of viral infection. Interferon & cellular immunolog. responses — BOTH]

7-19. INTERFERON

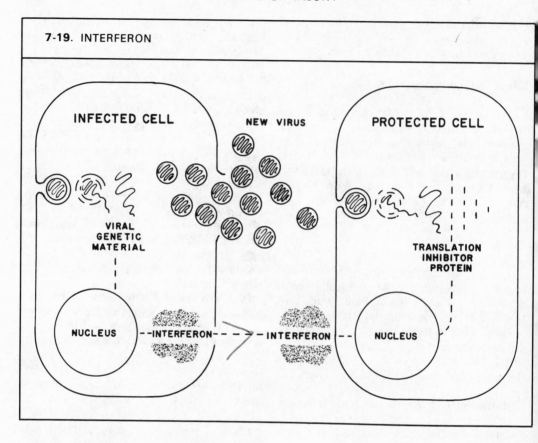

INFECTED CELL   NEW VIRUS   PROTECTED CELL

VIRAL GENETIC MATERIAL

TRANSLATION INHIBITOR PROTEIN

NUCLEUS   --INTERFERON-- --> --INTERFERON-- --   NUCLEUS

7-20. PROPHYLAXIS OF VIRAL INFECTION

1) PASSIVE IMMUNIZATION
   transfer of hyperimmune serum temporary and comparatively unreliable

2) ACTIVE IMMUNIZATION
   patient's own immune response is elicited to an innocuous form of the viral pathogen
   Killed—virulent
   live—attenuated

3) PRETREATMENT WITH INTERFERON
   experimental, not generally used interferon exhibits species specificity

"wild" form virus

Salk Vaccine

Sabin Vaccine used c live attenuated

Cell interference

Active Immunization

By far the most effective and generally used means of prophylaxis against viral infection is active immunization. A complete discussion of vaccines is beyond the scope of this subject and the student wishing to learn more about this important topic would do well to read one of the recent reviews.

4. Effect of Viral Infection on Immunologic Defenses

Perhaps because of their cycle of propagation within macrophages of the lymphoreticular system, an infecting virus will frequently depress the immunologic defenses of its host. This is usually a temporary effect, confined to the time around the acute illness. When viral infection is protracted, such as in the congenital rubella syndrome, immunologic deficiency may be quite pronounced. Infection *in utero* apparently prevents normal development of tissues mediating the immune responses and impairs the function of those which have completed development.

Additional Reading

Borden, E. C. and Carter, W. A. Viral chemotherapy: Its promises and problems. Medicine 51:189, 1972
Notkins, A. L. et al. Effect of virus infections on the function of the immune system. Ann. Rev. Microbiol. 24:525, 1970
Stokes, J., Jr. Recent advances in immunization against viral diseases. Ann. Int. Med. 73:829, 1970

CHLAMYDIAL (BEDSONIAL) DISEASE

LEARNING OBJECTIVE

To be able to list characteristics of the chlamydia and briefly describe the following chlamydial diseases:

    a) psittacosis
    b) lymphogranuloma venereum
    c) trachoma and inclusion conjunctivitis
    d) cat-scratch disease

Somewhat larger and more complex than the virus is the type of organism known as the chlamydia or Bedsonia. Because of their similarity to the virus, they were once thought to be a larger and more complex viral organism and were called "mantle" viruses in reference to their prominent sheath of protein. They are now known to be equipped with some faculties for independent (but still intracellular) metabolism, a feature that disqualifies them as a true virus.

1. Characteristics of the Chlamydia

Due in significant part to the pioneer work of Bedson with psittacosis, chlamydia have been shown to be far more complex than the virus; some authors have proposed calling them Bedsonia in recognition of his contribution. Like the virus the chlamydia is an obligate intracellular parasite. Their other distinguishing properties have been summarized as follows:

1. They are spherical, gram-negative, intracytoplasmic, bacteria-like organisms measuring 200 to 1,000 millimicrons.
2. They contain DNA and RNA.
3. They have a unique cycle of development *NOT* and, at one stage, divide by binary fission.
4. All share a common antigen.
5. They contain enzyme systems that allow the generation of useful energy.
6. They are sensitive to tetracyclines and, in some cases, to penicillin or sulfa drugs.

Chlamydiae are sometimes designated as the PLT group of organisms after the most prominent of the human diseases they cause (psittacosis, lymphogranuloma, trachoma). By far the most important of these is trachoma; it is the most common cause of progressive blindness in the world, being particularly prevalent in developing countries where poor personal and family hygiene are practiced.

Human chlamydial diseases are presented in tabular form in Illustration 7-21. The student should commit these to memory and be prepared to recognize them as diseases caused by this group of organisms. We will discuss psittacosis as an example.

not Typhus

7-21. CHLAMYDIAL (BEDSONIAL) DISEASES
1) PSITTACOSIS (ORNITHOSIS)
2) LYMPHOGRANULOMA VENEREUM
3) TRACHOMA
4) INCLUSION CONJUNCTIVITIS
5) CAT SCRATCH DISEASE (organism not isolated)

7-22. CHLAMYDIAL (BEDSONIAL) DIS-EASE

EXAMPLE
(PSITTACOSIS OR ORNITHOSIS)

1) ACQUIRED BY INHALATION OF CHLA-MYDIA IN DESSICATED URINE AND FECES FROM INFECTED BIRDS
    parrot
    pigeon
    sea gull

2) ATYPICAL PNEUMONIA WITH FEB-RILE ILLNESS
    intense headache
    leukopenia
    splenomegaly

3) CLINICAL COURSE MAY BE MILD OR SEVERE DEPENDING UPON AGE AND DEFENSE STATUS OF HOST: MAY BE FATAL IN AGED OR DEBILITATED PATIENTS

2. Psittacosis

Psittacosis is a disease of birds transmissable to man (Illustration 7-22). It is acquired by the inhalation of chlamydia in the dessicated urine and feces from a number of birds including the parrot, pigeon and seagull. Since the human usually has more opportunity to contract this disease from the parrot or parakeet it was once commonly known as "parrot fever," from which the term psittacosis is derived. The demonstration of its occurrence in other birds has suggested the newer term, ornithosis. The agent enters through the respiratory tract, penetrates the respiratory surface and becomes blood-borne. Shortly thereafter, the patient manifests atypical pneumonia accompanied by fever, intense headache, leukopenia and spleno-megaly. The clinical course of the disease depends, to a large extent, upon the defense status of the host and ranges from a mild illness to a rapidly fatal affliction. The mortality rate increases sharply among elderly patients where it may be as high as 20 per cent in untreated cases. Carrier states have been described in both the human and the bird.

Additional Reading

Johnson, W. T. & Helwig, E. B. Cat-scratch disease. Arch. Dermatol. 100:148, 1969
Werner, G. H. et al: Trachoma. Sci. Amer. Jan., 1964

RICKETTSIAL DISEASE

LEARNING OBJECTIVE

To be able to list the characteristics of the rickettsiae and briefly describe the following diseases:
    a) typhus
    b) Rocky Mountain spotted fever

Rickettsiae are a separate group of orga-nisms, at one time considered closely related to the virus, but now recognized as more akin to true bacteria. Unlike chlamydiae, they do not share a common antigen and reproduce only by binary fission. Most rickettsiae are obligate intracellular parasites, although one species has been cultivated in the absence of cells. As a group, their most unique feature is that they are spread by lice, fleas, ticks and mites, in which they multiply, usually without producing disease. When transmitted to an unnatural host such as man they cause a widespread, damaging infection accompanied by severe illness.

Many rickettsial diseases are primarily animal infections (zoonoses) with man being involved accidentally as the result of being bitten by the vector. Even epidemic typhus, a rickettsial disease of great historic significance, has been found as an infection of animals.

1. General Characteristics of Rickettsial Diseases

Human diseases caused by rickettsiae are presented in tabular form in Illustration 7-23.

7-23. RICKETTSIAL DISEASES

1) TYPHUS GROUP
   epidemic typhus
   endemic (murine) typhus

2) SPOTTED FEVER GROUP
   Rocky Mountain spotted fever
   Brazilian spotted fever
   fievre boutonneuse
   South African tick bite fever
   rickettsialpox

3) TSUTSUGAMUSHI GROUP
   scrub typhus
   others

4) Q FEVER

5) BARTONELLIOSIS
   (disease caused by a rickettsia-
   like organism)

7-24. RICKETTSIAL DISEASE (GENERAL CHARACTERISTICS)

1) ALL ARE ZOONOSES

2) ALL HAVE LICE, TICKS OR MITES AS VECTOR

3) ORGANISMS INOCULATED BY INSECT BITE AND DISSEMINATED WIDELY IN BLOOD
   invade capillary endothelial cells
   cells swell and proliferate
   thrombus develops
   neutrophil exudate forms causing focal necrosis

4) DISEASE IS FEBRILE WITH PROMINENT SKIN RASH
   comparatively high case fatality rates in some rickettsial diseases

---

The student should study these and be prepared to recognize common examples as diseases caused by this group of organisms.

Most rickettsial diseases exhibit similar general characteristics (Illustration 7-24). They are relatively uncommon, usually febrile and result in a rash. The rash, similar in all such diseases, is due to the localization of rickettsiae in the endothelium of very small blood vessels, particularly capillaries. Once they have invaded endothelial cells they produce a focus of cellular proliferation and acute inflammatory exudate that culminates in thrombosis and microhemorrhage. Some rickettsial diseases exhibit an alarmingly high mortality rate if untreated.

2. Typhus

Typhus is a typical rickettsial disease, severe, febrile and accompanied by a distinctive rash. It is seen in 2 forms, *endemic* or murine and *epidemic* or human. The latter is the most important in terms of its potential for epidemic

---

7-25. RICKETTSIAL DISEASE

(TYPHUS)

1) EPIDEMIC FORM IS MOST IMPORTANT (NUMERICALLY) OF THE RICKETTSIAL DISEASES
   historically significant
   still seen in groups where personal hygiene is neglected

2) CARRIED FROM MAN TO MAN BY INFECTED BODY LOUSE *& nothing else!*

3) 20 to 70 per cent MORTALITY IN EPIDEMIC FORMS

7-26. RICKETTSIAL DISEASE

EXAMPLE
(ROCKY MOUNTAIN SPOTTED FEVER)

1) ENDEMIC IN NORTH AND SOUTH AMERICA BUT CASES HAVE OCCURRED ELSEWHERE

2) SPREAD BY BITE OF INFECTED WOOD TICK

3) CLINICAL PICTURE SIMILAR TO TYPHUS EXCEPT THAT RASH IS MORE PROMINENT

4) RELATIVELY HIGH CASE FATALITY RATE (Average 20 per cent)

Although now under control in most technologically advanced nations, the typhus epidemic is always a hazard during war or other mass disaster. The disease is characterized by fever of sudden onset, accompanied by severe headache and a rash with appears between the fourth and eighth day of illness. Microscopic lesions occur throughout the body, but are most numerous in the skin, brain and spinal cord. Death may be caused by encephalitis, myocarditis or secondary bacterial pneumonia. Mortality has been reported to be 20-70 per cent in untreated cases of the epidemic form of typhus.

3. Rocky Mountain Spotted Fever

Rocky Mountain spotted fever is a febrile disease resembling typhus which is transmitted to man by the bite of the infected wood tick. It differs from typhus in that the rash appears earlier and tends to be more hemorrhagic-appearing. Like typhus, the fatality rate tends to run very high in untreated cases, the reported average being somewhere around 20 per cent (Illustration 7-26).

Additional Reading

Hazard, G. W. et al. Rocky Mountain spotted fever in the eastern United States. N. Engl. J. Med. 280:57, 1969
Rothschild, M. Fleas. Sci. Amer. 213:44, 1965

spread and fatal outcome. It is carried from man to man by the infected body louse, hence it tends to occur among groups of people in whom personal hygiene is neglected. An ideal substrate for the epidemic form of this disease is groups of refugees or armies forced to remain in the field for long periods of time. Typhus was said to have contributed significantly to the defeat of Napoleon.

Last ques. ans. E - all of above

#24 - not E

chapter 8

[handwritten: ques. #1 ans. E]

INFECTION WITH BACTERIA AND HIGHER ORGANISMS

[handwritten top right: Don't INVADE (Poison) / INVADE Sup. / INVADE DEEP / INVADE]

BACTERIA AS PATHOGENS

LEARNING OBJECTIVE

To be able to discuss the (convenient but imperfect) spectrum-like classification of diseases caused by bacteria, listing the examples that will be used in order of their position in this spectrum and mentioning how these diseases both conform to and deviate from this scheme

Of the many thousands of strains of bacteria and higher organisms only a very few are capable of causing human disease. Since these are members of several taxonomic groups, it is more convenient to arrange the material to be covered in this subject according to distinguishing characteristics of the infection rather than those of the causative organisms. Although this is not a system that would be useful to the bacteriologist, it does allow us to impose a kind of order on such a brief review of this complex subject. We will also take the liberty of selecting certain diseases as representative of specific pathogenetic mechanisms. The selection of a disease will be dictated by current significance, historic importance or because it represents the best example of a particular mechanism. Since most of this subject will be concerned with bacterial disease, we will confine our opening remarks to this kind of pathogen.

Disease caused by bacteria can be roughly classified according to the invasive behavior of the causative organism. Pathogenic bacteria that do *not* invade tend to produce a potent exotoxin, whereas at the other extreme are those that invade deeply and often produce endotoxin. This results in a spectrum-like distribution of diseases, ranging from exotoxin poisoning to widespread bacterial dissemination. Between the extremes of exotoxin producers and invaders we find a range in which

---

8-1. SPECTRUM-LIKE ARRANGEMENT OF EXEMPLARY BACTERIAL DISEASES

EXOTOXIN DISEASE

RANGE OF INTERMEDIACY *[handwritten: KNOW]*

- bacterial food poisoning
- cholera *[handwritten: agent doesn't invade; exotoxin in GI tract.]*
- tetanus *[handwritten: — must contaminate a wound]*
- diphtheria *[handwritten: — invades, superficial, doesn't need wound]*
- typhoid fever *[handwritten: — GI tract + spread SOMETIMES DEEP]*
- pyogenic coccal infections *[handwritten: DEEP INVADERS]*
- plague and tularemia *[handwritten: ENDOTOXIN]*
- syphilis* *[handwritten: ✳]*

DISEASE PRODUCED BY BACTERIAL INVASION

[handwritten: Bacterial invasion]

* In syphilis the causative organism becomes widely disseminated throughout the body. It is one of the best examples of the generalized infection and will be covered in detail in Subject 17.

---

bacteria demonstrate both, but tend to emphasize one or the other. As representatives of pathogens throughout this entire range we will consider the diseases listed in Illustration 8-1.

Additional Reading

Armelogor, G. J. Evolving response to human infectious disease. Bio. Science 20:271, 1970

Herrell, W. E. History of the development of antibiotics. Clin. Med. 77:10, 1970

Mudd, S. (ed.) Infectious Agents and Host Reactions. W. B. Saunders Co., Philadelphia, 1970

Neter, E. The immune response of the host: An aid to etiology, pathogenesis, diagnosis and epidemiology of bacterial infections. Yale J. Biol. Med. 44:241, 1971

EXOTOXIN PRODUCERS THAT DO NOT INVADE

LEARNING OBJECTIVE

To be able to outline the causative agent and pathogenetic mechanism responsible for each of the following kinds of diseases.

    a) food poisoning:
        staphylococcal food poisoning
        Clostridium perfringens food
          poisoning
        botulism
    b) non-invasive enteric pathogens:
        cholera

Our first group of bacterial pathogens are those devoid of the ability to invade the human body. These organisms produce disease by growing in human food or the gastrointestinal tract and producing exotoxin. As representative of this group of pathogens, we will consider the 2 categories of agents listed in Illustration 8-2.

1. Bacterial Food Poisoning

Bacterial food poisoning is a disease that results from the ingestion of food contaminated with exotoxin. These diseases are more accurately considered a form of poisoning rather than a type of infection.

Staphylococcal Food Poisoning

Staphylococcal food poisoning is a disease resulting from the ingestion of staphylococcal

---

8-2. EXOTOXIN PRODUCERS THAT DO NOT INVADE

1) BACTERIAL FOOD POISONING
    staphylococcal
    Clostridium perfringens
    botulism

2) NON-INVASIVE ENTERIC PATHOGENS
    cholera

---

enterotoxin. Conditions favoring such an incident are those in which warm food is contaminated with *Staphylococcus aureus* by a handler with an active superficial infection such as a pustule or furuncle. A common vehicle, for example, is potato salad prepared the night before and allowed to remain in the warm sun during a picnic. Under such conditions, staphylococci proliferate and an abundance of enterotoxin is produced. When such food is eaten severe enteric disturbance results. The syndrome of staphylococcal food poisoning typically includes nausea, severe cramping pains, diarrhea but not fever or other signs of acute infection.

Clostridium perfringens Food Poisoning

Clostridium perfringens food poisoning results from the ingestion of food containing large numbers of the cells of this organism. Although intact organisms must be eaten to produce the disease, no invasion of the gastrointestinal tract takes place. The incidence of food poisoning caused by *Clostridium perfringens* has increased alarmingly in the United States throughout the last decade. Outbreaks usually involve large numbers of individuals and are most commonly associated with beef or poultry dishes. The syndrome is less severe and of shorter duration than that produced by staphylococcal enterotoxin. Following an incubation period of 8 to 22 hours, there is the onset of cramping abdominal pain, diarrhea and prostration. Vomiting is rare (in contrast to staphylococcal food poisoning in which it is common) and no fever is present. Although staphylococcal food poisoning accounts for more outbreaks of such disease, the number of people affected per outbreak is much higher in *Clostridium perfringens* food poisoning. On this basis, *Clostridium perfringens* food poisoning now exhibits a higher over-all incidence than that caused by staphylococcus. The two are summarized in Illustration 8-3.

Botulism

Botulism is a severe food poisoning caused by ingestion of food contaminated with a potent neurotoxin formed during the growth of *Clostridium botulinum*. *Clostridium botulinum* is a spore-forming, soil-dwelling anerobe. The disease, botulism, is caused by the toxin and is

8-3. BACTERIAL FOOD POSIONING

(Staphyloccus and *Cl. perfringens*)

1) DISEASES CAUSED BY INGESTION OF BACTERIAL EXOTOXIN. MOST COMMON FORMS ARE CAUSED BY:
   Staphylococcus aureus
   *Clostridium perfringens**

2) ORGANISMS GROW IN CONTAMINATED FOOD ELABORATING ENTEROTOXIC SUBSTANCES

3) MAJORITY OF OUTBREAKS ASSOCIATED WITH BEEF AND POULTRY DISHES SERVED BY MASS FEEDING ESTABLISHMENTS

4) SYNDROME INCLUDES PROSTRATION, DIARRHEA AND ABDOMINAL PAIN: USUALLY TRANSIENT AND UNCOMPLICATED. NO FEVER

confined to GI tract

* The ingestion of intact organisms is apparently required for clostridium poisoning. However, no invasion is suspected.

---

completely independent of contact with the organism. *Clostridium botulinum* is widely distributed in nature and occurs in all soils, bottom sediments of streams, lakes and coastal waters, the intestinal tracts of fish and mammals and the gills and viscera of crabs and other shellfish. Sausages, meat products, canned vegetables and seafood products have been the most frequent vehicle for human botulism. In the usual case of botulism, the organism has found its way into canned food which has not been sufficiently heated to kill its spores. The container is then sealed and the anaerobic atmosphere created by the canning process permits the spores to germinate. Growing colonies that emerge from these spores produce botulinum toxin which is ingested with the food. Botulinum toxin has been estimated to be the single most poisonous substance (per gram of susceptible animal body weight) known to man. It takes very little of this toxin to turn canned food into a potent poison. If the food is heated adequately in cooking, the toxin may be denatured, but with an adequate dose of undenatured toxin there is the relatively sudden onset of central nervous system manifestations usually beginning as failure of coordinated movement, visual disturbance and, finally, loss of consciousness, coma and death due to respiratory arrest. Fifty per cent of cases serious enough to manifest central nervous system disturbance will prove ultimately fatal. Because of this strong potential for fatal outcome, botulism represents a considerably more serious (but fortunately more rare) example of food poisoning than either of the 2 discussed above (Illustration 8-4).

8-4. BACTERIAL FOOD POISONING

(Botulism) *MOST POISONING OF ANYTHING*

1) COMPARATIVELY RARE BUT POTENTIALLY FATAL FOOD POISONING RESULTING FROM INGESTION OF THE EXOTOXIN (NEUROTOXIN) OF *CL BOTULINUM*   *CNS* *
   spore-forming   *acts on neuro*
   soil-dwelling   *not entero*
   anerobe

2) VIABLE SPORES CONTAMINATE CANNED FOOD
   canned fish is most often involved

3) VEGETATIVE ORGANISMS GROW OUT AND PRODUCE POTENT TOXIN
   most poisonous substance known
   (per gram body weight of susceptible animal)

4) SUDDEN ONSET: CNS DISTURBANCES 50 per cent OF CLINICALLY APPARENT CASES ARE FATAL

2. Cholera

Cholera is a disease produced by the non-invasive enteric pathogen, *Vibrio cholerae,* a gram-negative, curved, rod-shaped, motile bacterium with a single polar flagellum. It occurs in 2 biotypes, the "classical" and the El Tor. The latter is responsible for a current pandemic of the disease which is thought to have reached a peak in 1970.

Vibrio cholerae is a single-host human pathogen. Traditionally, it is spread via contaminated drinking water. When taken into the human gastrointestinal tract the organism produces a toxin which causes massive loss of fluid and solutes from the gut wall, severe diarrhea, vomiting and abdominal pain. In classical cholera (cholera gravis), fluid loss can be so profound as to cause collapse and death within a day. Infection with the El Tor biotype, fortunately, is much milder and may even be confused with other acute enteric illnesses. Its rapid spread throughout the modern world is undoubtedly promoted by overpopulation, the great number of asymptomatic carriers that it generates and the broadcast effect of air travel (Illustration 8-5).

Additional Reading

Donadio, J. A. Botulism in the United States, 1899-1969. Am. J. Epidemiol. 93:93, 1971

Duffy, J. The History of Asiatic cholera in the United States. Bull. N.Y. Acad. Med. 47:1152, 1971

Fodor, T. et al. Food poisoning occurrences in New York City, 1969. Pub. Health Rep. 85:1013, 1970

Gangarosa, E. The epidemiology of cholera: Past and present. Bull. N.Y. Acad. Med. 47:1140, 1971

Gangarosa, E. J. Botulism in the United States. J. Infectious Dis. 119:308, 1969

Hendrix, T. The pathophipiology of cholera. Bull. N.Y. Acad. Med. 47:1169, 1971

Nakamura, M. and Schulze, J. *Clostridium perfringens* Food Poisoning. Ann. Rev. Microbiol. 24:359, 1970

8-5. NON-INVASIVE ENTERIC PATHOGENS

(Cholera)

1) DISEASE CAUSED BY THE PRESENCE OF

   Vibrio comma (cholerae)

   IN THE INTESTINAL TRACT

2) ORGANISM PRODUCES AN EXOTOXIN WHICH POISONS THE G.I. EPITHELIUM LEADING TO MASSIVE LOSS OF FLUID AND ELECTROLYTES

3) 50 per cent OF UNTREATED CASES ARE FATAL; HOWEVER, RESPONSE TO FLUID REPLACEMENT IS EXCELLENT   *CLASSICAL (SEVERE)*

4) MAN IS ONLY KNOWN RESERVOIR: TRANSMISSION THROUGH CONTAMINATED WATER AND FOOD

5) PANDEMIC OF MILDER FORM IS NOW DEVELOPING

   new (El Tor) biotype of organism
   overpopulation
   asymptomatic carriers
   air travel

KNOW DIFF. BETWEEN CLASSICAL & EL TOR

4.

PRODUCES ASYMTEMATIC CARRIER

EXOTOXIN PRODUCERS THAT INVADE SUPERFICIALLY

Not straight poisoning must get into b

LEARNING OBJECTIVE

To be able to describe the causative agent, pathogenesis, clinical course, and treatment or prophylaxis of the following diseases:

   a) tetanus

   b) diphtheria

The next group of organisms that we will examine are those having very little capacity for invasion yet requiring a location within the human body (however superficial) to be instrumental in disease. The 2 that we will consider extensively of this kind of disease are tetanus and diphtheria.

[handwritten margin note top: lodge in necrotized tissue]

1) Tetanus

In tetanus, just as in botulism, the actual disease is caused by a potent bacterial exotoxin. Like the organism of botulism, that of tetanus has no ability to invade. However, unlike botulism, in which the toxin is usually ingested in poorly prepared food, tetanus requires the actual intrusion of bacterial spores into the body through contamination of a wound.

Tetanus is caused by the organism, *Clostridium tetani,* a gram-positive, slightly motile, spore-forming bacillus, normally present in soil. The organism is especially prevalent in tropical and semi-tropical areas and is a constant danger in case of any wound, but particularly those sustained on a farm, battlefield or other situation in which soil contamination would be expected.

Throughout the world, today, the disease is seen in 3 circumstances:

1. Contaminated wounds of all kinds.
2. Among newborn children where the umbilical stump has been tied under unsanitary conditions (neonatal tetanus).
3. Among heroin addicts using poorly decontaminated equipment for drug injection.

Since the tetanus organism is an anerobe and can exist only as the spore in the atmosphere, it will enter the wound in the spore form. Given the 3 requirements of:

1. A relatively anerobic environment.
2. A small amount of necrotic tissue.
3. Soluble nutrients such as are usually present in wounds.

These spores germinate and the resulting vegetative organisms produce an exotoxin which is carried through the bloodstream to the central nervous system. This toxin is an extremely potent protein substance and only a very small amount is needed to cause disease. Clinically overt tetanus is usually seen 7 to 10 days following infection. It begins as trismus or spasms of the muscles mastication and in its mildest form is largely confined to this sign. Because trismus has long been recognized as the hallmark of tetanus the disease is often called "lock jaw." More severe cases do not stop with trismus, however, and may proceed to generalized spasmodic or even sustained convulsion. Despite its serious nature, there are usually no other signs or symptoms of tetanus. The patient does not manifest fever, leukocytosis or an increased erythrocyte sedimentation rate and no primary morphologic changes can be detected at autopsy.

About 50 per cent of all clinically apparent cases prove fatal, the prognosis usually correlating with the severity of the convulsive disorder. Those patients recovering do so without residual effect and, surprisingly, remain susceptible to another occurrence should they sustain another infection. As in the case of botulism, the only effective countermeasure is prevention; *overt tetanus cannot be successfully treated.* Prevention may be accomplished in 2 ways.

1. Treatment of the wounded and tetanus-liable patient with antitoxin or antibiotics or both.
2. Prior immunization with tetanus toxoid. The latter is the most effective and could, if applied throughout the world, practically eliminate tetanus.

[margin handwritten notes: 50% cases fatal before spores germinate / lethal if not failed & so failed prevented / 5]

8-6. EXOTOXIN PRODUCERS THAT INVADE SUPERFICIALLY

(Tetanus)

[handwritten: blood toxin]

1) DISEASE PRODUCED BY TOXEMIA WITH EXOTOXIN (NEUROTOXIN) OF *Clostridium tetani*

2) ORGANISM IS SPORE-FORMING SOIL-DWELLING ANEROBE

3) PUNCTURE WOUND (OR ANY WOUND) IS CONTAMINATED WITH SPORES WHICH GERMINATE AND PRODUCE TOXIN

4) AFTER 1 to 2 WEEKS STIFFNESS OF VOLUNTARY MUSCLES: CONVULSION

5) ACTIVE IMMUNIZATION WITH TOXOID IS MOST RELIABLE PROPHYLAXIS

[handwritten bottom notes: passive immunization for immediate treatment / denatured toxin stimulates antibodies ≈ 100% effective]

2. Diphtheria

Diphtheria is a highly communicable disease produced by the organism, *Corynebacterium diphtheriae*. The disease is usually transmitted by the inhalation of droplets expelled from an infected individual by sneezing or coughing. It causes a generalized but superficial infection of the pharyngeal wall, resulting in necrosis of the infected epithelium. Vessels immediately under the denuded surface release a fibrinous exudate which clots forming a fibrinopurulent membrane. This membrane actually forms a cast-like impression of the pharynx and upper respiratory tract. In many cases, it can be peeled off or is dislodged and coughed up. It may also occlude the airway, resulting in strangulation.

It has long been known that certain strains of *Corynebacterium diphtheriae* produced a potent toxin, whereas others were nontoxinogenic. In 1951, it was discovered that a bacteriophage could endow nontoxinogenic strains with the ability to produce toxin. Virulence and pseudomembrane formation are not dependent upon toxin formation, hence nontoxinogenic strains of this organism can cause a form of diphtheria with severe local damage.

Infection with toxinogenic strains, in addition to the characteristics described above, result in the release of a potent toxin into the blood stream. The most conspicuous effects of this toxemia are acute myocarditis and polyneuropathy. Acute myocarditis is the most common complication of diphtheria and is the usual cause of death. The toxin appears to interfere with the cardiac conduction system and death is usually associated with complete A-V block.

Although diphtheria attack rates and fatality rates have steadily declined in the United States over the past 25 years, outbreaks of diphtheria have been reported as recently as 1970. Immunization decreases the morbidity and mortality in diphtheria, but has little effect on the attack rate. The disease is still very prevalent in the eastern parts of the world; a recent publication reports 95 cases in 4 years, originating in a small town of southern Iran.

Additional Reading

Barksdale, L. *Corynebacterium diphtheriae* and its relatives. Bact. Rev. 34:378, 1970

Fusste, W. Prophylaxis against tetanus in wound management. Bull. Am. Coll. Surg. Sept.-Oct., 1967

van Heyningen, W. E. Tetanus. Sci. Amer. 218:69, 1968

La Force, F. M. et al. Tetanus in the United States (1965-1966). N. Engl. J. Med. 280:569, 1969

Mason, P. Tetanus in drug addicts. J. Am. Med. Assn. 205:118, 1968

Tahernia, A. C. and Moatamed, F. Diphtheria still lethal. Clin. Ped. 8:508, 1969

8-7. EXOTOXIN PRODUCERS THAT INVADE SUPERFICIALLY

(Diphtheria)

1) A COMMUNICABLE DISEASE (DROPLET TRANSMISSION) CAUSED BY *Corynebacterium, diphtheriae*

2) SUPERFICIAL INVASION OF URT: MUCOUS MEMBRANE IS DESTROYED AND FIBRINOPURULENT PSEUDOMEMBRANE FORMED

3) TOXIGENIC STRAINS PRODUCE POTENT EXOTOXIN THAT ENTERS BLOODSTREAM
   neuropathy
   myocarditis

4) POSSIBILITY OF RESPIRATORY OBSTRUCTION BY PSEUDOMEMBRANE

BACTERIA THAT ARE ABLE TO INVADE DEEPLY

LEARNING OBJECTIVE

To be able to discuss the causative agents, pathogenesis, clinical course, epidemiology, treatment and prophylaxis of the following diseases:

- a) staphylococcal and streptococcal infections as examples of those caused by pyogenic cocci
- b) typhoid fever

A number of pathogenic organisms invade the body with relative ease and may produce either exotoxin or endotoxin. These are, without a doubt, the most difficult to classify according to the system used in this subject. Rather than attempt to impose strict order on this group of pathogens, we will simply describe disease produced by 2 representative groups, the pyogenic cocci and the salmonella organisms.

1. The Pyogenic Cocci

The pyogenic cocci are a group of organisms, all of which cause infections characterized by the formation of copious amounts of pus. This group comprises the organisms listed in Illustration 8-8. Some of these organisms invade superficially, others deeply; some do both depending upon opportunity. Some produce exotoxin, some no toxin and others endotoxin. All exhibit a predilection for specific body locations. The staphylococcus, for example, is a constant normal inhabitant of the human skin. The streptococcus, pneumococcus and, in many cases, even the meningococcus is found in the oral cavity and pharynx of healthy individuals. Finally, the gonococcus is rarely found in other than infected individuals where it inhabits surfaces of the genitourinary tract and causes a superficial infection. In this subject we will discuss only the staphylococcus and streptococcus. The remaining 3 groups of organisms will be discussed as they are encountered in chapters covering the lung, the central nervous system and the genital systems.

Staphylococcus

The staphylococcus, particularly *Staphylo-*

8-8. BACTERIA THAT ARE ABLE TO INVADE DEEPLY

(The Pyogenic Cocci)

1) STAPHYLOCOCCUS

2) STREPTOCOCCUS

3) MENINGOCOCCUS

    principal disease (meningitis) will be considered in Chapter 15

4) PNEUMOCOCCUS

    principal disease (lobar pneumonia) will be considered in Chapter 16

5) GONOCOCCUS

    principal disease (gonorrhea) will be considered in Chapter 17

---

coccus aureus, is a very significant human pathogen. Although it is constantly present on the human skin and in the upper respiratory tract, it is able to cause disease only when host resistance has been compromised or when the organism is able to gain a portal of entry to deeper tissues. On the skin, the usual portal of entry is through a hair follicle. Staphylococcal infection of the hair follicle may result in a pustule, furuncle or, if the dermis is penetrated, a carbuncle. Staphyloccocal bronchitis and bronchopneumonia are common complications of many debilitating conditions whereas staphyloccal gastroenteritis (pseudomembranous enteritis) is sometimes seen as a complication of the post-surgical state. Osteomyelitis and endocarditis are also caused by staphylococci and will be considered under diseases of the skeleton and heart respectively. The ability for staphylococci to develop penicillin-resistant strains is well known. This, in turn, often causes life-threatening infections among debilitated patients in hospitals. Staphylococcal disease is summarized in Illustration 8-9.

Streptococcus

The second group of pyogenic pathogens

8-9. BACTERIA THAT ARE ABLE TO IN-VADE DEEPLY

(Staphylococcus)

1) *S. AUREUS* IS MOST SIGNIFICANT: FOUND AS COMMENSAL RESIDENT OF SKIN AND URT

2) USUAL P/E IS HAIR FOLLICLE

3) COMMONLY CAUSE
    furuncle (boil)
    carbuncle   *like a boil*
    osteomyelitis
    bronchitis, pneumonitis
    endocarditis
    various deep abscesses

that we will be considering is that of the streptococci. There are at least 30 identified major types of streptococci: however, not all of these are human pathogens. Those that do cause human disease are classified as beta hemolytic (Illustration 8-10). Streptococcal disease, quite in contrast to that caused by other pyogenic cocci, can develop in 2 ways. The great majority of such disease results from direct infection. Streptococcal infections of the oral pharynx, tonsils, middle ear, airway, skin and kidney are common and familiar examples. Another large and, in some ways, more serious, category of streptococcal disease results from post-infectious immunologic injury. In this pathogenetic mechanism, immune complexes formed between antibodies and streptococcal exotoxin become lodged in various structures resulting in 2 very prominent disease syndromes: 1) acute glomerulonephritis and 2) rheumatic fever. The former will be discussed in the chapter covering the urinary system and the latter will be discussed in that covering the heart. In both cases, complexes formed between streptococcal exotoxin and specific antibodies lodge in affected structures, fix complement and provoke severe inflammatory changes. In both diseases, the patient is suffering an essentially aseptic inflammatory

disorder of the involved organ. In fact, both usually occur some time after the provoking infection has been resolved.

2. Salmonella Infections

Salmonella organisms are gram-negative, motile bacteria that cause very characteristic enteric fevers (Illustration 8-11). The most important salmonella infection is typhoid fever (named for the similarity between its clinical appearance and that of typhus), an infection of serious proportions caused by the organism *Salmonella typhosa* (typhoid bacillus). Typhoid fever begins in the gastrointestinal tract and may remain confined there. The portal of entry for the typhoid bacillus is lymphoid tissue of the ileum. Affected lymphoid structures become grossly hyperplastic and ulcerate. Other lymphoid tissue throughout the body (including the spleen) also undergoes pronounced hyperplasia.

8-10. BACTERIA THAT ARE ABLE TO IN-VADE DEEPLY

(Streptococcus)

1) AT LEAST 30 MAJOR TYPES: ALL HU-MAN PATHOGENS ARE:
    beta hemolytic
    Lancefield Type A

2) STREPTOCOCCAL DISEASE ARE OF TWO KINDS
    direct infection
    postinfectious immunologic injury
       (glomerulonephritis)
       (rheumatic fever)

3) COMMONLY CAUSE
    pharyngitis, tonsilitis
    otitis media, mastoiditis
    scarlet fever
    cellulitis
    impetigo, erysipelas
    bronchitis, pneumonia

8-11. BACTERIA THAT ARE ABLE TO INVADE DEEPLY (SALMONELLA ORGANISMS)

1) SALMONELLA ORGANISMS CAUSE ENTERIC FEVERS

   most important salmonella infection is typhoid fever (*S. typhosa*)

2) TYPHOID FEVER ALWAYS TRANSMITTED VIA FECAL-ORAL ROUTE

   human carriers

   improper hygiene

3) P/E IS PEYER'S PATCH TISSUE

   become grossly hyperplastic and ulcerate

4) ACUTE DISEASE CONSISTING OF:

   mild to severe fever

   generalized lymphoid hyperplasia with soft splenomegaly

   diarrhea, rash

5) COMPLICATIONS INCLUDE INTESTINAL PERFORATION, HEMORRHAGE, BACTEREMIA WITH DISSEMINATED INFECTION AND SPLENIC RUPTURE

In addition, the acute illness includes fever, prostration, bloody diarrhea and a typical rash. Complications of typhoid fever include perforation of the intestine and hemorrhage. Typhoid bacteremia is often seen which may, in turn, give rise to pneumonia, sinusitis, meningitis and nephritis.

The typhoid infection is spread by human carrier and always transmitted by fecal contamination of food and drink. The carrier may be completely asymptomatic and the bacillus is thought to be harbored in the gallbladder. An active carrier constantly sheds virulent organisms in his stool. Such an individual becomes a public menace as a food handler or when placed in a situation in which improper sanitation permits fecal contamination of human food or water. This is often seen in areas where human waste disposal is not performed hygienically or where such waste is directed into a river which, in turn, flows into the ocean contaminating shellfish at its mouth. The most famous of all typhoid carriers was Mary Mallon, a cook who managed to avoid incarceration or treatment by constantly moving from job to job. In the course of her career she caused an estimated 10,000 cases of typhoid fever and an untold number of deaths. She died on November 11, 1938, having become a legend in her own lifetime as the notorious "Typhoid Mary."

Additional Reading

Arundell, F. D. Acne vulgaris. Ped. Clin. N. Amer. 18:853, 1971

Breese, B. B. Beta-hemolytic streptococcal infection. Am. J. Dis. Children 119:18, 1970

Smith, I. M. Death from staphylococci. Sci. Amer. 218:84, 1968

Wannamaker, L. W. Differences between streptococcal infections of the throat and of the skin. N. Engl. J. Med. 282:23, 78 (two parts), 1971

BACTERIA THAT USUALLY INVADE DEEPLY

LEARNING OBJECTIVES

To be able to discuss the causative agent, pathogenesis, epidemiology, clinical course, prophylaxis and treatment of the plague. To be able to describe the disease, tularemia, and note the position of syphilis as an example of a generalized infection. (Syphilis will be considered in detail in Chapter 17. It is mentioned here as the best example of a disease caused by an organism specialized to invasion and belonging at the very end of our spectrum)

Our final group of pathogenic organisms are those that are specialized to invasion. Some, like the plague bacillus, produce endotoxin;

others, like the agent of syphilis, produce no toxin. As examples of diseases in this category, we will use those produced by pasteurella organisms and the venereal disease, syphilis. Since syphilis will be considered in detail in Chapter 17, this learning objective will be devoted to the former and, in particular, to the historically important and always dangerous *plague.*

1. Diseases Caused by Pasteurella Organisms

The pasteurellae are gram-negative, aerobic, predominantly non-motile bacilli. In man, they produce the 2 diseases plague (P. pestis) and tularemia (P. tularensis).

Tularemia

Tularemia is a disease of rodents transmitted to man through contact with infected game animals. The handling, skinning and eating of diseased hares, rabbits and muskrats are the usual means of contracting the infection. Although capable of causing serious (and even fatal) disease, the organism of tularemia is not as virulent as that of the plague and usually controllable through the exercise of proper precautions in dealing with wild rodents.

Sylvatic Plague

Like tularemia, plague is essentially an infection of wild rodents. It is particularly prominent in India, Asia, South Africa, South America, western North America and Mexico. The disease is strongly endemic in these regions, being passed from animal to animal by fleas. Also like tularemia, infected animals are actually ill and many die from the infection. Plague endemic within a wild animal reservoir is called *sylvatic plague.*

Human Plague   Calif. ground Squirrel spreads CAUSE

On occasion, sylvatic plague is transmitted to the domestic rat. Since rats live in close contact with man, the death of many rats causes the rat flea to attempt to parasitize human beings. Its bite inoculates the organism which spreads rapidly through lymphatic channels causing inflammation and enlargement of lymph nodes (buboes) which may subsequently ulcerate to the surface. Hematogenous dissemination of the organism results in widespread hemorrhagic inflammatory lesions, particularly in the spleen, liver and lungs. Once established in the lung, the infection can be spread from man to man by droplet transmission (pneumonic plague). In a rapidly fatal form (septicemic plague), bacilli proliferate the blood stream, quickly overgrowing all attempts at defense. Although plague is now successfully treated with chemotherapeutic agents, before the advent of antibiotics it was 50 to 90 per cent fatal. Undoubtedly the most historically significant outbreak of plague occurred in 1348 to 1350. This epidemic was called the "Black Death," because it manifested an unusual incidence of the septicemic form of the infection which left corpses blackened. It is estimated to have caused the death of a quarter of the population of Europe. Major outbreaks have become increasingly rare in modern times, although as late as 1967, 5,000 cases reported in South Viet Nam.

8-12. BACTERIA THAT USUALLY INVADE DEEPLY

(Pasteurella Organisms)

1) PASTEURELLA ORGANISMS CAUSE:
   PLAGUE: spread by rat flea
   TULAREMIA: spread by contact with infected animal

2) BOTH DISEASES HAVE ANIMAL RESERVOIRS
   animals carrying the organism are suffering from the disease

(PLAGUE)

Rat flea parasitizes man, bite inoculates organism
Infection spreads along route of lymph drainage
Nodes enlarge and ulcerate forming buboes
50 to 90 per cent fatal before antibiotics
Historically significant as epidemic disease, the "Black Death"

2. Syphilis

Syphilis is a disease caused by the widespread dissemination of the causative agent (*Treponema pallidum*) in the body. It is always generalized and probably represents the best example of a common disease caused by an organism that specializes in invasion. It will be discussed in detail in Chapter 17.

Additional Reading

Braude, A. I. Bacterial endotoxins. Sci. Amer. 215:36, 1964

Kadis, S. et al. Plague toxin. Sci. Amer. 220:93, 1969

Langer, W. The black death. Sci. Amer. 215:114, 1964

Rats, Rats, Rats. The Sciences 7:1, 1967

Reed, W. P. et al. Bubonic plague in the Southwestern United States. Medicine 49:465, 1970

Young, L. S. et al. Tularemia epidemic: Vermont, 1968. N. Engl. J. Med. 280:1254, 1969

MYCOBACTERIAL INFECTION

LEARNING OBJECTIVE

To be able to discuss tuberculosis as representative of mycobacterial infection, mentioning the following:

  a) nature of the causative organism
  b) characteristics of the host response
  c) the Ghon complex
  d) secondary pulmonary tuberculosis
  e) miliary tuberculosis
  f) cavitation

Mycobacteria are rod-shaped, aerobic organisms that stain only with difficulty and cannot be classified as either gram positive or gram negative. Once stained, they resist discoloration, even when treated with acid, hence are described as "acid-fast." With regard to complexity, they occupy a position midway between bacteria and fungi. As might be expected, the character of the host response to mycobacterial infection differs considerably from that of infection with bacteria (Illustration 8-13). Although typical acute inflammation is seen in the opening stages of mycobacterial disease, granulomatous inflammation is far more prominent in succeeding stages. Mycobacteria cause 2 important human diseases, tuberculosis and leprosy. We will use the former as our example of mycobacterial infectious disease.

Tuberculosis is a chronic granulomatous infectious disease caused by human or bovine mycobacteria (*Mycobacterium tuberculosis* or *Mycobacterium bovis*). Infection may be established through either the respiratory or gastrointestinal route.

The organism produces neither exotoxin nor endotoxin. Its virulence is based on its ability to live within phagocytes where it not only resists digestion, but also is able to proliferate. Possibly because of its unusual waxy outer covering the tubercle bacillus elicits a strong cellular immunologic response and all effective host resistance seems to be based on cellular immunity.

The disease, tuberculosis, occurs in 2 stages (Illustration 8-14). Primary tuberculosis is the form that occurs upon first exposure to the tubercle bacillus. Primary exposure results in a combination of lesions known as the primary complex or Ghon complex which develops in the following steps:

8-13. MYCOBACTERIAL INFECTIONS

BACTERIA
  infections are common
  agents proliferate rapidly
  disease is usually acute
  toxins are usually involved

MYCOBACTERIA (tubercle and leprosy bacilli)
  characteristics of both

FUNGI
  infections are rare but increasing
  agents proliferate slowly
  disease is usually chronic
  no exotoxin or endotoxin

8-14. TUBERCULOSIS (CONSUMPTION, PYTHISIS)

1) CAUSED BY MYCOBACTERIUM TUBERCULOSIS (OR *M. BOVIS*)
- acid fast
- human and bovine strains are virulent in man
- no exotoxin or endotoxin
- elicits a strong cellular immune response

2) DISEASE OCCURS IN TWO STAGES
- Primary
  - focal pneumonitis
  - Ghon complex
  - immunization
- Secondary
  - tubercle formation
  - caseation

3) COMPLICATIONS
- pulmonary spread
- cavitation
- miliary dissemination
- spread by contact

HEMATOGEON DISSEMINATION

KNOW GHON COMPLEX

1) An inoculum of tubercle bacilli is (usually) inhaled and lodges at the periphery of the lung.
2) A focus of acute pneumonitis develops in which a typical acute inflammatory reaction is seen as the host response.
3) Products of the inflammatory site drain into regional (hilar) lymph nodes where they elicit a cellular immunologic response.
4) Sensitized lymphocytes are broadcast throughout the body and come upon tubercle bacilli at the site of primary infection. A granulomatous reaction ensues, which usually takes the form of a rather typical granuloma called a tubercle.
5) If the response proves adequate, the infection is brought under control, the remaining organisms killed and the tubercles (1 at the site of primary infection

and another in a regional node) heal and usually undergo calcification. The combination of healed, calcified tubercles at the site of primary infection (lung or gastrointestinal tract) and in regional nodes constitutes the Ghon complex.

Presence of the Ghon complex indicates that the patient has undergone a primary infection. It is presumed that immunologic sensitivity resulting from such an infection constitutes a degree of protection against further infection with the tubercle bacillus.

Once an individual has established cellular immunity to the tubercle bacillus, all further tuberculosis will occur as the secondary form. Secondary tuberculosis is caused by bacteria surviving the primary episode or by inhalation of a new inoculum. It may extend over a period of time and be very destructive as long as the active process continues. It begins with tubercle formation in the lung apex; if not arrested, these tubercles expand, accumulating caseous necrotic material at the center. The organism may become further distributed in lung parenchyma, initiating new tubercle formation. The combined effect of the spread of the organism and the expansion of individual tubercles results in the destruction of large amounts of lung parenchyma and suggested the earlier term "consumption" for this disease.

If the infection is arrested by adequate host resistance or proper treatment, the tubercles constituting the secondary disease may heal and calcify. These may remain quiescent or be reactivated later in life. If the active process continues unabated, various complications are possible (Illustration 8-14). These include further pulmonary extension, the erosion of tubercles into bronchi with the subsequent coughing up of their contents (cavitation), the erosion of tubercles into blood vessels with the subsequent hematogenous dissemination of the tubercle bacillus (miliary tuberculosis) or spread to other parts of the body by various other modes of contact.

Additional Reading

Faigel, H. C. Tuberculosis is alive and well in America. Clin. Pediat. 9:311, 1970

Mackaness, G. B. Cell-mediated immunity to infection. Hospital Pract. 5:73, 1970

Miller, F. J. W. B. C. G. vaccination. Practitioner 204:821, 1970

Scadding, J. G. Tubercular sensitivity in tuberculosis. Postgrad. Med. 47:694, 1971

MYCOTIC INFECTION

LEARNING OBJECTIVE

To be able to outline the causative agent, clinical course, epidemiology, prophylaxis and (where applicable) treatment of the following mycotic infections:

- a) candidiasis
- b) actinomycosis
- c) histoplasmosis
- d) blastomycosis
- e) coccidioidomycosis

Mycotic infections are those produced by fungi and yeasts; while still rare, these infections are now showing an absolute increase in incidence. This is probably due to a number of factors, among which is the increased use of antibiotics which cause wholesale elimination of bacteria serving to hold mycotic organisms in check as commensal inhabitants of the body. Also contributory is the recent increase in patients suffering from extremely debilitating conditions, including lymphoma, leukemia, disseminated solid tumors and long-term immunosuppressive therapy. Since most mycotic organisms are opportunistic agents of disease, debilitated patients provide a fertile substrate for infection. Characteristic of mycotic infections is that the organisms proliferates very slowly and produces no toxin. With few exceptions mycotic diseases are chronic and associated with granulomatous lesions, at least in later stages.

Mycotic diseases are conveniently classified into 2 large groups (Illustration 8-15). We will sample each of these, using examples listed.

1. Superficial Mycotic Infections

Superficial mycotic infections are those in which the organism rarely penetrates beneath the surface of the body. The usual lesion produced in these diseases is the ulcer, fissure or superficial inflammatory lesion. Examples include the common athlete's foot, ring-worm, barber's itch and a variety of other such diseases which are more of a nuisance than a threat. Somewhat more significant as a superficial mycotic infection is the disease Candidiasis.

8-15. MYCOTIC INFECTIONS

1) SUPERFICIAL (examples)
   dermatomycosis
   candidiasis

2) DEEP (examples)
   actinomycosis
   histoplasmosis
   blastomycosis
   coccidioidomycosis

8-16. SUPERFICIAL MYCOTIC INFECTION

(Candidiasis)

1) SUPERFICIAL INFECTION BY NORMALLY COMMENSAL FUNGUS
   Candida (Monilia) albicans

2) OCCURS ON ORAL MUCOUS MEMBRANES (THRUSH) VAGINAL SURFACE AND SKIN

3) HALLMARK OF WEAKENED RESISTANCE
   particularly that of cellular immunologic function

4) MAY BECOME SYSTEMIC IN EXTREME DEBILITATION

Candidiasis

Candidiasis or moniliasis (Illustration 8-16) is a disease caused by infection with the fungus, *Candida (Monilia) albicans*. This organism is constantly present on the skin and mucous membranes of the mouth and vagina. It is only when the patient begins to manifest weakened resistance that any degree of invasion can occur. In fact, chronic mucocutaneous candidiasis has come to be recognized as a hallmark of weakened defense, particularly that mediated by the cellular immunologic systems. Infection with *Candida albicans* is almost always superficial; when it occurs on the oral mucosa it is known as "thrush" and appears as a whitish, plaque-like deposit of fungus on the otherwise pink mucous membrane. This fungal plaque can usually be rubbed off, leaving a raw, reddish area exposed. The skin is often affected, particularly in moist, protected regions such as the perineum, axillae and infra-mammary areas. In extreme debilitation or as a complication of cardiac surgery, wider dissemination of the organism may occur. Esophageal, bronchopulmonary and systemic candidiasis have been seen in patients severely weakened by terminal malignancy, cardiac surgery, vigorous immunosuppression and a number of other such conditions.

2. Deep Mycotic Infections

Deep mycotic infections are those affecting lungs, gastrointestinal tract and other organs as well as superficial tissues. As examples, we will discuss the 4 listed in Illustration 8-15.

Actinomycosis

Actinomycosis is a disease caused by infection with the bacteria-like fungus, *Actinomyces bovis (israeli)*. It is more common in farm animals but, since the agent is capable of infecting man, the disease must be classified as a zoonosis. Characteristic of actinomycosis (quite in contrast to true mycotic disease) is the production of large amounts of pus. The organisms penetrate the body through a defect in the skin or mucous membrane and elicits copious pus formation. The pus dissects its way along tissue planes, forming large pools which erupt in draining sinuses to the surface of the skin. It contains tangled colonies of the organisms which are visible to the naked eye. Because of their characteristic color, these colonies are called "sulfur granules." Actinomycosis is most commonly seen in the general area of the head and neck, although it may occur elsewhere. In cervico-facial actinomycosis, the organism usually enters through a break in the oral mucosa, such as an ulcer or extraction wound. If untreated, the disease is extremely disfiguring; however, the agent is sensitive to antibiotics and usually responds quite readily. Most authorities now consider *Actinomyces bovis* a true bacterium rather than a fungus. This would explain the striking difference between this and other mycotic infections. Actinomycosis is reviewed in Illustration 8-17.

Histoplasmosis

Histoplasmosis is a disease resulting from infection with the fungus, *Histoplasma capsulatum*. As an infectious disease, it is unique in that it was not recognized as an important medical problem until after 1945. The reason is that histoplasmosis has no exclusive distinguishing characteristics, but closely mimics other well known diseases such as influenza and tuberculosis. The organism can be transmitted directly to humans from contaminated soil. The droppings of birds, such as pigeons, chickens, starlings and others seem to contain a substance which stimulates the growth of *Histoplasma capsulatum*. For this reason, the organism is quite prevalent in areas where large concentra-

---

8-17. DEEP MYCOTIC INFECTIONS

(Actinomycosis)

1) INFECTION BY BACTERIA-LIKE ORGANISM
   Actinomyces bovis (israeli)

2) MORE COMMON IN FARM ANIMALS THAN IN MAN

3) PRODUCES LARGE AMOUNTS OF PUS WHICH DISSECTS ALONG TISSUE CLEAVAGE PLANES ERUPTING TO THE SURFACE IN DRAINING SINUSES

   grossly visible, tangled colonies of the organism called "sulfur granules" are seen in the pus

4) COMMON SITE IS FACE AND NECK

tions of bird manure are found. This includes locations such as chicken houses and parks. It persists in the soil for some time after the birds have left. The disease is contracted by inhalation of spores. If there has been no previous exposure to the fungus, an acute inflammatory response will occur wherever the inoculum becomes arrested within lung parenchyma. Proliferation of the organism and its spread to regional nodes results in a strong cellular immunologic response and the appearance of skin sensitivity to histoplasmin, an extract of the organism. Healing of primary lesions results in the Ghon complex, much in the same manner as was seen in tuberculosis. The secondary form of the disease is granulomatous and associated with the formation of lesions resembling tubercles. The clinical picture of histoplasmosis assumes a bewildering number of patterns (Illustration 8-18). In its mildest form, it is easily confused with a number of unimportant respiratory infections. Diagnosis is usually confirmed by the histoplasmin skin test and the detection of small fibrotic or calcified lesions. Although histoplasmosis is a disease of worldwide distribution, histoplasmin skin sensitivity is most prevalent in river valley areas of temperate and tropical zones. Some areas such as Kentucky and Tennessee report attack rates as high as 95 per cent among young adults. Indeed, on a national basis, the prevalence of histoplasmin-positive skin reactivity may range as high as 15 to 20 per cent.

North American Blastomycosis

North American blastomycosis is a disease resulting from infection with *Blastomyces dermatitidis*. This agent is a yeast-like fungus which assumes a budding spherical form as a parasite and a filamentous, typically fungal configuration at room temperature. A similar disease, South American blastomycosis, is caused by the organism *Blastomyces brasiliensis*. North American blastomycosis is a rare disease, occurring at the rate of approximately 0.5 cases per 100,000 population per year. It is usually contracted by inhalation of the organism which first establishes a pulmonary infection and is then disseminated, usually to the skin, bones, viscera and meninges. Lesions are granulomatous, but also exhibit significant collections of neutrophils. Thus, the reaction

---

8-18. DEEP MYCOTIC INFECTIONS

(Histoplasmosis)

1) INFECTION WITH SMALL (2 to 4 μ) YEAST-LIKE INTRACELLULAR FUNGUS
   Histoplasma, capsulatum

2) USUALLY CONTRACTED BY INHALATION OF ORGANISM IN DRIED SOIL: PATHOGENESIS RESEMBLES TUBERCULOSIS

3) DISEASE OCCURS IN SPECTRUM OF SEVERITY FROM VERY MILD TO AN ACUTE, FULMINANT, FATAL FORM

4) SEEN THROUGHOUT THE WORLD BUT EXHIBITS AREAS OF VERY HIGH ENDEMICITY
   northeast, central and south central U.S.

---

appears to be a combination of acute and granulomatous inflammation. Organisms are found within giant cells and macrophages. The disease runs a rather protracted course and the disseminated form is usually fatal. Infection with *Blastomyces dermatitidis* is thought to occur only in the North American continent. The organism has been isolated from soil and is known to infect dogs. A cutaneous form of the disease occurs in wound contamination, but does not become generalized and is usually not fatal. North American blastomycosis is reviewed in Illustration 8-19.

Coccidioidomycosis

Coccidioidomycosis is a disease resulting from infection with the sporulating fungus, *Coccidioides immitis*. Like other fungal disease, it exhibits a pronounced geographic concentration, in this case the southwestern United States and, in particular, the San Joaquin Valley. The disease is contracted by the

8-19. DEEP MYCOTIC INFECTIONS
(North American Blastomycosis) 1) INFECTION WITH BUDDING YEAST-LIKE FUNGUS 　　*Blastomyces dermatitidis* 2) DISEASE IS CONTRACTED BY INHALATION OF ORGANISMS, PRIMARY INFECTION IS ALMOST ALWAYS PULMONARY 　　systemic dissemination results in lesions of *subcutaneous tissues* 　　nervous system 　　viscera 　　bones and joints 3) CONFINED TO NORTH AMERICA

8-20. DEEP MYCOTIC INFECTIONS
(Coccidioidomycosis) 1) INFECTION WITH SPORULATING FUNGUS 　　*Coccidioides immitis* 2) USUALLY CONTRACTED BY INHALATION OF ORGANISMS, PULMONARY INFECTION IS MOST COMMON 3) TWO FORMS ARE RECOGNIZED 　　mild, self-limiting febrile disease (San Joaquin Valley Fever) 　　fulminant, progressive fatal disease (rare) 4) HIGHLY ENDEMIC TO SOUTHERN CALIFORNIA 5) PULMONARY LESIONS RESEMBLE TUBERCULOSIS

inhalation of spores: however, entry through a wound is also thought possible. Clinical manifestations may be so mild as to go unnoticed or may amount to an acute, self-limiting, febrile attack with lesions largely confined to the lungs. On rare occasions, the organism becomes widely disseminated and the disease fulminant and fatal. As in the case of other deep mycotic infections, the original reaction is one of acute inflammation: however, primary exposure will generate a strong cellular immunologic response and all subsequent lesions will be granulomatous. Morphologically, pulmonary lesions resemble those of tuberculosis except that some vestiges of acute inflammation may persist along with the granuloma. Although known as "San Joaquin Valley fever" because of its strong endemicity, outbreaks of coccidioidomycosis have been reported from other areas. Illustration 8-20 summarizes important items of information regarding this disease.

Additional Reading

Coodley, E. L. "Actinomycosis:" Clinical diagnosis and management. Postgrad. Med. 46:73, 1969

Furculow, M. L. Histoplasmosis. Clinical Notes on Resp. Dis. Summer, 1967

Furculow, M. L. et al. Prevalence and incidence studies of human and canine blastomycosis. Am. J. Epidem. 92:121, 1970

Obenour, R. A. North American blastomycosis. J. Tenn. Med. Assn. 62:324, 1969

Taschdjian, C. L. Opportunistic yeast infections with special reference to candidiasis. Ann. N.Y. Acad. Sci. 174:606, 1970

Teel, K. W. et al. A localized outbreak of coccidiodomycosis in southern Texas. J. Pediat. 77:65, 1970

Williams, R. J. et al. Candida septicemia. Arch. Surg. 103:8, 1971

HUMAN PARASITOLOGY

LEARNING OBJECTIVE

To be able to describe characteristics of the following 4 groups of human parasites and discuss the specific diseases mentioned in some detail.

- a) protozoa
- b) round worms or nematodes
- c) flat worms:
    - cestodes
    - trematodes
- d) arthropods

Parasitism is a phenomenon that is widespread in nature. Whereas infectious diseases are all valid examples of parasitism, the medical use of the term, parasitology, has come to be confined to infections caused by protozoa and higher organisms. Illustration 8-21 is a list of the principal divisions of organisms usually included in this subject. Within each of these main divisions are numerous subdivisions, each of which is responsible for a separate human disease. We will consider the first 2 of these categories, selecting only 1 or 2 specific diseases for detailed discussion.

1. Parasitic Protozoa

Protozoa are responsible for a number of very important human diseases. Members of this group of pathogens are listed in Illustration

---

8-21. HUMAN PARASITOLOGY

1) PARASITIC PROTOZOA

2) ROUNDWORMS (NEMATODES)

3) FLATWORMS:
    cestodes (tapeworms)
    trematodes (flukes)

4) ARTHROPODS

8-22. PARASITIC PROTOZOA

1) INTESTINAL AND ATRIAL
    Entamoeba histolytica (ameoba)
    Balantidium coli (ciliate)
    Trichomonas and Giardia (flagellates)

2) BLOOD AND TISSUE
    Plasmodium (3 species)
    Leishmania (3 species)
    Trypanosoma (3 species)
    Uncertain classification (pneumocystis, sarcocystis toxoplasma)

8-22. Note that they can be subdivided into 2 large groups. Although all of these organisms are important as agents of human disease, we will single out the first member of each large group for further discussion.

Amebiasis

Amebiasis is a disease resulting from infection with the ameba, *Entameba histolytica*. The disease is contracted by ingestion of the microscopic, encysted organisms as shown in Illustration 8-23. Once in the gastrointestinal tract, the trophozoite or feeding form emerges and burrows into the gut wall, causing ulceration of the mucosa and extensive damage to deeper tissue. If such damage becomes extensive, the patient manifests dysentery which may become so severe as to cause death. Complications include perforation of the gut wall as well as the spread of amebae to the liver and beyond where collections of the organisms cause the formation of "abscesses." Even with apparent cure, the patient may harbor the organism and excrete its encysted form, acting as a highly infective carrier of the disease.

Malaria

Malaria is probably the most prevalent serious infectious disease in the world. A different form of the disease is caused by each of 4 species of sporulating protozoa (Illustra-

repeated. The synchronous release of many merozoites is the event causing the sudden onset of chills and fever so characteristic of malaria. These attacks correspond to the interval required for 1 asexual cycle and differ among the 4 species of Plasmodium that cause human malaria. In all species, a few of the intracellular organisms develop into sexual forms (gametocytes), which remain in the blood stream when released with the merozoites. If taken into the stomach of an anopheles mosquito with a blood meal, these undergo a sexual cycle and the resulting spores are passed to the next human bitten.

2. Nematodes (Roundworms)

Nematodes or roundworms are the second of our 4 classes of human parasites. They are divided into 2 large categories as shown in Illustration 8-25. We will discuss only the first disease in the first category (trichinosis) as our example of this kind of human illness.

Trichinosis is a disease produced by infection with the roundworm, *Trichinella spiralis*. At one time, this disease was strikingly prevalent in

---

8-23. HUMAN PROTOZOAL DISEASES

(Amebiasis)

1) INFECTION WITH PATHOGENIC-AMEBA
   Entamoeba histolytica

2) MAN IS BOTH RESERVOIR AND VECTOR

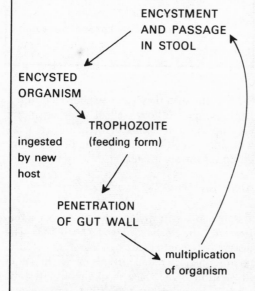

ENCYSTMENT AND PASSAGE IN STOOL

ENCYSTED ORGANISM

TROPHOZOITE (feeding form)

ingested by new host

PENETRATION OF GUT WALL

multiplication of organism

3) COMPLICATIONS INCLUDE INTESTINAL PERFORATION AND LIVER "ABSCESSES"

8-24. HUMAN PROTOZOAL DISEASES

(Malaria)

1) INFECTION WITH ONE OF FOUR SPECIES OF SPORULATING PROTOZOA
   Plasmodium vivax (most common)
   Plasmodium malariae
   Plasmodium falciparum
   Plasmodium ovale (very rare)

2) ORGANISM COMPLETES ASEXUAL PHASE OF LIFE CYCLE IN MAN AND SEXUAL PHASE IN ANOPHELES MOSQUITO WHICH SERVES AS ITS VECTOR

3) RELEASE OF ORGANISMS AND DEBRIS FROM EXHAUSTED ERYTHROCYTES AT END OF EACH CYCLE CORRESPONDS TO PAROXYSM OF CHILLS AND FEVER

---

tion 8-24). All 4 of these parasites undergo the asexual phase of their life cycle in man and the sexual phase in the Anopheles mosquito, which serves as the common vector. The most prevalent form of malaria is caused by *Plasmodium vivax*, the least prevalent by *Plasmodium ovale*. The organism is injected into man by the bite of the infected female mosquito. After 7 to 10 days, it begins to parasitize circulating red blood cells, in which it grows out as a large schizont. This form then divides into several merozoites which are simultaneously released from many infected erythrocytes. Each of these then goes on to penetrate a new blood cell and the cycle is

---

8-25. NEMATODES

1) INTESTINAL
> hookworm   (Ancyclostoma   and   Necator)
> *Ascaris lumbricoides*
> *Enterobius vermicularis*
> *Trichinella spiralis*
> *Trichuris trichïura*
> *Strongyloides stercoralis*

2) BLOOD AND TISSUE
> Filiariae   (several   species)

---

the United States, but the closer control of pork production, along with increased awareness of the need for thorough cooking of pork, has caused its sharp decline. The pig is usually infected by eating garbage scraps containing infected pork or by eating infected rats. The human is infected by eating pork muscle containing encysted larvae of the parasite. The larvae are freed in the process of digestion. They mature in the intestinal mucosa where, as adults, they copulate and the females give birth to a new generation of larvae. The new larvae then begin a migration throughout the body, an event that often causes acute illness. They eventually reach voluntary muscle and they become encysted. This cycle is recapitulated in Illustration 8-26.

3. Cestodes and Trematodes (Flatworms)

Cestodes (tapeworms) and trematodes (flukes) are often considered together as "flatworms." Their life cycles and modes of infection are quite different and all are very complicated. Since an adequate discussion of either of these classes of parasites is beyond the scope of this learning objective, we will do no more than mention and list them here (Illustration 8-27).

4. Arthropods

A number of arthropod species also exist primarily or exclusively as human parasites. Again, they will only be listed here (Illustration 8-28).

8-26. NEMATODE INFECTION

(Trichinosis)

1) DISEASE CAUSED BY INFECTION WITH *TRICHINELLA SPIRALIS*

2) WORM COMMON IN RATS,
> pigs and other carnivorous mammals are commonly infected by eating rats or garbage containing uncooked pork

3) MAN IS INFECTED BY EATING POORLY COOKED, CONTAMINATED PORK

4) LARVAE EMERGE, BURROW INTO INTESTINAL WALL, MATURE, COPULATE AND GIVE RISE TO A SECOND GENERATION OF LARVAE
> visceral larval migrans
> encystment

8-27. FLATWORMS   (CESTODES   AND   TREMATODES)

1) CESTODES (TAPEWORMS)
> *Taenia solium* (pork)
> *Taenia saginata* (beef)
> *Diphyllobothrium latum* (fish)
> *Hymenolepis nana* (man-man)
> *Hymenolepis diminunata* (rat-man)
> Others

2) TREMATODES (FLUKES)
> *Schistosoma* (3 species)
> > veins
> *Fasciolopsis buski*
> > intestine
> *Clonorchis sinensis*
> > liver
> *Paragonimus westermani*
> > lung

8-28. ARTHROPODS

1) MYRIOPODA
   poisonous centipeds

2) ARACHNIDA
   spiders
   scorpions
   ticks
   mites

3) INSECTA
   lice
   fleas
   bugs
   flies
   mosquitos
   roaches

Additional Reading

Alvarado, C. A. and Bruce–Chwatt, L. J. Malaria. Sci. Amer. 206:86, 1962

Bick, R. L. and Anhalt, J. E. Malaria transmission among narcotic addicts. California Med. 115:56, 1971

Brown, H. W. Antihelminthics, new and old. Clin. Pharmacol. Therap. 10:5, 1969

Elsden, R. Amebiasis as a world problem. Bull. N.Y. Acad. Med. 47:438, 1971

Fuchs, F. Congenital toxoplasmosis: A prospective study of 4,048 obstetric patients. Am. J. Obstet. Gynec. 111:197, 1971

Harbottle, J. E. Trichinosis in the United States, 1969. J. Infectious Dis. 122:568, 1970

Juniper, K. Amebiasis in the United States. Bull. N.Y. Acad. Med. 47:448, 1971

March, C. H. et al. Man versus arthropods. G. P. 36:115, 1967

Remington, J. S. and Gentry, L. O. Acquired toxoplasmosis: infection versus disease. Ann. N.Y. Acad. Sci. 174:1006, 1971

Sodeman, W. A. Amebiasis. Am. J. Digest. Dis. 16:51, 1971

Vawter, G. F. Pneumocystis carinii. Ann. N.Y. Acad. Sci. 174:1048, 1971

Zimmerman, W. J. et al. The changing status of trichiniasis in the U.S. population. Public Health Rep. 83:957, 1968

part 3

diseases of development and function

chapter 9
DISORDERS OF DEVELOPMENT

PRINCIPLES OF DEVELOPMENTAL DISEASE

LEARNING OBJECTIVE

To be able to discuss the concept of the gene both as a structure and as a unit of inheritance, using each of the following terms in its correct context:

  a) **clinical stages of human development**
  b) **regulator gene, operon, allele**
  c) **transcription, translation**
  d) **chromosome, homologous pair**
  e) **mitosis, meiosis**

Every individual of every species is largely an expression of information contained in his genes. Adequate genes, together with their successful expression as full development, is the very cornerstone of health. Developmental disease results when either the genes (or chromosomes) are faulty or development is frustrated. With this subject we will consider a sample of both genetic and extragenetic causes for developmental disease, looking first at diseases caused by a defective genetic apparatus and finally at those resulting from the improper expression of good genes. Since some background will be necessary, the following discussion is offered as a minimal preparatory review of principles that underlie these subjects.

1. The Significance of Genes and Chromosomes

In a very real sense there is only one life on earth. In this sense life is a system for conveying a high degree of molecular order through time. This molecular order is represented by germ plasm or the collection of all of the genes that go into the determination of all forms of life on earth. Each individual carries the germ plasm of his species for a limited time, following which it is relayed to a new generation of individuals.

Genetic information for the development of a complete individual is contained primarily within the nucleus of the fertilized ovum. This collection of genetic information is usually termed the individual's *genome* or *genotype*, in that it determines to a great extent what he *can* be given optimal conditions for further development. The genome, of course, lacks information for certain variable factors that are added (or withheld) either *in utero*, or later through culture and environment. Important as they are, good genes are only the first installment on a healthy body and mind.

In the course of carrying the human germ plasm through his lifetime, an individual passes through several clearly defined developmental periods. (Illustration 9-1). The duration of

---

9-1. DEVELOPMENTAL PERIODS

1) **EMBRYONIC PERIOD**
   conception to 8 weeks post-conception

2) **FETAL PERIOD**
   8 weeks post-conception to 40 weeks post-conception disorders of development (congenital or latent)

3) **PERINATAL PERIOD**
   labor to 1 day after birth

4) **INFANCY**
   to 1 year after birth

5) **CHILDHOOD**
   to end of puberty

6) **ADULTHOOD**

---

these periods, as well as the form and function of the emerging individual, are all determined by genetic information.

All genetic information exists in the form of specific sequences of nucleotide base units that make up the DNA of the chromosomes of an individual's first cell. In effect, the information is "coded" into the primary structure of this material. This means of information storage has come to be known as the genetic code. The significance of the genetic code is truly worthy of reverence. It represents our most basic insight into life as a process. All life on earth uses this same code!

In the genetic code, a group of 3 nucleotides is called a *codon* and specifies the position of 1 amino acid in a protein molecule that will go into the developing individual. The gene, in turn, is made up of a sequence of codons. Each gene dictates the structure of a whole single protein molecule through the scheme depicted in Illustration 9-2. *The structure of all proteins of the human body are expressions of information stored in the genes while the "use" of genetic information always involves the synthesis of protein.*

Genes apparently exist as 2 kinds, *structural genes* and *control genes*. A structural gene specifies the amino acid sequence of a protein molecule, whereas its corresponding control

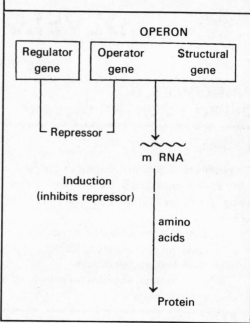

9-3. HYPOTHESIS FOR THE GENETIC CONTROL OF PROTEIN SYNTHESIS

genes regulate the rate at which this protein is synthesized. Control genes are further divided into *operator genes* and *regulator genes*; the former actually start and stop the synthetic activity of the structural gene, whereas the latter regulate the process by synthesizing a repressor substance which inhibits the control gene as long as it is present. The "turning on" of an operator gene and control gene (operon) is accomplished by "turning off" the associated regulator gene. Many hormones act as derepressors in that they suppress the regulator gene and allow the operator gene to start structural gene synthetic activity. You may have to read that whole paragraph over again to get the picture, or, better still, look at Illustration 9-3, where an attempt is made to show this as a diagram.

Try thinking of the gene as a tiny protein factory. The regulator gene represents the management, the operator gene the foreman and the structural gene the workers.

Each cell of an individual contains all of the genes of the original cell (zygote). This enormous fund of information is passed on intact to

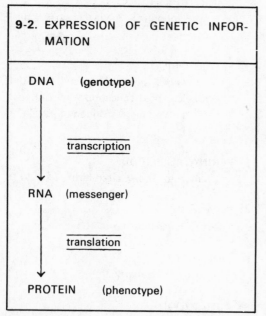

9-2. EXPRESSION OF GENETIC INFORMATION

each new cell as part of the complex process of mitosis. Although each cell of the body retains all of the genetic potential of the original normal adult, it will use only that tiny part of the information needed for its own specialized function. Genes that are not used are "turned off" or repressed and only under the comparatively rare circumstances of a cell's giving rise to a gamete is the derepression of all genes seen.

Genes are organized into structural units called chromosomes. Chromosomes are gene sequences, long strands of DNA that drift loosely in the fluid component of the nucleus of each cell. A single chromosome may carry as many as a thousand genes and it is through the precise replication of each chromosome that genes are duplicated and transferred to daughter cells. In all higher plants and animals, chromosomes exist not as single structures but as homologous pairs (Illustration 9-4). Every chromosome has a near-twin counterpart. Although not identical, this second chromosome is very similar and contains genes that correspond to those of the first. Genes that occupy corresponding positions on homologous chromosomes are called *alleles*.

9-5. REPLICATION OF GENETIC MATERIAL

During replication the normally double-stranded DNA separates and complementary chains are synthesized

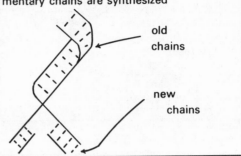

old chains

new chains

In effect each normal somatic cell has twice the number of chromosomes (and genes) that it actually needs. Because of this double dose it is said to be *diploid* or 2n with regard to chromosome number.

2. Meiosis

Some (but comparatively few) cells are destined to become gametes and participate in reproduction. When a somatic cell becomes a germ cell or gamete (as it does in spermatogenesis), it undergoes meiosis or reduction division giving up half of its chromosome complement to each daughter cell (Illustration 9-5). Although each of the daughter cells will receive one of the chromosomes of each homologous pair, representatives of each pair are mixed on a random basis in the daughter cells. In this way, the now haploid (n) sperm can combine with a haploid (n) ovum giving rise to a diploid (2n) zygote which can then develop into a new individual with an entirely novel combination of genes. This opportunity to experiment with new gene combinations is the ultimate advantage of the sex drive, Madison Avenue notwithstanding.

3. Mitosis

Very few somatic cells will end up as germ cells, however, and most will divide by mitosis.

9-4. HOMOLOGOUS PARING OF CHROMOSOMES

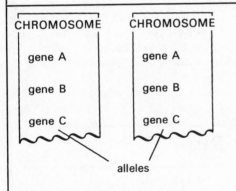

CHROMOSOME	CHROMOSOME
gene A	gene A
gene B	gene B
gene C	gene C

alleles

HOMOZYGOSITY
    alleles identical

HETEROZYGOSITY
    alleles different: only one will express its information (dominant): the other is nonexpressed (recessive)

9-6. MEIOSIS AND MITOSIS

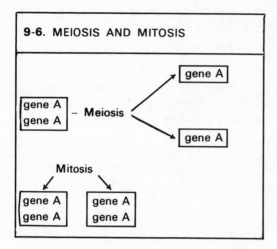

CHROMOSOMES AND KARYOTYPE ANALYSIS

LEARNING OBJECTIVE

To be able to discuss the arrangement of genes into chromosomes and the use of chromosome patterns in karyotype analysis, mentioning the following:

- a) ploidy, autosome, sex chromosome
- b) homologous pairing of chromosomes and its significance
- c) visualization of chromosomes and the karyotype
- d) the Lyon Hypothesis and the Barr body (sex chromatin)
- e) major categories of genetic disease

When a cell divides by mitosis both sets of chromosomes are exactly duplicated (Illustration 9-6), following which they become tightly coiled. At telophase the duplicates are transmitted to 1 daughter cell and the originals remain with the other. At the completion of the mitotic cycle, 2 new diploid cells exist where only 1 had previously been.

Under normal conditions, a daughter cell receives exactly the same set of chromosomes (and genes) that its parent cell possessed before the mitotic cycle began. In this way a whole adult human body is built up from its first single cell and each cell gets a full complement of genetic information.

Each normal diploid human cell contains 46 chromosomes (Illustration 9-7). Of these, 44 are called *autosomes* and exist as 22 homologous pairs whereas 2 are paired only in the female and are called *sex chromosomes* (Illustration 9-8). Sex chromosomes carry a variety of genetic information, only part of which is that determining the sex of an individual. The female possesses 2 of 1 kind called the X chromosome whereas the male has 1 X and 1 Y chromosome.

Note that in the female the sex chromosomes are a homologous pair (XX) while in the male they are not matched (XY). This fact is very important in the understanding of disease states associated with sex chromosome inheritance.

Additional Reading

Dyer, K. F. How man's genes have evolved. Science J. 6:27, 1970

Goldstein, S. Somatic cell genetics. Canad. Med. A. J. 105:738, 1971

McKusick, V. Human genetics. Ann. Rev. Gen. 4:1, 1970

Ochoa, S. The chemical basis of heredity: The genetic code. Bull. N.Y. Acad. Med. 40: , 1964

Shikes, R. H. Heredity, differentiation and development. In Principles of Pathobiology. LaVia, M. and Hill, R. B. Jr. (ed.) Oxford University Press, N.Y., 1971

Whittle, J. R. S. Background genetics. Postgrad. Med. 48:195, 1972

9-7. PLOIDY

SOMATIC CELLS = diploid (2n)

GAMETES   = haploid (n)

- - - - - - - - - - - - - - - - - -

ALSO CONSIDER:

    euploid, aneuploid, polyploid

9-8. CHROMOSOMES OF THE NORMAL HUMAN CELL

1) EACH NORMAL HUMAN CELL IS EQUIPPED WITH

22 pairs, autosomes
1 pair, sex chromosomes

- - - - - -

46 pairs, total (diploid or 2n)

2) AUTOSOMES OCCUR IN HOMOLOGOUS PAIRS: SEX CHROMOSOMES OCCUR AS A HOMOLOGOUS PAIR IN THE FEMALE ONLY

XX = female
XY = male

3) IN CHROMOSOME "SHORTHAND" THE NORMAL HUMAN KARYOTYPE IS EXPRESSED AS:

46, XX   (female)
46, XY   (male)

1. The Karyotype

During the mitotic cycle at the stage following their duplication, chromosomes become tightly coiled preparatory to movement of the 2 exact duplicates (chromatids) into each of the daughter cells. At this stage they can be easily stained and visualized as discrete structures within the nucleus. If a mitotic cell is arrested at metaphase, flattened on a slide and stained, the chromosomes will appear something like that seen in Illustration 9-9.

If these chromosomes are now photographed, cut out and carefully arranged in pairs on the basis of their size and the location of their centromere, the resulting pattern reveals the chromosome complement of the cell and (usually) that of all the cells of the individual from whom it was taken. The pattern of chromosomes so obtained is called the *karyotype* (Illustration 9-10). Karyotype analysis is now used routinely to detect morphologic defects in chromosomes such as abnormalities of number or structure. Defects such as these, known as *cytogenetic defects*, are associated with very serious disease.

2. Significance of Sex Chromosomes

Much is yet to be learned about the function of the sex chromosomes. But, even at this stage of our knowledge, it appears that the X chromosome is far more important as a vehicle of identifiable, specific traits than the Y. In fact, all known heritable features with the exception of male sex characteristics, stature and the possible additional exception of hairy ear rims are carried on the X chromosome.

This puts the male in a decidedly disadvantageous position. He has only one X chromosome and all of its genes must be perfectly functional or he will suffer from a deficiency of some important protein normally supplied by an X-linked gene. The female on the other hand can easily tolerate a recessive (non-functional) gene on one of her X chromosomes, since chances are that its allele on the other member of the pair will be normal and supply as much of the product of that gene as needed.

3. The Lyon Hypothesis

Recently it has become apparent that the X chromosome is unique in even another respect. It has been discovered that, in each somatic cell of the female, 1 X chromosome becomes inactivated. Insofar as any given cell is concerned, it seems to be a matter of chance as to whether the maternal or paternal X assumes this state, but early in the development of the embryo 1 or the other will take over exclusive function and the 1 remaining will undergo condensation and cease to operate. This phenomenon has come to be known as the Lyon hypothesis.

At the time of inactivation, 2 populations of cells arise in the developing female, 1 using maternal X-related genes and the other paternal X-related genes. Further, all progeny of each

9-9. METAPHASE CHROMOSOMES

Cell arrested at metaphase, flattened and stained. Since the mitotic cycle was stopped before the daughter chromosomes separated each unit actually consists of an original chromosome and its exact duplicate (called chromatids at this stage) joined at the centromere.

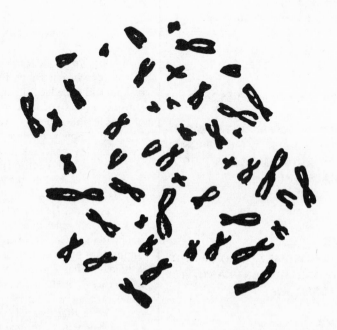

type of cell will maintain the same inactive X (Illustration 9-11).

In effect the normal female is a random mosaic of cells expressing either her father's or her mother's X-related genes. In this way, all genes carried on both X chromosomes are given an opportunity to operate in the female. Some authorities believe that this may account for the female's apparent superior resistance to disease.

4. The Barr Body

At the time of X inactivation in the female, the chromosome to be turned off undergoes condensation and becomes fixed at the periphery of the nucleus. In this position, it can be easily visualized after the cell has been flattened and stained (Illustration 9-12). This little blob of sex chromatin at the nuclear periphery is called the *Barr body* after the investigator who first described its association with sexual differentiation.

A Barr body is easily demonstrated by simply scraping cells from the buccal mucosa, applying them to a slide and staining them. The number of Barr bodies at the periphery of any cell will equal the number of X chromosomes minus 1.

5. Major Categories of Developmental Disease

The whole subject of developmental disease includes information from both the structural and population approach to the gene as well as a great deal from non-genetic teratologic developmental stages. Some genetic defects such as those described above can be visualized, whereas others can only be appreciated through observation of the pattern of their transmit-

9-10. KAROTYPE OF NORMAL MALE (46, XY)

9-11. THE LYON HYPOTHESIS

1) EARLY IN EMBRYOLOGIC DEVELOPMENT OF THE FEMALE 1 X CHROMOSOME OF EACH SOMATIC CELL BECOMES INACTIVATED

   matter of chance as to whether this is maternal or paternal X

2) ALL PROGENY OF A CELL MAINTAIN THE SAME INACTIVE X

3) ERGO: THE FEMALE IS A RANDOM MOSAIC OF CELLS EXPRESSING EITHER MATERNAL OR PATERNAL X

9-12. THE BARR BODY (SEX CHROMATIN)

1) THE INACTIVATED X BECOMES CONDENSED AT THE NUCLEAR PERIPHERY AS THE BARR BODY

2) THE NUMBER OF BARR BODIES = THE NUMBER OF X CHROMOSOMES MINUS 1

9-13. MAJOR CATEGORIES OF GENETIC DISEASE

1) DISEASES CAUSED BY CYTOGE-NETIC DEFECTS

usually quite severe: defect in chromosome number or structure can be demonstrated, manifested congenitally

2) DISEASES CAUSED BY SINGLE-GENE DEFECTS

traceable to single defective gene inherited in a regular Mendelian pattern: congenital or latent

3) POLYGENIC DISEASE

tend to occur with greater frequency in consanguinous groups: based on contributions from several defective genes: congenital or latent

4) TERATOLOGIC DISEASE

congenital defects resulting from improper embryologic development

DISEASES CAUSED BY CYTOGENETIC DEFECTS

LEARNING OBJECTIVE

To be able to compare and contrast additions, deletions, translocations and mosaicism as categories of cytogenetic disease, classifying each of the following as one of the 4 and describing the syndrome, itself, in some detail:

a) Down's syndrome
b) Klinefelter's syndrome
c) the Philadelphia chromosome
d) Turner's syndrome

Cytogenetic defects are abnormalities of the number or structure of chromosomes. They are known to be responsible for a significant amount of disease, most of which results in fetal wastage. Approximately 20 per cent of fetuses dying spontaneously *in utero* have shown cytogenetic abnormalities whereas the incidence among newborns with obvious congenital malformations is about 4 per cent. In infants appearing normal at birth, the corresponding incidence is estimated at 0.5 per cent. Although cytogenetic defects are most often incompatible with life, a few permit the individual to live, usually under severe disability.

It must be emphasized that *most* cytogenetic defects are not inherited diseases; they represent malformations of the chromosome complement based on a mechanical disorder of mitosis, either during gametogenesis in the parent or early embryologic development in the offspring. Patients manifesting cytogenetic defects are commonly the children of normal-appearing parents. One type of cytogenetic defect (translocation) can be inherited, however, and introduces the possibility of the parent acting as a carrier for this disorder.

In general, cytogenetic defects are classified as either *additions, deletions, translocations* or *mosaicism* (Illustration 9-14). We will consider only the first 2 of these. The third, translocations, is significant in that it is the only 1 of the 4 that is commonly passed on from parent to child.

tance. Considering all approaches, the major categories of developmental diseases are those listed in Illustration 9-13. In subsequent learning objectives we will consider each of these disease categories in greater detail.

Additional Reading

Bergsma, D. (ed.) Chicago Conference Standardization in Human Cytogenetics. Birth Defects, Original Article Series. Vol. II (2), Dec., 1966

Davidson, R. G. The Lyon hypothesis. J. Pediat. 65:765, 1964

Redding, A. and Hirschhorn, K. Guide to human chromosomes defects. Birth Defects Original Article Series. Vol. IV (4), Sept., 1968

Sager, R. Genes outside the chromosomes. Sci. Amer. 212:71, 1965

Smith, D. W. Genetic basis for clinical disorder. South. Med. J. 4:(Suppl. 1.) 4, 1971

9-14. CYTOGENETIC DEFECTS

1) ADDITION

　　an extra chromosome (autosome or sex chromosome)

2) DELETION

　　all or part of a chromosome is missing

3) TRANSLOCATION

　　part of one chromosome is found attached to another: some examples are heritable

4) MOSAICISM

　　the individual consists of some cells with cytogenic defects and some without

1. Autosomal Addition Defects

By far, the cytogenetic defect seen most commonly in a *living* human being is the extra chromosome or addition. The only autosomal addition defects compatible with life are single additions of chromosome numbers 13, 18 and 21. The occurrence of a single extra chromosome is called *trisomy*.

Trisomy 21 gives rise to a disease known as Down's syndrome or mongolism, a condition described long before its chromosomal basis was appreciated (Illustration 9-15). The person with Down's syndrome exhibits a characteristic set of features among which are Mongoloid facies, mental retardation and a predisposition to congenital heart disease and leukemia. The incidence of Down's syndrome increases sharply as the maternal age exceeds 40, a trend shown in Illustration 9-16.

Although most cases of Down's syndrome are based on trisomy 21, a small number of

9-15. DOWN'S SYNDROME (TRISOMY G, TRISOMY 21 or MONGOLISM)

9-16. RELATIONSHIP OF DOWN'S SYNDROME TO MATERNAL AGE		
MATERNAL AGE	RISK OF OCCURRENCE	RISK OF RECURRENCE
20–30	1 : 1500	1 : 500
30–35	1 : 750	1 : 250
35–40	1 : 600	1 : 200
40–45	1 : 300	1 : 100
45 up	1 : 60	1 : 20

examples have been described as a result of translocation defects. These latter, of course, can be inherited (50 per cent rate) and are independent of the mother's age. Life expectancy of individuals afflicted with Down's syndrome has been greatly extended through modern therapeutic measures. Approximately one-half die by age 5, usually of pneumonia or heart disease. About 1 in 5 now survive to the age of 30, hence certain individuals with Down's syndrome are fully capable of becoming parents.

2. Sex Chromosome Additions

The presence of additional sex chromosomes occurs with much greater frequency and variety than that of autosomes. All show increased incidences with increasing maternal age and all are compatible with long life. The 3 examples that we will use by no means exhaust the catalog of those reported, but will serve to point out certain features of this type of defect. Because of a pre-empting effect of the Y chromosome on gonadal differentiation whenever a Y chromosome is present, the individual will be phenotypically male regardless of the number of accompanying X chromosomes.

Klinefelter's Syndrome (47, XXY)

Klinefelter's syndrome is the most common of all addition defects. Although male, the individual with Klinefelter's syndrome will be sterile and may exhibit an appearance that ranges from normal to obviously eunuchoid. He is usually somewhat tall and may manifest a degree of gynecomastia. Because of the presence of 2 (or more) X chromosomes the patient with Klinefelter's syndrome will also exhibit a Barr body (Illustration 9-17).

Triplo-X (or Multiple-X) Syndrome (47, XXX)

The individual with 3 or more X chromosomes will be phenotypically female, but will exhibit a high incidence of multiple congenital anomalies. Such an individual may be fertile: however, the syndrome often includes a degree of mental retardation.

XYY Syndrome (47, XYY)

Some investigators believe that a higher incidence of the XYY karyotype is to be found among tall, overly aggressive males with pronounced criminal tendencies. This idea is still somewhat controversial and has received a great deal of attention in recent literature.

3. Autosomal Deletions

The second major category of cytogenetic defects is the deletion, a condition in which all or part of a single chromosome is missing from the karyotype. Like additions, deletions have been demonstrated in autosomes and sex chromosomes: however, the deletion of an entire autosome is apparently not compatible with life. All autosomal deletions found in *living* human beings will be those of the partial deletion type discussed below.

9-17. KLINEFELTER'S SYNDROME (47, XXY)

Cri-du-Chat Syndrome

The Cri-du-chat syndrome is a disorder resulting from the deletion of a short arm of a B-group chromosome. Infants with this condition suffer from both mental and growth retardation, as well as various other malformations. Their cry has a high piercing quality resembling that of a cat, hence the rather fanciful term by which this syndrome is known.

The Philadelphia Chromosome

An unusual example of the deletion of an autosome is seen in the occurrence of the Philadelphia chromosome, a partially deleted autosome 21. The Philadelphia chromosome occurs in individuals suffering from chronic myelocytic leukemia: however, it can be seen only in the neoplastic cells of the actual tumor. It is not seen in normal cells of the host and the condition itself almost never runs in families.

4. Deletions of Sex Chromosomes

Total deletion of the X chromosome is never seen in a living individual, since this condition is incompatible with life. Total deletion of the Y chromosome, however, is tolerated and gives rise to a disease known as Turner's syndrome (45, X).

The individual with Turner's syndrome is phenotypically female, but of short stature and always sterile. She may also exhibit multiple congenital anomalies and, of course, no Barr body will be observed in a buccal smear preparation (Illustration 9-18).

9-18. TURNER'S SYNDROME (45, X)

Additional Reading

Barr, M. L. et al. The triplo-X female. Canad. Med. A.
J. 101:247, 1969

Federman, D. D. Abnormal Sexual Development. W.
B. Saunders Co., Philadelphia, 1968

German, J. Studying human Chromosomes today. Am.
Scientist 58:182, 1970

Parker, C. E. The XYY Syndrome. Am. J. Med.
47:801, 1969

Summitt, R. L. Autosomal abnormalities: A review. G.
P. XXXVI: 96, 1967

SINGLE-GENE AUTOSOMAL DEFECTS

LEARNING OBJECTIVE

To be able to describe inheritance following dominant, co-dominant and recessive autosomal patterns and classify each of the following according to the inheritance pattern manifested, discussing each in some detail:

a) hereditary spherocytosis
b) sickle cell disease and hereditary alpha 1 antitrypsin deficiency
c) phenylketonuria
d) cystic fibrosis
3) Gaucher's disease (as an example of a lysosomal storage disease)

A gene, in addition to serving as a unit of heritance, is actually a tiny protein factory. Each gene performs an indispensable service in the over-all operation of the human body. To maintain health all genes must respond normally, producing a protein that functions adequately as either a structural element or a component of metabolism.

To understand genetic disease, one must first realize that *some genes are defective.* Defective genes either fail to respond to demand signals or do so with the production of a deformed kind of protein. These defective genes may be carried on either autosomes or sex chromosomes; they cannot be demonstrated as chromosomal abnormalities, but they are part of all cells of an individual and will be made part of those of a certain number of the next generation (Illustration 9-19).

Defective genes, like normal genes, are inherited according to Mendelian laws and the pattern of their inheritance is described by specifying their locus and the mode of their expression (Illustration 9-20).

1. Diseases Inherited as Autosomal Dominant Genes

Some genes are always expressed in the phenotype, even if present as a single allele. Such genes are said to be dominant. Many examples of normal protein polymorphism in the human are inherited according to a domi-

---

9-19. DISEASES CAUSED BY SINGLE GENE DEFECTS

1) DEFECTIVE GENES
   not manifested as chromosome abnormalities
   inherited according to Medelian laws

2) INHERITANCE PATTERN DESCRIBED BY SPECIFYING:
   gene locus
   autosomal
   sex-linked
   gene expression
   dominant
   co-dominant
   recessive

9-20. EXPRESSION OF SINGLE GENE DISEASES

1) DOMINANT
   expressed if present
   gene functions well but produces a protein that does not perform optimally
   diseases inherited as dominant traits are usually less severe than those inherited as recessive traits

2) CO-DOMINANT
   expressed to an intermediate degree if present as one allele and full degree if present as both

3) RECESSIVE
   not expressed if dominant allele is present
   represents non-functional gene or gene that synthesizes non-functional protein

nant pattern. Most are carried on autosomes and give rise to innocuous conditions. The "male pattern baldness" and the A and B blood group antigens are examples of such normal polymorphism.

Diseases inherited as dominant genes are those in which the gene produces a protein variant that does not permit the individual to function with a full measure of success. They are usually relatively mild defects, since they are always expressed and have persisted throughout many generations. Obviously, a lethal dominant gene would quickly disappear from a population. An example of a disease inherited as an autosomal dominant gene is *hereditary spherocytosis.*

Hereditary Spherocytosis

Hereditary spherocytosis is an inherited disorder of the erythrocyte membrane. Red blood cells became sphere-shaped, indicating a heightened degree of fragility. Spherocytes are destroyed at an abnormally high rate by the spleen: hence, there is a greater than normal rate of hemolysis. It is especially common in people of northern European origin and usually

---

9-22. HEREDITARY SPHEROCYTOSIS

1) INHERITED DISORDER OF RED BLOOD CELLS BASED ON MEMBRANE DEFECT
   autosomal dominant

2) CELLS ASSUME ROUNDED SHAPE (BICON*VEX* DISC) AND ARE MORE FRAGILE

3) HIGH RATE OF HEMOLYSIS LEADS TO:
   jaundice
   pigment stones in gallbladder
   hyperplastic bone marrow
   reticulocytosis
   splenomegaly

9-21. EXAMPLES OF DISEASES INHERITED AS SINGLE-GENE DEFECTS

1) AUTOSOMAL DOMINANT
   normal protein polymorphism
   structural protein defects
   hereditary spherocytosis

2) AUTOSOMAL CO-DOMINANT
   sickle cell disease
   α_1 antitrypsin deficiency

3) AUTOSOMAL RECESSIVE
   inherited enzyme deficiencies
   PKU and Gaucher's disease
   cystic fibrosis

4) SEX-LINKED RECESSIVE
   hemophilia A

---

manifested first as jaundice and splenomegaly. As in other types of hemolytic anemia, the afflicted individual is predisposed to the formation of pigment gallstones. Splenectomy usually results in permanent remission of this disease: hence, the spleen is now thought to play an active part in its etiology (Illustration 9-22).

2. Diseases Inherited as Autosomal Co-dominant Genes

A co-dominant gene is one that is partly expressed, if present as a single allele, and fully expressed, if present as both. This mode of expression suggests that the product of such a gene is maintained at a critical level by its constant production and that both alleles must be functioning in order to supply this product at an adequate rate. The phenomenon of co-dominance gives rise to the possibility for 2 degrees of disease; if both alleles are defective, the disease will be seen in its most severe form, whereas if only 1 allele is defective an intermediate form will be seen. As our examples of diseases inherited as co-dominant genes, we will consider *sickle cell disease* and *hereditary alpha-1 anti-trypsin deficiency.*

Sickle Cell Disease

Sickle cell disease is a form of hemolytic anemia based on the production of an unusual kind of hemoglobin (hemoglobin S). This hemoglobin differs from normal hemoglobin (hemoglobin A) in the substitution of only a single amino acid in 1 of the 3 chains that make up the protein component of the molecule. Erythrocytes carrying hemoglobin S assume a very distinctive cresent or "sickle" shape when de-oxygenated. Since oxygen is usually transferred from erythrocyte to tissue in capillary-sized vessels, severe sickling leads to vascular obstruction, tissue anoxia, microinfarction and fibrosis. Erythrocytes carrying hemoglobin S are also unusually fragile and exhibit a shorter than normal lifespan. The disease is seen almost exclusively in members of the black race. The patient homozygous for the sickling gene suffers from a very severe disease characterized by anemia and progressive generalized fibrosis. Such individuals usually do not live beyond

---

9-23. SICKLE CELL DISEASE

1) INHERITED DISORDER OF RED BLOOD CELLS BASED ON VARIANT FORM OF HEMOGLOBIN (HbS)

    autosomal co-dominant
    hemoglobinopathy

2) HETEROZYGOUS FORM SEEN IN 8 PER CENT OF BLACK PERSONS: NOT DISABLING

    homozygous form is more rare, severely disabling, results in early death

3) RBC's CARRYING HbS ASSUME BIZARRE SHAPES (RESEMBLING SICKLES) WHEN DEOXYGENATED

    cells are fragile and have shorter lifespan

    sickle cells obstruct microcirculation

---

early adulthood. In the heterozygote about 60 per cent of the hemoglobin will be normal and the disease far less severe. In fact, among West Africans, where this gene seems to have originated, it appears to offer some degree of resistance to malaria (Illustration 9-23).

Alpha-1 Anti-Trypsin Deficiency

Alpha-1 anti-trypsin is a globulin (occurring in the alpha electrophoretic fraction of serum) that inhibits the action of trypsin *in vitro*. The gene directing the synthesis of this protein has been shown to exist in a number of variants that are co-dominant in any combination. Homozygosity for a defective gene can result in an alpha-1 anti-trypsin level of 15 per cent of normal; in the heterozygote this same level will be about half normal. In severe alpha-1 anti-trypsin deficiency a non-specific, chronic pulmonary disease develops at a relatively early age. This disease consists of a primary panlobular emphysema. Females are affected more often than males. Predisposition to pulmonary disease in the heterozygote is less than that seen in the homozygote, but is thought to be still greater than in normal individuals. Very low levels of alpha-1 anti-trypsin have also been associated with the occurrence of peptic ulcers and a form of juvenile cirrhosis.

3. Diseases Inherited as Autosomal Recessive Genes

Diseases inherited as autosomal recessive genes are based on the unfortunate circumstance of being endowed with a double dose of a gene that either does not function or produces a crippled form of protein. In effect, the patient with a disease of this kind is deprived of an enzyme or some other important protein component of his body. Diseases inherited as recessive genes tend to be more severe than those inherited as dominant genes. The responsible gene can be located on either an autosome or the X-chromosome: however, we will defer discussion of the latter until the following learning objective. As our examples of autosomal recessive diseases we will consider *inherited enzyme deficiencies* and *cystic fibrosis*.

Inherited Enzyme Deficiencies

A recessive gene is one that does not function. It may be a mutated control gene that fails to respond to demand signals or a mutated structural gene that produces a non-functional product: but, whatever the reason, the patient inheriting such a gene experiences a deficiency of a single protein. Such deficiencies can cause injury in 2 ways, through the accumulation of a material that would normally have been the substrate of the missing enzyme or through the shortage of a material that would have been its product. In many cases, the accumulation or shortage of this material damages essential tissue and these conditions are often associated with mental deficiency and premature death. Although a number of these kinds of disorders have been described we will use only 2 as examples, *phenylketonuria* and *Gaucher's disease* (Illustration 9-24).

Phenylketonuria is a disease characterized by extreme mental deficiency and the urinary excretion of phenylpyruvic acid. The signs and symptoms of this disease are related to faulty conversion of phenylalanine, a normal component of the diet, to tyrosine due to a lack of the enzyme, phenylalanine hydroxylase (Illus-

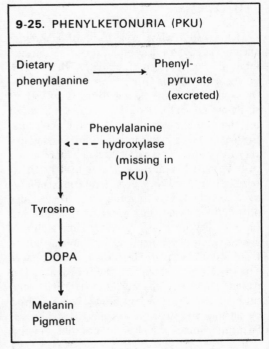

9-25. PHENYLKETONURIA (PKU)

Dietary phenylalanine → Phenyl-pyruvate (excreted)

Phenylalanine ⤎ - - - hydroxylase (missing in PKU)

Tyrosine

DOPA

Melanin Pigment

tration 9-25). The accumulation of phenylalanine is toxic to the brain. The disease is most prevalent among Caucasians where the frequency is reported to be 1 in approximately 20,000 live births. Although rare, this disease results in such severe mental deficiency that all states have now passed some form of legislation requiring a screening program. Treatment consists of the restriction of phenylalanine-containing foods. Patients detected and treated early (less than 1 month of age) will demonstrate an IQ in the range of 80 to 90 whereas untreated phenylketonurics average 67.

Gaucher's disease is an example of the deficiency of a lysosomal enzyme. More than 40 such enzymes have now been identified and deficiency diseases based on 12 of these have been reported. In all such diseases, a lysosomal degradative enzyme is missing and a macromolecular substrate accumulates within secondary lysosomes in certain cells. In Gaucher's disease, a lipid material (kerasin) collects in phagocytic cells. The disease runs a long and comparative benign course of 20 to 30 years, during which time the spleen and liver gradually increase in size due to the accumulation of this material (Illustration 9-26).

9-24. INHERITED ENZYME DEFICIENCIES (INBORN ERRORS OF METABOLISM)

1) BOTH ALLELES ARE NON-FUNCTIONAL OR CODE FOR NON-FUNCTIONAL ENZYME

2) MANY SUCH CONDITIONS ARE ASSOCIATED WITH MENTAL RETARDATION

3) WE WILL USE ONLY TWO OF THE MANY POSSIBLE EXAMPLES
   Phenylketoneuria (PKU)
   Gaucher's disease (as example of lysosomal storage kind of inherited enzyme deficiency)

9-26. GAUCHER'S DISEASE

1) DEFECTIVE GENE OR PRODUCT IN SYNTHESIS OF A SINGLE LYSOSOMAL ENZYME

2) LIPID (KERASIN) ACCUMULATES PRINCIPALLY IN MACROPHAGES (GAUCHER CELLS)

3) HEPATOSPLENOMEGALY, LYMPHADENOPATHY AND BONE LESIONS

4) COURSE OF THE DISEASE MAY BE 20 YEARS OR MORE

9-27. CYSTIC FIBROSIS

1) MOST COMMON AUTOSOMAL RECESSIVE DEFECT OF MAN

2) ACTUALLY A DIFFUSE EXOCRINOPATHY

3) MOST DAMAGING FEATURE IS VISCOUS MUCIN
   mucoviscidosis

4) SYNDROME INCLUDES
   recurrent URT infections
   bronchopneumonia
   obstruction of pancreas
   malabsorption
   male sterility

Cystic Fibrosis

Cystic fibrosis is the most common single autosomal recessive defect of man. It is a generalized condition in which all exocrine glands produce a pathologically altered secretion. The most damaging feature of the disease is the production of a thick, viscid mucin which obstructs ducts and bronchioles. The lungs are usually most seriously involved, but the pancreas, and less commonly the liver and salivary glands, may be affected. A constant feature of this disease is that sweat glands produce a secretion with a greatly increased electrolyte concentration. Deterioration of lung parenchyma secondary to bronchiolar obstruction leads to repeated episodes of bronchopneumonia and is the usual cause of early death. Obstruction of pancreatic ducts leads to cyst formation and pancreatic fibrosis (hence the name of the disease), as well as a serious deficiency of pancreatic secretion. This may lead, in turn, to malabsorption and a deficiency of fat soluble vitamins. The male afflicted with cystic fibrosis is sterile due to obstruction of seminiferous tubules: however, the female is fertile and with modern supportive treatment can live to childbearing age. Features of cystic fibrosis are summarized in Illustration 9-27.

Additional Reading

Berman, J. L. Phenylketonuria. Am. Family Phys. 3:112, 1971

Blaskovics, M. E. and Nelson, T. L. Phenyloketonuria and its variations. Calif. Med. 115:42, 1971

Gordon, H. Mendelian inheritance autosomal patterns. Postgrad. Med. 52:149, 1972

Jaffe, E. R. Hereditary hemolytic disorders. Bull. N.Y. Acad. Med. 46:397, 1970

Pinsky, L. Inborn errors of metabolism: Principles and their applications. Canad. Med. A. J. 106:677, 1972

di Sant' Agnese, P. A. Unmasking the great impersonator—cystic fibrosis. Today's Health, Feb., 1969

Sherwood, L. M. Clinically important variants of human hemoglobin. N. Engl. J. Med. 282:144, 1970

Varpela, E. and Saris, N. E. Hereditary alpha antitrypsin deficiency. Ann. Clin. Res. 3:46, 1971

Westerman, M. P. The common hemoglobinopathies. G. P. 2:86, 1970

SINGLE-GENE
SEX-LINKED DEFECTS

LEARNING OBJECTIVES

To be able to compare and contrast patterns of inheritance exhibited when genes are located on the X chromosome with those seen when the gene locus is an autosome, discussing the following in detail:

    a) differences between the 2 patterns and the reason for these differences

    b) examples of X-linked traits

    c) the syndrome of hemophilia-A

Sex chromosomes differ from autosomes in a number of ways. Although the Y-chromosome carries genetic determinates of male gonadal differentiation and stature, all other sex-linked traits, both normal and abnormal, are carried on the X-chromosome; the X-chromosome functions in sexual determination and carries many genes determining functions unrelated to sex. One region, for example, includes genes for color blindness, hemophilia, and the enzyme, glucose-6-phosphatase dehydrogenase.

Sex chromosomes are homologous only in the female. The female (XX) may be either homozygous or heterozygous for a sex-linked gene, whereas the male (XY) can be only hemizygous. Thus, both good and bad X-linked genes are always expressed in the male; the male transmits his X-linked genes to all of his daughters and there is no father-son inheritance (Illustration 9-28).

About 60 X-linked human genes have been identified. Their association with the X-chromosome is known because of the occurrence of rare non-functional (recessive) alleles which, when present in the hemizygous male, cause a severe developmental or functional disorder (Illustration 9-29). One of the most important of these is *hemophilia-A.*

Hemophilia-A (Illustration 9-30) is an inherited disorder of the intrinsic coagulation mechanism based on the absence of clotting factor VIII. A comparable disease based on the absence of factor IX (Christmas disease or hemophilia-B) is also seen in the male; however, hemophilia-A accounts for 80 per cent of such bleeding disorders. The individual afflicted with

---

9-28. SEX-LINKED INHERITANCE

1) ALL IDENTIFIED TRAITS ARE X-LINKED (NORMAL OR ABNORMAL)
    possible exception is hairy ear rims

2) DOMINANT OR RECESSIVE

3) FEMALE (X-X) MAY BE EITHER HOMOZYGOUS OR HETEROZYGOUS: MALE CAN BE NEITHER (X-Y)
    whether dominant or recessive a sex-linked trait is always expressed in the male

4) NO FATHER-SON TRANSMISSION
    father transmits only Y chromosome to son

5) ABOUT 60 X-LINKED TRAITS IN MAN
    most are abnormal, most recessive

9-29. EXAMPLES OF UNFAVORABLE X-LINKED TRAITS

1) AGAMMAGLOBULINEMIA
    Bruton type

2) HEMOPHILIA-A

3) COLOR BLINDNESS

4) GLUCOSE-6-PHOSPHATASE DEFICIENCY

5) A FORM OF MUSCULAR DYSTROPHY

POLYGENIC DISEASES

+---+
| 9-30. HEMOPHILIA-A |
+---+
| 1) SEX-LINKED RECESSIVE |
| |
| 2) INHERITED DISORDER OF INTRINSIC |
| COAGULATION MECHANISM |
| BASED ON ABSENCE OF FACTOR |
| VIII |
| |
| 3) COAGULATION TIME PROLONGED |
| BUT BLEEDING TIME NORMAL |
| rebleeding phenomenon is seen |
| |
| 4) SEVERE HEMORRHAGE FOLLOWS |
| TRIVIAL INJURY |
| |
| 5) SPONTANEOUS HEMORRHAGE INTO |
| JOINT SPACES (HEMARTHROSIS) IS |
| CHARACTERISTIC SIGN |
+---+

LEARNING OBJECTIVE

To be able to discuss the inheritance of a trait according to a polygenic pattern and describe the implication of this phenomenon in the study of disease, mentioning the following:

a) the recognition of a polygenic component in the epidemiology of a disease

b) some examples of diseases with strong or weak polygenic patterns

---

hemophilia-A has inherited a deleterious X-linked gene from his mother. This gene either produces an inadequate amount of factor VIII or a poorly functioning form of this protein. The effect is to interrupt the intrinsic coagulation cascade, prolonging the time required for clot formation. Since platelet function is unaffected, bleeding will cease within a normal interval following injury: however, with disintegration of the platelet patch and the failure of fibrin formation, bleeding resumes soon thereafter. This phenomenon, characteristic of disorders of the intrinsic coagulation mechanism, is known as "rebleeding." Also typical of hemophilia is prolonged hemorrhage following even trivial injury. Perhaps the most characteristic sign of this condition is the occurrence of spontaneous hemorrhage into joint spaces (hemarthrosis).

Additional Reading

Childs. B. Genetic origin of some sex differences among human beings. Pediatrics 35:798, 1965

McKusick, V. The royal hemophilia. Sci. Amer. Aug. 1965

We cannot see genes; indeed there is some doubt that we would recognize one, even if we could. There are 2 reasons why we have come to think that such a thing as a gene even exists:

1. Some genes exert an all-or-none control over observable characteristics in the phenotype.
2. Each parent organism can possess 2 alternative forms (alleles) of these all-or-none genes and will distribute them in a random way among their progeny.

Traits such as eye color and enzyme deficiencies inherited in this way are called single-gene or monogenic traits. Although they are the easiest to study, they account for only a small number of features, most traits being the result of cooperation among many genes. These latter are known as polygenic traits or, in the case of defects, polygenic diseases. The most interesting of human traits, i.e. physique, intelligence, temperament and the predisposition to disease are all highly polygenic. Man undoubtedly has hundreds of thousands of genes contributing to polygenic traits, whereas only a few hundred are recognized as monogenic.

When a disease (or susceptibility to a disease) is inherited as a polygenic trait, the pattern of its inheritance will not be predictable. At best it might be said to have a "strong" or "weak" tendency to occur among related individuals. Some very common diseases exhibit this polygenic hereditary component (Illustratration 9-31). Inheritance of such conditions depends upon a person's receiving a constellation of many genes from 1 or both of his parents.

9-31. POLYGENIC TRAITS (OR DIS-
EASES)

1) A CHARACTERISTIC (OR DISEASE)
INHERITED AS THE RESULT OF CO-
OPERATION AMONG MANY GENES

2) "STRONG" OR "WEAK" TENDENCY
TO OCCUR AMONG RELATED INDI-
VIDUALS

3) NO PREDICTABLE INHERITANCE
PATTERN

4) SOME COMMON DISEASES EXHIBIT
HEREDITARY (POLYGENIC) PREDIS-
POSITION
    carcinoma of breast
    tuberculosis
    peptic ulcer
    diabetes mellitus

TERATOLOGIC DISEASE

LEARNING OBJECTIVE

To be able to explain the concept of the
teratologic defect, listing several examples of
known teratogens and citing specific examples
of teratologic disease caused by:
    a) drugs
    b) virus

Teratology is the study of factors related to
developmental defects arising *during the embryonic period of development*. Some kinds of
teratologic diseases are inherited, others are
caused by cytogenetic defects and an even
larger group occur as the result of interference
with embryologic development in a genetically
adequate and potentially normal individual.
The last are caused by extrinsic factors and the
agents producing them are called *teratogens*.
    A wide variety of physical agents (ionizing
radiation, trauma, maternal stress, maternal age,
nutritional inadequacy, chemicals, drugs, hormones and infectious agents) have been shown
to act as human teratogens.

9-32. CONGENITAL MALFORMATIONS

1) SOME CONGENITAL MALFORMA-
TIONS EXHIBIT STRONG POLYGENIC
INHERITANCE
2) EXAMPLES:
    congenital heart disease
    fusion defects

Some congenital anomalies of development also
exhibit a polygenic pattern of inheritance
(Illustration 9-32). These include such common
defects as congenital heart disease and cleft
palate.

Additional Reading

Kennedy, W. P. Epidemiologic aspects of the problem
of congenital malformations. Birth Defects Original
Article Series III (No. 2.) Dec., 1967
Neel, J. V. Familial factors in adenocarcinoma of the
colon. Cancer 28:46, 1971

9-33. TERATOLOGIC DISEASE

1) CONGENITAL DEFECT: OCCURS DUR-
ING EMBRYOLOGIC STAGE OF DE-
VELOPMENT
    caused by endogenous (genetic)
    or exogenous factors

2) WIDE VARIETY OF AGENTS CAN ACT
AS TERATOGEN
    most common are:
        intrauterine infections (such
        as rubella)
        drugs (such as thalidomide)

3) RARELY A SINGLE DEFECT

Perhaps the most clearly defined example of intrauterine infection as a teratogen is seen in the relationship between maternal rubella infection and the incidence of congenital abnormalities. The clinical syndrome includes a variety of malformations including congenital heart disease.

But the event providing most impetus to the renewed study of teratology was the recent thalidomide tragedy among European, Japanese and Canadian children. Anomalies of the limbs (phocomelia) were reported to result from use of the drug during the 2-week period of gestation when limb morphogenesis was in process.

Additional Reading

Clegg, D. J. Teratology. Ann. Rev. Pharmacol. 11:409, 1971

Lenz, W. How can the teratogenic action of a factor be established in man? South. Med. J. 64: (Suppl. 1), 41, 1971

Maeck, J. van S. and Phillips, C. A. Rubella vaccine program: Its implications in obstetric practice. Am. J. Obstet. Gynec. 112:513, 1972

Morris, J. M. Postcoital antifertility agents and their teratogenic effect. Contraception 2:85, 1970

Wilson, J. L. Developmental pharmacology: A review of its application to clinical and basic science. Ann. Rev. Pharmacol. 12:423, 1972

liveborn children exhibit developmental disease within the first year of life. The tragedy of developmental disease, as well as emerging prospects for the genetic improvement of the human race, has prompted a renewed interest in human genetic intervention. Proposals have followed 1 of 2 lines of thought. The more conservative suggests a prophylactic approach in an attempt to slow the incidence of developmental anomalies, whereas the more venturesome propose programs of actual "genetic engineering" aimed at improvement of the human race through eugenics.

Either approach, of course, must contend with limitations of the human genetic situation (Illustration 9-34). Almost all contemporary mutations are retrograde and no selective mechanism exists to purge sublethal mutant genes as they occur. Further, genes cannot yet be added or subtracted from the human gene pool directly. At best, given the status of today's technology, our efforts must be confined to those 2 listed in Illustration 9-35.

Although the situation might be favorably influenced by the primary prevention of mutation, the greatest problems will be encountered in the detection and humane containment of

PROSPECTS FOR HUMAN GENETIC IMPROVEMENT

LEARNING OBJECTIVE
To be able to compare and contrast the aims of "genetic engineering" to those of genetic counseling, mentioning the limitations of each and explaining both of the following in some detail:

  a) amniocentesis for the detection of enzyme deficiency or cytogenetic defects

  b) the goals of early detection of genetic disease

Disorders of human development are common examples of disease. Two to 5 per cent of

---

9-34. THE HUMAN GENETIC SITUATION

1) ALL HUMAN GENES EXIST AS SETS WITHIN LIVING MEMBERS OF THE HUMAN RACE (except for the comparatively few haploid sets that are frozen in sperm banks)
   (concept of the gene "pool")

2) ALMOST ALL MUTATIONS ARE RETROGRADE

3) NATURAL SELECTION IS NOT FULLY OPERATIVE IN MODERN SOCIETY

4) GENES CANNOT (YET) BE ADDED OR SUBTRACTED FROM A SET

9-35. AVENUES OF HUMAN GENETIC IMPROVEMENT*

1) PRIMARY PREVENTION OF MUTATION
    radiation hygiene
    suppression of chemical mutagens

2) DETECTION AND HUMANE CONTAINMENT OF DNA LESIONS ONCE THEY OCCUR WITHIN THE GENE POOL
    prospects are viable only for single-gene defects or cytogenetic defects
    even single-gene disease is difficult to detect because of heterozygous state
    screening programs require an enormous investment of time and money

* Joshua Lederberg

9-36. GENETIC COUNSELING

1) DETECTION OF CHROMOSOME ANOMALIES THROUGH SELECTIVE SCREENING

2) IN A FEW CASES THE HETEROZYGOUS CARRIERS OF RECESSIVE MUTATIONS CAN BE DETECTED AND PROSPECTIVE PARENTS ADVISED OF THE RISK
    voluntary avoidance of pregnancy
    monitoring of pregnancy

Know

9-37. LIMITATIONS AND PROBLEMS OF GENETIC INTERVENTION

1) DIFFICULTY IN DETECTING MUTANT GENES AND CYTOGENIC DEFECTS

2) LACK OF UNDERSTANDING OF POLYGENIC CHARACTERISTICS: INABILITY TO INFLUENCE THEM

3) INABILITY TO ADD OR REMOVE GENES FROM HUMAN SETS
    prospect for use of virus is remote

4) SOCIAL AND MORAL LIMITATIONS

bad genes. First of all, one must dismiss entirely (at least for the forseeable future) any prospect for the amelioration of polygenic disease. This leaves cytogenic defects and single gene defects as the only areas in which a reasonable return might be expected for any effort invested.

Since the aim of any such program would be to prevent the occurrence of the genetically disordered individual, heavy reliance would have to be placed upon screening programs intended to detect chromosomal anomalies *in utero* and the heterozygous carriers of recessive mutations (Illustration 9-36). Such programs, in order to be economically feasible, would have to be highly selective. Amniocentesis might be performed on certain high-risk populations of pregnant women whereas inexpensive screening tests might be devised for the more generalized interception of heterozygotes carrying recessive genes for the alpha-1 anti-typsin and cystic fibrosis.

Although the limitations and problems of genetic intervention are formidable (Illustration 9-37), the more limited ambitions or genetic counseling or prophylaxis would constitute a reasonable beginning.

Additional Reading

Davis, B. B. Prospects for genetic intervention in man. Science 170:1279, 1970

Dishotsky, N. I., et al. LSD and genetic damage. Science 172:431, 1971

Gerbic, A. B., et al. Amniocentesis in genetic counseling. Am. J. Obstet. Gynec. 109:765, 1971

Lederberg, J. Genetic engineering, or the amelioration of genetic defects. Pharos of A.O.A. 34:9, 1971

Legator, M. S. Chemical mutagenesis comes of age. W. E. Key Lecture, AIBS Annual Mtg., 1970

Sinsheimer, R. L. Genetic engineering: The modification of man. Impact of Science on Society XX:279, 1970

chapter 10
DISEASES OF THE ENDOCRINE SYSTEM

functioning tumor

THE PITUITARY

LEARNING OBJECTIVE
To be able to describe the location, structure and normal function of the pituitary. To be able to broadly compare and contrast syndromes of pituitary hyperfunctionion and hypofunction using the following diseases as examples:

  a) **the acidophilic tumor and gigantism/acromegaly**
  b) **basophil and chromophobe tumors and Cushing's disease**
  c) **post-partum pituitary necrosis (Sheehan's syndrome)**
  d) **craniopharyngioma**
  e) **diabetes insipidus**

The pituitary is an endocrine gland shaped like a small bean. It is situated at the base of the skull in intimate contact with the primitive brain through the hypothalamus (Illustration 10-1). The pituitary is divided into 2 primary sections, the anterior and posterior lobes, by a smaller intervening layer, the pars intermedia. The anterior lobe differs from the posterior lobe in the nature of the secretion produced. Illustration 10-2 is a list of all pituitary secretions arranged according to their source.

An important concept in understanding pituitary physiology is to realize its strategic location, both anatomically and functionally, between the primitive areas of the brain and the even more primitive endocrine system. In Illustration 10-3, this unique position of the pituitary is represented diagrammatically. Endocrine products stimulated by pituitary tropic hormones exert a feedback control over the pituitary by inhibiting its activity as they reach adequate levels in the circulating blood. Thus, there are 2 means of influencing pituitary activity, through the hypothalamus and

through prevailing blood levels of products of endocrine organs it controls.

As we will do with most endocrine glands, diseases of the pituitary will be considered as diseases of hyperfunction and hypofunction.

1. Pituitary Hyperfunction

Functional cells of the pituitary are classified into 3 principal types: the acidophil (30 to 40 per cent), the basophil (5 to 10 per cent), and the chromophobe (50 per cent). Most diseases based on pituitary hyperfunction result from a functioning tumor and most of these tumors are benign.

The Acidophilic Tumor

Because acidophils normally produce HGH (human growth hormone) a functioning tumor of acidophils is usually associated with either *gigantism* or *acromegaly*. If the tumor occurs in youth while epiphyseal growth centers are still active, the afflicted individual grows to gigantic height. If, on the other hand, it occurs in adulthood after growth centers have closed it results in acromegaly. In acromegaly, enlargement will occur in those areas that are still able to grow in response to hormonal stimulation. Since all such growth, whether normal or abnormal, results from interstitial growth of cartilage, acromegaly is characterized by 3 prominent changes, elongation of the nasal septum, linear growth of the ramus of the mandible and generalized enlargement of the acral (joint) areas of the body. In addition to cartilagenous overgrowth, there is also a coarsening and enlargement of all features of the body due to exaggerated subperiosteal bone growth. Since HGH is diabetogenic the patient in acromegaly will frequently show some degree of insulin resistance, if not overt diabetes mellitus.

Endocrine products exert feedback

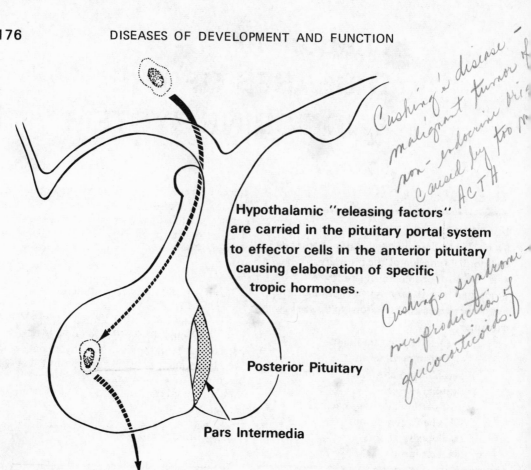

Hypothalamic "releasing factors"
are carried in the pituitary portal system
to effector cells in the anterior pituitary
causing elaboration of specific
tropic hormones.

Posterior Pituitary

Pars Intermedia

*Cushing's disease -
malignant tumor of
non-endocrine origin
caused by too m—
ACTH*

*Cushing's syndrome -
overproduction of
glucocorticoids.*

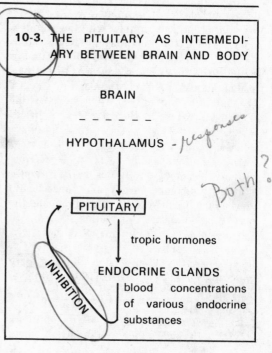

10-2. PITUITARY SECRETIONS

Anterior lobe	Posterior lobe
HGH (STH)	Oxytocin
TSH	ADH (vasopressin)
ACTH*	– – – – – – – –
FSH	MSH (in some species)
LH (ICSH)	
LtH	

     * ACTH has some MSH activity

10-3. THE PITUITARY AS INTERMEDIARY BETWEEN BRAIN AND BODY

BRAIN

– – – – – –

HYPOTHALAMUS *- responses*

Both?

PITUITARY

tropic hormones

INHIBITION

ENDOCRINE GLANDS
blood concentrations
of various endocrine
substances

10-4. DISEASES OF THE PITUITARY

1) HYPERFUNCTION
   acidophilic adenoma
   basophilic adenoma
   some chromophobe tumors

2) HYPOFUNCTION
   chromophobe adenoma
   craniopharyngioma
   other destructive lesions

10-5. PITUITARY HYPERFUNCTION

1) ACIDOPHILIC ADENOMA
   ⬇
   GIGANTISM (growing)
   ACROMEGALY

2) BASOPHILIC ADENOMA
   ⬇
   CUSHING'S DISEASE

Basophil and Chromophobe Tumor

Benign or malignant tumors of pituitary basophil and chromophobe cells are very rare. When they occur they are often associated with a number of clinical syndromes, the characteristics of which depend upon the hormonal products of the neoplasm. Among these is Cushing's disease caused by an overproduction of ACTH. Since ACTH stimulates the adrenal cortex, most of the actual clinical picture of Cushing's disease is due to products of the adrenal and not to those of the pituitary tumor itself. The physical signs of Cushing's syndrome are outlined in Illustration 10-7. Interestingly, it has recently come to light that most spontaneous Cushing's disease is produced not by pituitary tumors but by malignant tumors of non-endocrine origin. The oat-cell carcinoma of bronchial epithelium for example, commonly produces an ACTH-like material that gives rise to the typical picture of Cushing's disease.

2. Pituitary Hypofunction

Pituitary hypofunction results from any of a number of factors that damage or destroy pituitary tissue. A complete list of the more

10-6. CUSHING'S DISEASE

1) First described 1932 by Harvey Cushing: Once incurable and fatal

2) Functional pituitary neoplasm basophilic adenoma) produces excess of ACTH causing overstimulation of adrenal: variety of clinical types

TYPICAL CUSHING'S SYNDROME	spectrum ⟶	ADRENO-GENITAL SYNDROME

10-7. PHYSICAL SIGNS OF CUSHING'S SYNDROME (TYPICAL)

1) "BUFFALO" HUMP

2) OBESITY CONFINED TO TRUNK

3) "MOON" FACE

4) ABDOMINAL STRIAE

5) HYPERPIGMENTATION
   primary ACTH excess

6) NEUTROPHILIA WITH LYMPHOPENIA

7) HYPERTENSION AND DIABETES ARE COMMON

10-8. PITUITARY HYPOFUNCTION

1) ANTERIOR

⇩

PANHYPOPITUITARISM

2) POSTERIOR

⇩

DIABETES INSIPIDUS

hypofunct. of pit
ANS. PREGNANCY & PARTUITION

significant of these would be (Robbins and Angell):

1. Post-partum pituitary necrosis (Sheehan's syndrome)
2. Non-functioning tumors that compress or invade the pituitary
3. Congenital disorders
4. Therapeutic ablation of the pituitary

Since the pituitary is possessed of great functional reserve, most of the gland must be destroyed before a syndrome of insufficiency (panhypopituitarism) is noticed.

Destruction of the posterior pituitary, a relatively uncommon occurrence, gives rise to a syndrome based on the shortage of ADH. Without ADH, the kidneys are unable to concentrate urine and the individual must pass gallons of dilute fluid each day to discharge metabolic wastes. The condition is known as diabetes insipidus (Illustration 10-8).

Additional Reading

Beck, J. S. and Melvin, J. M. O. Chronic adenohypophysitis in a Rhesus monkey immunized with extracts of human placenta. J. Path. 102:125, 1970

Robbins, S. and Angell, M. Basic Pathology. W. B. Saunders Co., Philadelphia, 1971

Welbourn, R. B. et al. The natural history of treated Cushing's syndrome. Brit. J. Surg. 58:1, 1971

DISEASES OF THE ADRENALS

LEARNING OBJECTIVE

To be able to describe the location, structure and normal function of the adrenals and compare diseases resulting from hyperfunction and hypofunction, using the following syndromes as examples:

a) Cushing's syndrome
b) primary hyperaldosteronism (Conn's syndrome)
c) pheochromocytoma
d) Waterhouse-Friderichsen syndrome
e) Addison's disease

The adrenal glands are flattened, humble-appearing structures covering the superior pole of each kidney. Their unimpressive size fails to reflect their critical function in both health and disease; they are absolutely necessary for life and essential for an adequate response to any kind of injury. Each gland consists of 2 parts: the medulla, derived from neural crest and essentially similar to sympathetic nerve tissue, and the cortex, composed of lipid-carrying cells that produce a variety of steroid hormones.

10-9. DISEASE OF THE ADRENAL (EXAMPLES)

1) HYPERFUNCTION
   CORTEX:
   Cushing's syndrome (primary)
   adrenogenital syndrome
   primary hyperaldosteronism
   MEDULLA:
   pheochromocytoma

2) HYPOFUNCTION
   CORTEX:
   Waterhouse-Friderichsen syndrome
   Addison's disease
   MEDULLA:
   not a significant disease

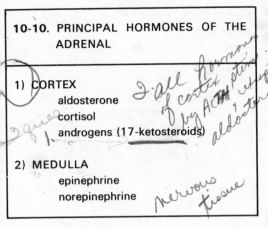

10-10. PRINCIPAL HORMONES OF THE ADRENAL

1) CORTEX
   aldosterone
   cortisol
   androgens (17-ketosteroids)

2) MEDULLA
   epinephrine
   norepinephrine

(handwritten annotations:) I all hormones of cortex given by ACTH except aldosterone / 2 given / 1. / nervous tissue

Whereas the medulla is controlled by sympathetic nerve impulses, the cortex appears to be wholly regulated by humoral factors. Synthesis of all products of the cortex with the exception of aldosterone is stimulated by ACTH.

1. Adrenal Hyperfunction

Cortex

Hyperfunction of the adrenal cortex occurs as a variety of different-appearing clinical conditions, the details of which are dictated by the hormone or hormones being overproduced. Overproduction of glucocorticoids resulting in Cushing's syndrome, for example, occurs most often as the result of overstimulation of the cortex by ACTH of pituitary or extrapituitary origin. Overproduction of aldosterone gives rise to a condition known as primary hyperaldosteronism or Conn's syndrome, in which there is excessive sodium retention, potassium loss and moderate hypertension. This condition most often results from a tumor primary to the adrenal cortex. The third form of adrenocortical hyperfunction, the adrenogenital syndrome, occurs as the side effect of an inherited enzyme deficiency which results in the overproduction of androgens secondary to a failure of the feedback inhibition of the pituitary; it is rarely due to a functioning tumor.

Medulla

A tumor of the adrenal medulla is known as a pheochromocytoma. Most of these will overproduce catecholamines and give rise to severe hypertension. This is one of the few correctable causes of hypertension, the others being a tumor of the cortex producing aldosterone and various diet-related conditions.

2. Adrenal Hypofunction

Cortex

Hypofunction of the adrenal cortex occurs in 2 clinical forms, acute and chronic. It can be seen as the former in cases where trauma destroys a significant portion of the adrenal and in the Waterhouse-Friderichsen syndrome in which there is hemorrhagic destruction of the adrenals associated with meningococcal bacteremia or other forms of septicemia. Acute adrenal failure is manifested as sudden circulatory collapse, prostration and death unless treatment is instituted promptly. Chronic adrenal failure (Addison's disease) is associated with a more protracted kind of adrenal destruction such as one would see in idiopathic atrophy of the adrenal cortex, tuberculosis or metastatic cancer. It is usually first noticed as weakness and fatigability, deepening pigmentation of the skin and oral mucosa and hypotension.

One of today's most common causes of adrenal insufficiency syndromes stems from improper use of adrenocortical steroid analogs as drugs. Long-term therapy with 1 of these agents results in atrophy of the adrenal cortex and dependence upon the exogenous source. Injudicious withdrawal of the drug at this stage can lead to an acute or chronic insufficiency syndrome.

Medulla

Adrenal medullary insufficiency is not a significant disorder.

Additional Reading

Forsham, P. H. Abnormalities of the adrenal cortex. Clinical Symposia, Vol. 15, No. 2. Ciba Pharmaceutical Co., Summit, N. J., 1963

Forsham, P. H. The adrenal gland. Clinical Symposia, Vol. 15, No. 1. Ciba Pharmaceutical Co., Summit, N. J., 1963

(handwritten margin note:) cause hemorrhagic destruction of adrenal

DISEASES OF THE THYROID

LEARNING OBJECTIVE

To be able to describe the location, structure and normal function of the thyroid and compare diseases resulting from hyperfunction and hypofunction, using the following as examples:

- a) Grave's disease
- b) cretinism
- c) myxedema
- d) classification of goiter and its association with thyroid function

10-11. DISEASES OF THE THYROID

1) HYPOFUNCTION

⇨

CRETINISM (child)
MYXEDEMA

2) HYPERFUNCTION

⇨

GRAVES' DISEASE

The thyroid is an endocrine gland located in the neck at approximately the origin of the trachea. It is composed of acinar structures called follicles that are lined by a single layer of cuboidal to columnar epithelium and normally filled with a material called colloid. Also a component of the thyroid is the parafollicular or C. cell, which in recent years has been shown to be the source of calcitonin. The thyroid controls the rate of body metabolism through the secretion of iodine-containing hormones needed for normal physical, sexual and mental development and function. The thyroid responds to a thyrotropic hormone (TSH) from the pituitary and is the only major organ of the body using iodine in any significant quantity. The amount of protein-bound iodine in the blood is directly related to the degree of thyroid activity. As we have done in our treatment of other endocrine glands, we will consider diseases of the thyroid as those of hyperfunction and hypofunction: however, in the case of the thyroid, we must add the additional category of the condition of enlargement known as goiter (Illustration 10-11).

1. Thyroid Hyperfunction

Hyperthyroidism is a condition of increased metabolism and autonomic nervous activity brought on by overproduction of thyroid hormones. It is caused by functional tumors of the thyroid or, more commonly, by an idiopathic primary hyperplasia of the entire thyroid gland. Idiopathic hyperplasia leads to a particularly severe form of hyperthyroidism, usually accompanied by protrusion of the eyes (exophthalmos), a syndrome known as Grave's disease.

Whether or not it is seen as the complete form of Grave's disease, hyperthyroidism will usually be associated with an enlargement of the thyroid (goiter), elevation of body temperature, increased heart rate and systolic blood pressure, intolerance for heat, marked weight loss, extreme irritability and generalized hyperplasia of lymphoid tissue. There is an absolute lymphocytosis, superficial lymph nodes being palpable; the thymus and spleen may be enlarged.

In Grave's disease, there is diffuse lymphocytic infiltration of the thyroid gland, a feature now thought to indicate autoimmune etiology. In most patients with Grave's disease, there is a circulating immunoglobulin of the IgG class which fixes to some component of the thyroid acinar cell and causes long-acting stimulation of mitosis and hormone synthesis. This antibody has come to be known as LATS (long-acting thyroid stimulator).

2. Thyroid Hypofunction

Cretinism

Deficient thyroid function in a newborn child results in a condition known as *cretinism*. No signs of thyroid inadequacy can be noticed at the time of birth, because the child has been maintained *in utero* by the mother's thyroid hormones. The assuming of independent existence causes the child to begin reliance on his own thyroid secretions and, should the gland fail to function properly, cretinism will develop. Cretinism is characterized by failure in the development of the mind combined with an over-all slowing of the processes of growth. The cretin is typically short, mentally incompetent and exhibits coarse hair and facial features. The tongue is enlarged resulting in almost constant drooling. The abdomen is protuberant and the disposition markedly lethargic. It is important that thyroid inadequacy be detected as soon as possible after birth since, if allowed to progress, certain aspects of cretinism, including mental deficiency, become irreversible.

Myxedema

When thyroid hypofunction occurs in the adult the condition is called *myxedema*. The term refers to the fact that interstitial deposition of a gelatinous mucoprotein substance (myx-) occurs within tissues throughout the body. This is accompanied by other signs of hypothyroidism including slowed mental processes, weakness, lethargy, intolerance of cold, coarse hair and enlargement of the tongue with slurring of the speech. In women there is also interruption of the menstrual cycle. Hypothyroidism in the adult may result from destructive inflammatory diseases such as Hashimoto's thyroiditis (to be discussed later) or as primary idiopathic myxedema, in which one sees a more subtle and diffuse lymphocytic infiltration of the thyroid. Both are thought to be of autoimmune etiology and may even be different stages of the same disease.

3. Goiter

Any enlargement of the thyroid is known as *goiter* or *struma*. Goiter occurs in 4 general types as listed in Illustration 10-12.

The colloid goiter is almost always caused by dietary iodine deficiency. It is usually associated with euthyroidism (normal thyroid activity) and is becoming increasingly rare because of the now wide-spread practice of iodizing table salt. This kind of goiter may be diffuse and symmetrical or multinodular and assymetrical, the latter usually being the larger.

A goiter caused by diffuse hyperplasia of the thyroid has been discussed under hyperthyroidism. Bear in mind that this is the type associated with Grave's disease.

Inflammatory enlargement of the thyroid is seen most commonly as Hashimoto's thyroiditis

---

10-12. GOITER (STRUMA)

1) SIMPLE (endemic, iodine deficiency, colloid)

2) DIFFUSE

3) NODULAR

4) INFLAMMATORY
   example: Hashimoto's thyroiditis

5) NEOPLASTIC

(struma lymphomatosa). This disease is characterized by massive lymphocytic infiltration leading to inflammatory destruction of the thyroid. It occurs with 30 times the frequency in women as it does in men. Hashimoto's thyroiditis is often associated with mild hypothyroidism and, indeed, may actually be the very same disease as primary idiopathic myxedema, intercepted in an earlier, more destructive phase. It is generally acknowledged to be an autoimmune phenomenon and the antigens are believed to be thyroglobulin as well as 2 that are cell-associated.

True neoplastic goiters (thyroid tumors) may be either benign or malignant. Benign neoplasms frequently show follicular architecture and are usually functional, whereas the malignant varieties are more often highly cellular and either weakly functional or non-functional. One malignant tumor of thyroid origin, the medullary carcinoma, is thought to take the origin in the parafollicular or C-cells. These tumors may synthesize a variety of endocrine products, among which are calcitonin, ACTH and prostaglandins.

DISEASES OF THE PARATHYROIDS

LEARNING OBJECTIVE

To be able to outline the role of the parathyroids in calcium homeostasis contrasting diseases resulting from hypofunction and hyperfunction, using the following syndromes as examples:

    a) clinical appearance of parathyroid insufficiency

    b) primary hyperparathyroidism

    c) secondary hyperparathyroidism

A constant serum calcium concentration of 10 mg/dl is absolutely necessary for many of the normal processes of life. Among body functions known to be sensitive to calcium ion concentration are the transmission of nerve impulses, the contraction of muscle, the coagulation of blood and the formation of bone and tooth substance. To assure that a proper serum concentration is always maintained the body employs an elaborate calcium control mechanism, one important component of which are the 4 small parathyroid glands located in the neck behind the thyroid. Because of this intimate and exclusive association with calcium homeostasis, diseases of the parathyroid glands are essentially diseases of calcium metabolism. The parathyroid glands respond directly to low blood calcium concentrations by secreting parathormone (PTH). Insofar as is known, the pituitary does not exert any direct control over the activity of these glands.

As discussed in Chapter 3 serum and extracellular fluid are supersaturated with respect to the components of bone mineral. Figuratively speaking, calcium is "pumped" into the general circulation and a calcium "pressure" is maintained in all tissues. This calcium-concentrating mechanism is some common part of a variety of cells that respond to parathyroid hormones. In the kidney, tubular cells resorb calcium from the glomerular filtrate; at the wall of the gut, cells respond by absorbing calcium from food; bone cells answer by resorbing older bone.

1. Parathyroid Hypofunction

If the parathyroid glands are removed or destroyed, the concentration of serum calcium will drop to around 7 mg/dl. Without the parathyroid glands the body has no functioning calcium pump. Tetany is soon seen and death usually ensues in untreated cases. The most common cause of hypoparathyroidism is accidental removal of the parathyroids during thyroidectomy.

2. Parathyroid Hyperfunction

Hyperparathyroidism is classified as either primary or secondary. The former refers to any disease originating in a parathyroid gland that leads to increased output of hormone, whereas the latter denotes diseases originating elsewhere that cause the parathyroids to overproduce PTH.

The most common cause of primary hyperparathyroidism (80 to 85 per cent) is an adenoma of a single gland. These tumors occur at all ages and favor males only slightly. Depending upon size and functional ability they lead to a wide range of clinical manifestations.

Secondary hyperparathyroidism is most often due to chronic kidney disease with failure of calcium resorption from the glomerular filtrate. This leads to chronic blood calcium shortage and constant production of PTH. Whereas the serum calcium concentration will be elevated in primary hyperparathyroidism, it will most often be normal in the secondary disease.

The manifestations of overproduction of PTH, whatever the cause, are referrable to 1 of

---

10-13. DISEASES OF THE PARATHYROIDS *diseases of Ca⁺ metabolism*

1) HYPOFUNCTION

    ▽

    HYPOCALCEMIA
    TETANY

2) HYPERFUNCTION   (primary-secondary)

    ▽

    OSTEOPOROSIS
    OSTEITIS FIBROSA CYSTICA
    von Recklinghausen's disease

2 major effects of this hormone: 1) elevated serum calcium levels (in the primary disease) and 2) bone resorption (in both forms of the disease) (Hypercalcemia may lead to metastatic calcification of the kidneys, blood vessels, lungs and stomach while exaggerated resorption leads to diffuse rarefaction of bones and, in far advanced, severe cases, focal replacement of large areas of bone with soft, hemorrhagic giant-cell lesions. This latter condition is called osteitis fibrosa cystica or von Recklinghausen's disease of bone.)

WRONG ANS.
Something to do c FACE

Additional Reading

Copp, D. H. Endocrine regulation of calcium metabolism. Ann. Rev. Physiol. 32:61, 1970
Haymovits, A. and Rosen, J. F. Calcitonin: Its nature and role in man. Pediatrics 45:133, 1970
Straus, F. H. and Paloyan, E. The pathology of hyperparathyroidism. Surg. Clin. N. Amer. 49:27, 1969

DIABETES MELLITUS

LEARNING OBJECTIVE

To be able to describe the endocrine functions of the pancreas, broadly comparing juvenile and maturity-onset diabetes. With regard to the former, to be able to discuss each of the 4 stages of its progress mentioning the following:

  a) **insulin status of the patient at each stage**
  b) **metabolic manifestations at each stage**
  c) **atherosclerosis and complications**
  d) **microangiopathy, retinopathy and renal changes**

Diabetes is a word that very literally means any condition characterized by the discharge of an excessive amount of urine. The term, diabetes mellitus, denotes this condition with the added feature of the presence of sugar in the urine. Since the single term, diabetes, is now generally accepted to mean diabetes mellitus, we shall use it in such a manner throughout this discussion.

10-14. DIABETES

Any condition characterized by the discharge of excess urine

- - - - - - - - - - - - - - - - - -

DIABETES MELLITUS (sugar diabetes)
DIABETES INSIPIDUS (failure to concentrate urine)

10-15. DIABETES MELLITUS

1) INSULIN DEFICIENCY FORM (JUVENILE OR "BRITTLE")
   onset before 30
   strong hereditary component (presumably polygenic)

2) FUNCTIONAL FORM (ADULT OR MATURITY-ONSET)
   onset usually about 40 but may be later
   higher incidence in female
   obesity appears to be associated
   hereditary component is weak or absent

Despite the very obvious metabolic changes associated with diabetes, the basic nature of the defect in this disease is essentially unknown. Many authorities now believe that the primary cause has very little to do with the metabolic changes and is somehow associated with generalized deterioration of capillary basement membranes.

Diabetes is seen in 2 forms as listed in Illustration 10-15. Insulin-deficiency (hereditary) diabetes starts early in life (before 30) whereas adult or maturity-onset diabetes begins later (usually after the age of 40). The latter is a comparatively mild disease; it usually does not require insulin treatment, nor will it be associated with severe, irreversible lesions. Most of the following description, and particularly that of far-advanced chronic lesions, applies to the juvenile form of this disease.

The pathogenesis of diabetes follows the 4 stages listed in Illustration 10-16.

1. Prediabetes

Prediabetes is the first stage in the pathogenesis of diabetes mellitus. In this stage there is no detectable derangement of glucose metabolism. Some investigators feel that functional or even morphologic changes can be demonstrated in capillary basement membranes at this early stage: however, glucose metabolism is essentially normal. Diabetes is thought inherited according to a polygenic pattern and the genetic component of diabetes is such that a person's liability increases in rough proportion to the number of cases of diabetes in his family group. Thus, if both parents are diabetic, there is an unusually pronounced predisposition to diabetes (50 per cent or higher depending upon criteria), whereas if the family history is negative, there is a greatly reduced risk. The prediabetic, then, would be a person with a strong predisposition who has not yet begun to manifest clinical signs of the disease.

Metabolic change

10-16. CLINICAL STAGES OF DIABETES MELLITUS

1) PREDIABETES

2) SUBCLINICAL DIABETES

3) LATENT DIABETES (chemical diabetes)

4) OVERT DIABETES (acute diabetes)

USUAL TIME OF DIAGNOSIS

5) GRADUAL ONSET OF CHRONIC LESIONS

10-17. PREDIABETES

1) GENETIC PREDISPOSITION BUT NO OVERT METABOLIC SIGNS

2) NO ABNORMALITY OF GLUCOSE TOLERANCE

Note: The results of some investigations would suggest that the microvascular disease that will later develop into the typical lesions of chronic diabetes is often detectable at this very early stage

---

2. Subclinical Diabetes

The assigning of stages to the natural history of diabetes must, of necessity, be arbitrary. The onset of the second stage of diabetes is usually accepted as being heralded by the appearance of abnormalities in glucose metabolism. Such abnormalities can only be detected through the use of the glucose tolerance test while the individual is either pregnant or under stress (spontaneous or simulated through the use of exogenous glucocorticoid).

3. Latent Diabetes (Chemical Diabetes)

In the third stage of the pathogenesis of diabetes, an abnormality of glucose metabolism can be detected by the glucose tolerance test *without* stress or pregnancy. The fasting blood sugar is usually normal, but may be slightly elevated.

4. Overt Diabetes (Acute Diabetes)

In the fourth stage, the patient manifests unprovoked signs of abnormal glucose metabolism. There is persistent hyperglycemia, glycosuria and ketosis in the untreated case. The patient must be supplied with exogenous insulin at this stage, as he is now beginning to show a constant effect of the slow destruction of his insulin-producing cells. Throughout the course of the disease to this stage the pancreatic islets have been undergoing gradual deteriora-

<table>
<tr><td>

10-18. SUBCLINICAL DIABETES

1) NO OVERT METABOLIC SIGNS

2) ABNORMAL GLUCOSE TOLERANCE IS DETECTABLE *ONLY WHEN PREGNANT OR UNDER STRESS*

    stress may be simulated by administration of adrenocortical hormone or analog

</td><td>

10-19. LATENT DIABETES (CHEMICAL) DIABETES

1) NO OVERT METABOLIC SIGNS

2) ABNORMAL GLUCOSE TOLERANCE DETECTABLE AT ANY TIME

    without stress or its hormonal simulation

</td></tr>
</table>

tion and have been replaced with hyaline and fibrous tissue; the effects of this are now observable as a critical shortage of insulin.

Without insulin, cells that normally consume most circulating blood glucose are no longer able to do so. This leads to an increased blood sugar level and the mobilization of fat for use as an energy source. Fat mobilization leads to ketosis (accumulation of ketones), while the high level of blood sugar "spills over" into the urine as glycosuria. These 3 signs (hyperglycemia, ketosis and glycosuria) as shown in Illustration 10-19 are the cardinal signs of diabetes. At this same time the patient begins to notice excessive urination, weight loss and an exaggerated tendency to eat and drink. Because of these now-obvious metabolic changes most diabetes is first seen by the physician at this stage.

5. Chronic Lesions of Diabetes

Characteristic of juvenile diabetes is the comparatively early onset of chronic disease. Most of the chronic lesions of diabetes are traceable to the deterioration of blood vessels. These blood vessel changes can be roughly classified as either *atherosclerotic* or *microangiopathic* (Illustration 10-20).

Atherosclerosis in Diabetes

In the chronic diabetic, atherosclerosis and its usual complications (ischemic heart disease, cerebral vascular disease, peripheral vascular insufficiency and aortic aneurysm) show an earlier onset and a more severe course than in the non-diabetic. This condition as seen in the

---

10-20. OVERT DIABETES (ACUTE DIABETES)

1) OVERT METABOLIC SIGNS (UNPROVOKED)

    hyperglycemia
    ketosis
    glycosuria

2) USUAL TIME OF DIAGNOSIS

    polyuria
    polydipsia
    polyphagia
    weight loss

3) CHRONIC LESIONS OF DIABETES SHOW GRADUAL ONSET FOLLOWING THIS STAGE

NOTE: It is not clear whether chronic lesions are the result of the metabolic imbalance or if they are of other etiology

---

diabetic is not qualitatively different, but appears earlier and exhibits more severe complications.

Microvascular Disease in Diabetes

One of the most distinctive of the vascular lesions of diabetes is that occurring in capillary and pre-capillary-size vessels. Although this

10-21. CHRONIC LESIONS OF DIABETES

1) APPEARANCE OF IRREVERSIBLE TISSUE CHANGES

2) PRINCIPAL SITES
   blood vessels
   kidneys
   eyes
   peripheral nerves

10-22. BLOOD VESSEL DISEASE IN DIABETES

1) LARGE VESSELS: Exaggerated atherosclerosis of early onset leading to:
   myocardial infarct
   CVA
   peripheral vascular insufficiency
   aortic aneurysm
   hypertension

2) MICROVASCULATURE
   diabetic macroangiopathy—gradual widening of capillary basement membranes

10-23. MICROVASCULAR DISEASE IN DIABETES

1) DIABETIC RETINOPATHY

2) DIABETIC GLOMERULOSCLEROSIS
   diffuse sclerosis
   K-W disease

3) GENERALIZED CAPILLARY DISEASE
   basement membrane thickening

condition may be found in the non-diabetic, it is described as being of very early onset (pre-diabetics may show it) and more generalized distribution (all tissues except fat) in the diabetic. It takes the form of hyaline thickening of the basement membranes and accounts for destructive changes in the kidneys, eyes and other organs. Microvascular lesions in the kidneys are seen as diffuse and nodular sclerosis of the glomerulus leading to renal failure. The incidence of eye lesions correlates closely with those of the kidney and are seen as basement membrane thickening, microaneurysms and fibrosis of the retina and other parts. Advanced lesions of the eye lead to blindness.

As recently as 1920, the diagnosis of diabetes meant premature death from metabolic imbalance. With the advent of insulin therapy control of the metabolic disorder became possible and the person with diabetes was granted additional decades of productive life. Today, 75 to 80 per cent of mortality in diabetes results from vascular disease of the heart, kidneys or extremities. Although insulin is still indispensable in the metabolic defect in juvenile-onset diabetes, there is no evidence that it retards vascular deterioration. In fact, the relationship between pancreatic islet cell destruction and vascular deterioration has not yet been definitely established. It is tempting indeed to consider that both of these changes might be caused by some yet-undiscovered factor which is the true ultimate cause of the disease.

Additional Reading

Barker, W. F. Peripheral vascular disease in diabetes. Med. Clin. N. Amer. 55:1045, 1971

Fajans, S. F. What is diabetes? Med. Clin. N. Amer. 55:793, 1971

Felig, P. Pathophysiology of diabetes mellitus. Med. Clin. N. Amer. 55:821, 1971

Mann, R. J. "Honey urine" to pancreatic diabetes: 600 B.C.-1922. Mayo Clin. Proc. 46:56, 1971

Rimoin, D. L. Inheritance in diabetes mellitus. Med. Clin. N. Amer. 55:807, 1971

Trautmann, J. C. and Kearns, T. P. Diabetes and the eye. Postgrad. Med. 45:133, 1969

Williamson, J. R. et al. Microvascular disease in diabetes. Med. Clin. N. Amer. 55:847

Pit. — acromegaly & giantism / Hyper
diabetes — hypo

Adrenals — adrenogenital syn.
Cushing's syndrome
Conn's syndrome
Addison's
Waterhouse-Friedrickson

Thyroid - Grave's - hyper
Cretinism > hypo
myxedema

Parathyroid - tetany - hypo
osteoporosis, osteitis fibrosa / hyper
Von Recklinghausen's disease

chapter 11
NUTRITIONAL DISEASE

THE INADEQUATE DIET IN EARLY LIFE

LEARNING OBJECTIVE

To be able to compare and contrast effects of nutritional inadequacy in the child and adult, using the following syndromes as examples of the former:

a) kwashiorkor
b) nutritional marasmus
c) rickets (calciferol deficiency)
d) infantile scurvy (ascorbic acid deficiency)

11-1. NUTRITIONAL DISEASE

1) INADEQUATE DIET
   in early life during growth and development
   in adult life
2) MALABSORPTION
   pancreatic insufficiency
   acholia
   parasitism
   enterogenous factors
3) FAILURE OF RETENTION OR UTILIZATION
   repeated vomiting
   renal disease
   enteropathy
   inherited enzyme deficiency
   metabolic inhibition

Diseases associated with nutrition are among the most difficult to eradicate, even though most respond readily to simple alterations of the diet. The reason is that, outside the laboratory, most are linked to political, cultural or emotional problems that require more complicated treatment than the simple manipulation of food intake. Malnutrition, for example, is a problem of somatic health, but the conditions of poverty and ignorance that usually cause it are signs of a malfunctioning society. Obesity is clearly an organic nutritional problem, but the compulsion to over-eat is based on neurotic needs that have little to do with what is eaten. For almost every bona fide nutritional disease there is a contributory factor somewhere in the patient's social or emotional status and the disease is usually shared by others of the same status. Perhaps it will eventually be found that this is also true of most other diseases, but the relationship to nutritional disease is obvious (and frustrating) even today.

Our first category of nutritional disease is that of inadequacy. Nutritional inadequacy can result from a number of quite different causes (Illustration 11-1), many of which we will mention in subsequent learning objectives. Malnutrition during any of the stages of early development or childhood leads to more severe consequences than a comparable condition in the adult. The child needs food to grow as well as function. He passes through brief intervals of life during which proper nutrition permits full development, whereas deprivation results in delayed maturation or perhaps even permanent damage. Severe malnutrition during pregnancy, for example, can result in fetal death, premature parturition or, at the very least, a small, poorly developed infant. Serious malnutrition during childhood is known to produce delayed physical maturation and smaller adult size and may even result in irreversible impairment of the mind.

Several distinct syndromes are seen in the severely undernourished child (Illustration 11-2). We will consider each in the order presented.

1. Kwashiorkor (Protein Starvation in Infancy)

Kwashiorkor (protein starvation in infancy) is seen among impoverished people of developing countries. It occurs mainly in children, 1 to

---

11-2. THE INADEQUATE DIET IN EARLY LIFE

1) KWASHIORKOR
   protein starvation in infancy

2) NUTRITIONAL MARASMUS
   calorie starvation in infancy

3) RICKETS
   calciferol deficiency

4) INFANTILE SCURVY
   ascorbic acid deficiency

11-3. KWASHIORKOR

1) FAILURE TO GROW

2) SKIN RASH, GRAYING OR REDDEN-ING OF HAIR

3) FATTY DEGENERATION OF LIVER
   hepatomegaly *— enlargement of liver*

4) HYPOPROTEINEMIA
   edema
   ascites *— most prominent sign*

5) ANEMIA

6) DIARRHEA

7) APATHY AND EXTREME WEAKNESS
   SHOCK IN ADVANCED STAGES

---

3 years of age, whose diets are grossly deficient in protein. The most common circumstances are those in which a child is weaned from breastmilk to a starchy staple food such as bananas, which, although adequate in calories, is devoid of protein. The usual signs of kwashiorkor are listed in Illustration 11-3. Shock is always a danger in advanced cases, but response to protein therapy is prompt and complete. Incidently, the term is taken directly from the African Ga dialect words for "first" and "second" where it is intended to mean a disease of the first child when he is displaced from the breast by the second.

2. Nutritional Marasmus

lack of food

In contrast to kwashiorkor, nutritional marasmus is usually seen in children under 1 year of age. It is common in nearly all developing countries and most often based on the simple lack of food. It may begin with premature cessation of breast feeding due to death of the mother, but more often it is simply the mother's desire to bottle-feed the baby because of her impression that this method is more advanced or sophisticated. Over-dilution of the formula in an effort to stretch a meager income leads to underfeeding of all nutrient material and incipient starvation. Gastrointestinal infection because of poor hygienic measures in *diarrhea* the preparation of the formula is a common complication at this stage and the infant slips rapidly into severe nutritional marasmus.

11-4. NUTRITIONAL MARASMUS (CAL-ORIE STARVATION IN INFANCY)

1) FAILURE TO GROW

2) WASTING

3) USUALLY COMPLICATED BY INTESTI-NAL INFECTION AND MULTIPLE VI-TAMIN DEFICIENCIES

---

3. Rickets (Calciferol Deficiency in Childhood)

Although rickets or its adult counterpart, osteomalacia, are widely regarded as nutritional inadequacies resulting from the lack of vitamin D, there are perhaps better reasons for considering them hormonal deficiencies. Calciferol is actually a hormone produced by the skin through ultraviolet radiation of 7-dehydro-cholesterol. The skin liberates calciferol into the blood stream when exposed to ultraviolet light. When children are kept out of sunlight, they will suffer a deficiency of this skin hormone. In this sense, then, rickets is more of

hormonal deficiencies

a deficiency of sunlight than it is a dietary problem.

Although calciferol is the natural hormone produced by irradiated skin, it is not the only sterol that will work. Several products of irradiated plant sterols will perform quite well in place of calciferol and can be administered in the diet. These are known collectively as vitamin D. Technically, of course, vitamin D is not really a vitamin, since it compensates for the lack of a hormone and is not an essential component of the normal human diet. The value of seeing this disease in its true prospective is more than just one of scientific precision. Indeed, the relationship between human migrations of prehistory, skin pigmentation and calciferol production could be such that it will someday add a whole new insight to our appreciation of the racial differentiation of mankind.

Calciferol promotes the transport of calcium across intestinal epithelium into the blood stream. It is absolutely necessary to assure an adequate rate of calcium absorption. The child with rickets cannot absorb calcium from his food and is actually suffering from a shortage of body calcium, regardless of the amount ingested in the diet (within limits). The principal signs of the disease are the skeletal changes listed in Illustration 11-5. Others, such as slow growth and gastrointestional disturbances are also present, but, by in large, the rachitic child appears healthy and well nourished.

4. Infantile Scurvy (Ascorbic Acid Deficiency in Infancy)

Scurvy is a disease resulting from the dietary deficiency of vitamin C (ascorbic acid). Like other nutritional deficiencies syndromes, it is more common and far more severe in the growing child than in the adult. Ascorbic acid is a factor necessary for the synthesis of collagen and its associated mucopolysaccharides. As could be predicted, the effect of such a fundamental disorder is disastrous, particularly in the rapidly growing infant. Capillary walls become exceedingly fragile and connective tissue structures begin to deteriorate. A list of the prominent signs of infantile scurvy is provided in Illustration 11-6. The pain associated with subperiosteal hemorrhage is said to be the most prominent sign of this disease.

11-5. RICKETS (CALCIFEROL DEFICIENCY IN THE GROWING CHILD)

1) CALCIFEROL OR VITAMIN D ENHANCES INTESTINAL ABSORPTION OF CALCIUM AND PHOSPHORUS

2) CALCIFEROL DEFICIENCY
   rickets (childhood)
   osteomalacia (adult)

hormone produced by skin

3) GENERALIZED ACCUMULATION OF UNCALCIFIED BONE MATRIX

4) RICKETS IS MORE SEVERE BECAUSE OF GROWTH COMPONENT
   swelling of longbone epiphyses
   swellings at costochondral junctions ("rachitic rosary")
   softening of skull (craniotabes)
   generalized osteoporosis with frequent bowing of legs

irradiated plant sterols

11-6. INFANTILE SCURVY (ABSCORBIC ACID DEFICIENCY IN THE INFANT)

1) WIDESPREAD HEMORRHAGES
   petechiae
   epistaxis
   hematuria
   melena

2) TENDERNESS OF LIMBS DUE TO PAINFUL SUBPERIOSTEAL HEMORRHAGE

3) ANEMIA — *because of hemorrhage*

4) FAILURE OF HEALING — *inability to synthesize tropocollagen*

5) TENDENCY TO CARDIAC FAILURE AND SUDDEN DEATH

form interstitial cement substance of endothelial membrane

Although it is rarely seen in either form today, infantile scurvy is more common than its adult counterpart. It tends to occur in infants 2 to 12 months of age who are bottle fed with a formula containing little or no vitamin C. Recovery is usually complete when vitamin C therapy is instituted, but, as in the case of other such diseases, relapse can be prevented only by correcting the environmental conditions that led to the original disease.

Additional Reading

Arbeter, A. et al. Nutrition and Infection. Fed. Proc. 30:1421, 1971

Barnes, R. H. Nutrition and man's intellect and behavior. Fed. Proc. 30:1429, 1971

Cravioto, J. and De Licardie, F. The long-term consequences of protein-calorie malnutrition. Nutrition Rev. 29:107, 1971

Kallen, D. J. Nutrition and society. J. Am. Med. Assn. 215:94, 1971

Latham, M. C. Scope manual on nutrition. Kalamazoo, The Upjohn Co., 1970

Loomis, W. F. Rickets. Sci. Amer. 223:77, 1970

Majumder, S. K. Vegetarianism: Fad, faith or fact. Am. Scientist 60:175, 1972

Turner, J. S. The Chemical Feast. New York, Grossman, 1970

Weick, M. T. A history of rickets in the United States. Am. J. Clin. Nutrit. 20:1234, Nov., 1967

VITAMIN MALNUTRITION

LEARNING OBJECTIVE

To be able to compare and contrast disease states resulting from deficiency and over-sufficiency (where applicable) of the following vitamins:
    a) **vitamin A**
    b) **vitamin K**
    c) **vitamin B$_1$ (thiamine)**
    d) **niacin (nicotinic acid)**
    e) **vitamin B$_{12}$ (cyanocobalamin)**

In considering vitamin nutrition as the basis for disease, one must be mindful of the possibility for 2 conditions, deficiency (hypo-

---

11-7. VITAMINS IN NUTRITION

1) DEFICIENCY
    avitaminosis

2) OVERSUFFICIENCY*
    hypervitaminosis

– – – – – – – – –

*(Only significant for lipid soluble vitamins)

---

vitaminosis or avitaminosis) and over-sufficiency (hypervitaminosis). Illustration 11-7 summarizes this concept. Note that hypervitaminosis is significant only in the case of lipid-soluble vitamins; these can accumulate in the body to toxic levels whereas excess water-soluble vitamins are simply "washed out" as urinary solutes.

Lipid or fat-soluble vitamin toxicity may occur as either an acute episode or a chronic, habit-related disease. The chronic form is often associated with the ill-advised therapeutic use of one of these agents. In this learning objective we will consider only a few of the many possible diseases associated with vitamin deficiency and toxicity states.

1. Vitamin A

Vitamin A is a fat-soluble substance that is absolutely essential for maintaining the integrity of highly specialized epithelium and for normal growth and health. Incipient deficiency of this vitamin is experienced as gradual failure of night vision but, since the human liver stores enough vitamin A for approximately 1 year, the more advanced signs of hypovitaminosis A are quite slow in onset and occur much later than night blindness.

One of the most striking signs of the serious deficiency of vitamin A is metaplasia of highly specialized epithelium to the more resistant stratified squamous type. One also sees overproduction of keratin by epithelia that are normally stratified squamous, but are not given

2. Vitamin K

Vitamin K is a lipid-soluble substance necessary for the synthesis of clotting factors II ✳ (prothrombin), VII (stable factor), IX (Christmas factor) and X (Stuart factor) by the liver. Although found in almost all human foods, it is present in such extremely small amounts that dietary sources alone cannot provide adequate maintenance. The most significant source of ✳ vitamin K in human nutrition is that synthesized by gastrointestinal flora.

Because the gut of the newborn is sterile, the very young infant has no primary source of vitamin K. It is now generally believed that this accounts for most cases of fatal intracranial hemorrhage seen in the perinatal period, especially in premature infants. In the adult, vitamin K deficiency results from any of a number of conditions that cause failure to absorb fats and their subsequent excretion in the stool (steatorrhea). A deficiency-like syndrome in the adult results from the use of ✳ vitamin K analogs as anticoagulant drugs. Such drugs are often used to prevent recurrent thrombosis in patients recovering from myocardial infarction.

Being a lipid-soluble vitamin there is the usual potential for toxicity and, indeed, excessive doses of synthetic vitamin K have been reported to lead to hemolytic anemia and kernicterus in the infant.

Characteristics of vitamin K-related syndromes are outlined in Illustration 11-9.

3. Vitamin B₁ (Thiamine)

Thiamine is a water-soluble substance that functions in the conversion of carbohydrates to energy. The body is unable to store thiamine and a continued dietary supply is necessary for health. It is found in human foods of both animal and vegetable origin, but is easily destroyed by pressure cooking or frying. The most prominent spontaneous example of serious thiamine deficiency is the disease, *beriberi*. It occurs almost exclusively among rice-eating peoples of the world. Actually, the outer coat of the rice grain would act as a rich source of thiamine, but this is discarded in the refining process and only the starchy inner grain is eaten. Attempts to subsist on unsupplemented

---

11-8. VITAMIN A

1) LIPID SOLUBLE

2) ESSENTIAL FOR EPITHELIAL INTEGRITY

3) AVITAMINOSIS

   squamous metaplasia of colum. and trans. epithelium

   - - - - - - - - - - - -

   follicular keratosis

   - - - - - - - - - - - -

   1. night blindness, earliest change

   - - - - - - - - - - - -

   xerophthalmia, keratomalacia, loss of sight

4) HYPERVITAMINOSIS
   acute and chronic

[handwritten annotations: drying of eye; corneal & conjunctival membrane becomes inflected + ulcerated]

---

to the production of a horny surface. The most disturbing effects of advanced vitamin A shortage are seen in the eye as *xerophthalmia* (dry eye). In untreated cases, this leads to *keratomalacia*, in which the abnormally keratinized corneal and conjunctival membrane becomes ulcerated and infected. Deterioration to this stage is irreversible and the person will be blind in the affected eye. Keratomalacia is almost unknown in more technologically advanced nations, but is a common cause of blindness in Asia and the Middle East where it is usually associated with nutritional marasmus.

The medical literature contains 17 case reports of chronic vitamin A intoxication, most resulting from the administration of large doses over protracted periods for the management of a variety of dermatologic conditions. In all cases, there is a typical erythematous rash accompanied by increased intracranial pressure, bone pain, fatigue and anorexia.

[handwritten: acute Vₐ toxicity rare]

11-9. VITAMIN K

1) LIPID SOLUBLE

   principal source is intestinal bacteria—*not diet*

2) ESSENTIAL FOR HEPATIC SYNTHESIS OF CLOTTING FACTORS II, VII, IX, X

3) DEFICIENCY LEADS TO COMPLEX COAGULATION DEFECT AND HEMORRHAGIC DIATHESIS (MOST COMMON CAUSE OF CEREBRAL HEMORRHAGE IN THE NEWBORN)

4) DEFICIENCY RESULTS FROM: lack of intestinal bacteria (infant), ingestion of inhibitor substance, failure to absorb lipid (steatorrhea), as seen in:

   sprue
   celiac disease
   cystic fibrosis
   idiopathic steatorrhea

11-10. VITAMIN B$_1$ (THIAMINE)

1) ESSENTIAL FOR OXIDATIVE METABOLISM *muscular weakness + heart failure*

2) DEFICIENCY SEEN MOST COMMONLY AS BERIBERI AMONG RICE-EATING PEOPLE

3) SIGNS INCLUDE

   peripheral neuritis   *WERNICKE-*
   extreme weakness   *KORSAKOF SYN*
   enlargement and gradual failure of heart

11-11. VITAMIN B$_2$ (RIBOFLAVIN)

1) ESSENTIAL FOR OXIDATIVE METABOLISM

2) PURE RIBOFLAVIN DEFICIENCY IS RARE

3) SIGNS INCLUDE

   stomatitis
   angular cheilosis
   burning of eyes
   failure of vision
   atrophic glossitis

---

diet of refined rice leads to the rapid onset of beriberi.

A second example of thiamine deficiency is seen in alcoholism and known as the *Wernicke-Korsakoff syndrome*. Although it does not resemble beriberi in detail, both conditions respond readily to treatment with thiamine.

Classical beriberi begins with the gradual onset of lethargy and extreme muscular weakness. Signs of cardiac failure are common and ankle edema may be seen very early in the course of the disease. Peripheral neuritis is also present. The untreated case progresses to generalized edema, prostration and death from circulatory collapse. The syndrome shows a startling response to thiamine, the edema usually clearing within a few days. Thiamine deficiency is outlined in Illustration 11-10.

4. Vitamin B$_2$ (Riboflavin)

Although known to be essential for oxidative metabolism, riboflavin deficiency is rarely encountered as an uncomplicated spontaneous human disease. The signs of riboflavin deficiency are usually seen as part of a dietary problem involving the entire B complex. Riboflavin deficiency leads to an erosive stomatitis with fissuring lesions at the corners of the mouth (angular cheilosis). Atrophy of the lingual mucosa leads to a reddish appearing painful tongue (atrophic glossitis). Other signs include a scaling dermatitis distributed over the face and eye changes manifested as a burning sensation with gradual failure of vision. Characteristics of riboflavin deficiency are outlined in Illustration 11-11.

inflam of mout

5. Niacin (Nicotinic Acid)

Just as thiamine deficiency is linked to a diet of refined rice, a deficiency of niacin is seen where the diet consists primarily of corn. Niacin deficiency leads to the disease, pellagra, a condition once quite common in the southern United States and Mexico.

Niacin and its amide are water-soluble vitamins present in many human foods of both vegetable and animal origin; the human body enjoys an additional source in that it is able to convert the amino acid, tryptophan, to niacin. Although corn contains some niacin, it is present in a bound form and unavailable for absorption. Since corn contains very little tryptophan, both sources of niacin are denied a person subsisting largely on a corn diet.

The disease, pellagra, is conveniently summarized in the three "D's," dermatitis, diarrhea and dementia. Skin lesions occur on areas of the body exposed to sunlight and, when fully developed, appear as dry, scaly, cracked or fissured areas. Frequently, the lesions of pellagra are seen in conjunction with those of riboflavin deficiency in which angular cheilosis, stomatitis and an enlarged, red, painful tongue (atrophic glossitis) may be seen.

Digestive signs of pellagra include abdominal pain and diarrhea, while alteration of nervous function may be manifested as anxiety, emotional instability, loss of memory or even frankly demented behavior. At one time it was common for victims of pellagra to be mistakenly committed to mental institutions.

Niacin deficiency is summarized in Illustration 11-12.

6. Vitamin B$_{12}$ (Cyanocobalamin)

Vitamin B$_{12}$ or cyanocobalamin is a water-soluble, cobalt-containing substance that functions in metabolic reactions in which chemical groups are reduced. It is essential for the metabolism of all cells, but particularly cells of the bone marrow. In the human diet, it is obtained primarily from food of animal origin and a significant amount can be stored by the liver.

A peculiar feature of vitamin B$_{12}$ metabolism is that it cannot be absorbed directly from food without the presence of a material secreted by stomach epithelium called "intrinsic factor" (Illustration 11-13).
of Castle

11-12. NIACIN (NICOTINIC ACID)

1) ESSENTIAL FOR OXIDATIVE METABOLISM

2) DEFICIENCY SEEN AS PELLAGRA AMONG PEOPLE SUBSISTING LARGELY ON CORN

3) CHARACTERISTIC THREE "D'S"
   dermatitis
   dementia — ? _disturbed pattern of behavior_
   diarrhea

11-13. VITAMIN B$_{12}$ (CYANOCOBALAMIN)

1) ESSENTIAL FOR MATURATION OF ERYTHROCYTES AND FUNCTION OF PERIPHERAL NERVOUS SYSTEM

2) DEFICIENCY SEEN AS PERNICIOUS ANEMIA _& peripheral neuritis_

3) ACTUALLY A FAILURE TO ABSORB B$_{12}$ DUE TO LACK OF "INTRINSIC FACTOR" OF CASTLE (normally secreted by stomach) _mucoprotein_

So long as intrinsic factor is produced by the stomach, adequate amounts of vitamin B$_{12}$ are absorbed. Should the production of intrinsic factor be discontinued, absorption of vitamin B$_{12}$ stops and, when liver stores are depleted, the patient begins to manifest signs of vitamin B$_{12}$ deficiency. Since this vitamin is so critically needed by bone marrow to complete the maturation of erythrocytes, 1 of the most prominent features of its shortage is the appearance in the marrow and peripheral circulation of large, poorly adapted red blood cells. This cell has a very short life span and its

---

11-14. PERNICIOUS ANEMIA

1) MEGALOBLASTIC ANEMIA —

2) PERIPHERAL NEURITIS

3) ATROPHIC GLOSSITIS
    sore, inflamed tongue with papil-
    lary atrophy

4) REDUCED PRODUCTION OF HCl *& digestive*
    secondary to atrophic gastritis *engymes*

---

patient with too little functioning epithelium and infestation with the fish tapeworm, *Diphyllobothrium latum*, simply uses up a great deal of vitamin B_{12} in the intestine.

Additional Reading

Jolly, M. Vitamin A deficiency: A review (Parts I and II). J. Oral Therap. Pharmacol. 3:364 and 3:439, 1967
Muenter, M. D. et al. Chronic vitamin A intoxication in adults. Am. J. Med. 50:179, 1971
Rivlin, R. S. Riboflavin metabolism. N. Engl. J. Med. 283:463, 1970
Stadtman, T. C. Vitamin B_{12}. Science 171:859, 1971

rapid destruction leads to a kind of anemia known as *pernicious anemia*. The patient with pernicious anemia shows a variety of clinical signs, a list of which is provided in Illustration 11-14.

The disease was described as "pernicious," because, at the time of its first detailed description in 1849, it was invariably fatal. It was not until approximately 50 years ago that a successful treatment using a combination of meat and normal gastric juice was begun by Castle; the therapeutic component in the meat was called *extrinsic factor* and that in normal gastric juice, *intrinsic factor*. Extrinsic factor, of course, was later shown to be vitamin B_{12}

It is important to realize that pernicious anemia is actually a disease of the stomach. Atrophy of the gastric epithelium (atrophic gastritis) and its subsequent failure to produce intrinsic factor is the very basis for all that happens later. Today, treatment is carried out by simply injecting vitamin B_{12}, bypassing the need for its absorption. This corrects the anemia and other reversible manifestations of the disease, but the stomach remains atrophic. Since insufficient hydrochloric acid is produced, peptic digestion is inhibited. Also, a point of very critical concern, the patient with long-standing atrophic gastritis is strongly predisposed to the development of carcinoma of the stomach.

Conditions other than atrophic gastritis can lead to a pernicious anemia-like syndrome; for example, radical gastrectomy may leave the

Thought to be autoimmune attack

MINERAL MALNUTRITION

LEARNING OBJECTIVE

To be able to review the classification of elements as proposed by Hardwick and discuss the difficulty involved in establishing normal requirements for essential trace elements.

The possibility for variety in nutritional disease is legion. Any single or combined deficiency of the 40 or so essential organic and/or inorganic nutrients is imaginable and probably exists somewhere in the world.

A major component of essential human nutrients are the chemical elements. These can be grouped, first of all, into those of major importance such as calcium, phosphorus, sodium, chloride, potassium and magnesium, and into a second group usually called trace elements. Those classified as major nutrients are required in significant amounts, whereas those functioning as trace elements may be required in such extremely small amounts that their role as essential nutrients may actually be in question. Finally, there is a group consisting of all remaining elements which, at least, insofar as it is now known have no biologic role.

Hardwick has suggested a classification for trace elements as outlined in Illustration 11-15.

11-15. TRACE ELEMENTS IN NUTRITION (HARDWICK)*

GROUP I
non-essential elements
no known biologic role

GROUP II
essential elements required as components of demonstrated reactions of living tissues
iron, copper, zinc, molybdenum, iodine, cobalt, manganese, sclenium
Only trace amts.

GROUP III
essential elements with unknown metabolic roles
fluoride, bromine, barium, strontium: recent evidence would suggest the addition of vanadium and perhaps lithium to this group. (Author)

* Hardwick, J. L. Caries-resistant Teeth. London, Little, Brown & Co., 1965

Great amts. needed —
40 or so organic +
inorganic essential nutrients

chemical elements needed
in lrg. amts.
Ca
Ph
Na
Cl
K
Mg

NUTRITIONAL DEFICIENCIES SECONDARY TO OTHER DISEASE

LEARNING OBJECTIVE

To be able to compare and contrast nutritional deficiency based on malabsorption and the failure of retention of metabolites using the following syndromes as examples:
a) pancreatic insufficiency
b) acholia
c) intestinal parasitism
d) celiac disease and sprue
e) Crohn's disease (regional enteritis)

A concept of key importance to the diagnostician is the possibility for nutritional deficiency secondary to other disease. The quantity and composition of the diet, while perhaps of major importance in the over-all picture of human nutrition, is not the sole determinant of its adequacy. An individual must not only eat, but must also absorb and retain nutrients to maintain health.

We will consider secondary nutritional diseases under 2 main headings, *malabsorption* and *failure of retention or utilization.*

1. Malabsorption

Malabsorption occurs secondary to a number of very different diseases, some of which are listed in Illustration 11-16. We have encountered the first of these in our discussion of pernicious anemia, in which atrophy or resection of the stomach leads to a deficiency of "intrinsic factor."

Pancreatic Insufficiency

Pancreatic insufficiency results from the failure of the pancreas to produce or release digestive enzymes. The most common condition associated with pancreatic insufficiency is obstruction of the pancreatic duct as seen with an occluding tumor or in cystic fibrosis. Another common cause is diffuse parenchymal disease such as hemorrhagic pancreatitis. Among enzymes provided by the pancreas are lipases which initiate the digestion of fats. In

mucin obstructs duct

11-16. MALABSORPTION

1) GASTRIC ATROPHY OR RESECTION

2) PANCREATIC INSUFFICIENCY

3) ACHOLIA (LACK OF BILE)

4) INTESTINAL PARASITISM

5) INTESTINAL MALABSORPTION SYNDROMES
    sprue
    celiac disease
    intestinal lipodystrophy
    Crohn's disease

11-17. GASTRIC ATROPHY OR RESECTION

1) A VARIETY OF NUTRITIONAL ALTERATIONS ARE POSSIBLE

2) MOST SERIOUS RESULTS FROM FAILURE TO SECRETE "INTRINSIC FACTOR" OF CASTLE

3) MAY LEAD TO P.A.

the absence of pancreatic lipases fats are not reduced to absorable form and proceed through the intestinal tract to be excreted intact in the stool (steatorrhea). Since the production of bile is not impeded, normal stool pigmentation is seen in steatorrhea resulting from pancreatic insufficiency. Something like this same kind of absorptive difficiency is seen with a lack of bile, except, of course, the fat will not be accompanied by bile pigment and will be partially formed into soaps. Lack of bile (acholia) can result from obstruction of the biliary outflow tract such as might result from a tumor or impacted gallstone. Bile emulsifies fat, whereas pancreatic enzymes are necessary for its digestion. Lack of either factor prevents fat absorption as well as the absorption of fat soluble vitamins.

Intestinal Malabsorption Syndromes

A number of cases for malabsorption are traceable to diseases originating in the intestine. Celiac disease, for example, is an affliction in which there is marked atrophy of the villi and microvilli of the jejunum. Although the pathogenesis of celiac disease is somewhat obscure, it is thought to be an unusual immunologic reaction to wheat or rye gluten. Celiac disease is morphologically indistinguishable from a tropi-

11-18. PANCREATIC INSUFFICIENCY

1) OBSTRUCTION OF PANCREATIC DUCT, CYSTIC FIBROSIS OR SEVERE DIFFUSE PANCREATIC DISEASE

2) RESULTS IN COMPLEX ABSORPTIVE PROBLEM INCLUDING STEATORRHEA
    (fat in stool in form of neutral lipid: bile pigment is present)

11-19. ACHOLIA

1) OBSTRUCTION OF BILIARY TRACT OR SEVERE DIFFUSE LIVER DISEASE

2) RESULTS IN STEATORRHEA AND LIPID-SOLUBLE VITAMIN DEFICIENCIES
    (fat in stool as soaps: no pigment)

cal disease called sprue: however, whereas celiac disease apparently results from a immunologic abnormalitiy, sprue is thought to be caused by an infectious agent. Celiac disease is usually diagnosed in young to middle-aged adults, but may be seen in children. It is now generally accepted that the childhood and adult forms are phases of the same condition. Clinical signs are variable, but always include steatorrhea and weight loss. Depending upon the duration and severity of the disease, the patient may also manifest deficiencies of vitamins, calcium and other metabolites. Treatment consists of adopting a gluten-free diet, which usually results in the immediate reversal of enteric changes.

Our second example of enterogenous malabsorption is Crohn's Disease or regional enteritis. Crohn's disease is a chronic, granulomatous, segmental inflammatory disease usually affecting the terminal ileum. There also may be extraenteric changes such as arthritis and skin lesions. Although the etiology of Crohn's disease is unknown, many authorities believe that it represents some kind of immunologic abnormality, or perhaps an obscure infection combined with an unusual immunologic response. Lesions are thought to begin in lymph nodes adjacent to the gut and eventually spread

---

11-21. FAILURE OF RETENTION OR UTILIZATION

1) REPEATED VOMITING

2) RENAL DISEASE ✓

3) ENTEROPATHY — *lose protein thru walls of intestines*

4) INHERITED ENZYME DEFICIENCY

5) METABOLIC INHIBITION — *by drugs*

complication — intestinal obstructions

through its entire thickness (transmural inflammation). Manifestations of malabsorption become apparent only when intestinal involvement has become extensive.

2. Failure of Retention or Utilization

Regardless of the adequacy of one's diet or absorptive abilities, adequate nutrition is also dependent upon retention and utilization of nutrient material. It must be at least mentioned that a variety of disease states (Illustration 11-21) can lead to secondary nutritional deficiency through the loss or metabolic inhibition of a nutritional factor. A thorough consideration of each of these would be beyond the scope of this discussion.

Additional Reading

Finkelstein, J. D. Malabsorption. Med. Clin. N. Amer. 52:1339, 1968
Ginsberg, A. Alterations in immunologic mechanisms in diseases of the gastrointestinal tract. Am. J. Digest. Dis. 16:61, 1971
Hall, C. A. Autoimmune mechanisms and the gastrointestinal tract. Med. Clin. N. Amer. 52:1285, 1968
Knowlessar, O. D. and Phillips, L. D. Celiac disease. Med. Clin. N. Amer. 54:647, May, 1970

11-20. INTESTINAL MALABSORPTION SYNDROMES (EXAMPLES)

1) SPRUE
   tropical
   probably infectious
   intestinal atrophy
   steatorrhea

2) CELIAC DISEASE
   sprue-like but not infectious
   intolerance to gluten *protein component of wheat n rye*
   infants and adults

3) INTESTINAL LIPODYSTROPHY
   Whipple's disease

4) CROHN'S DISEASE *REGIONAL*
   advanced stages *ENTERITIS*

1) SEGMENTAL
2) TRANSMURAL (THRU WALL OF INTESTINES INTO REGIONAL NODES)

MAJOR HEALTH PROBLEMS INVOLVING NUTRITION

LEARNING OBJECTIVE

To be able to discuss the association between diet and:
   a) atherosclerosis
   b) dental caries

It is always more practical to prevent chronic disease than to attempt its cure; most chronic disease is not amenable to cure or it would not be classified as chronic. A majority of scientific opinion now favors an association between diet and 2 very different forms of chronic disease, *atherosclerosis* and *dental caries*. We will use these as examples of the role of nutrition in major health problems.

1. Atherosclerosis

There is growing conviction among authorities that diet is an important factor in the development of atherosclerotic cardiovascular disease (ACVD). Since complications of this condition will kill 40 per cent of American males alive today, and since diet is one of the most flexible factors implicated in this disease, the concept must be given serious consideration. Atherosclerosis is a condition in which the walls of the aorta and its medium-sized muscular branches (including cerebral and coronary arteries) become distended, fibrotic and ultimately calcified as a result of the subendothelial deposition of cholesterol and other fats; it has been mentioned in Chapter 3 and will be treated in Chapters 15 and 16. Atherosclerosis is undoubtedly a multifactoral disease (Illustration 11-22). Recent reports indicate that there are at least 3 components to the involvement of nutrition in atherosclerosis (Illustration 11-23).

The first dietary component apparently has its roots in an improper diet during adolescence or perhaps even younger. Early dietary patterns and habits determine how and what is eaten in later life as well as whether or not an individual will smoke. It is now apparent that American males, 20 years of age or even younger, are beinning to manifest ACVD. Traditionally, this disease has been considered one of males in their 40's, 50's or older, since it

---

11-22. ATHEROSCLEROSIS (A MULTI-FACTORIAL DISEASE)

1) HEREDITY

2) DIET

3) HYPERTENSION

4) CIGARETTE SMOKING

5) OBESITY

6) SEDENTARY LIFE PATTERN

7) CULTURE

8) ENVIRONMENT

9) ANXIETY

10) DIABETES

11-23. DIET AND ATHEROSCLEROSIS

1) IMPROPER EATING HABITS IN ADO-LESCENCE

2) IMPROPER DIET AS ADULT

3) POSSIBLE REQUIREMENT FOR TRACE ELEMENTS, MOST NOTABLY LITHIUM

---

is at these ages that coronary and cerebral *complications* of atherosclerosis appear. But recent autopsy studies have shown that the atherosclerosis causing these serious problems has its onset in the second decade of life or earlier, a feature that sets American males sharply apart from comparable groups in other cultures. It thus appears that forces within an individual's environment that will contribute to his experiencing ACVD in middle life actually begin to operate during adolescence or even pre-adolescence. This suggests that efforts toward the prevention of atherosclerosis must be directed toward much younger age groups, if the disease is to be controlled.

The second dietary subfactor in atherosclerosis is improper diet as an adult. Judging from the condition of arteries of males in more technologically retarded countries one must conclude that ACVD is *not* the inevitable consequence of advancing age. It is only in the United States and, to a lesser extent, in other more technologically advanced nations that the ravages of atherosclerotic disease reach such serious proportions in older men. This amounts to a rather specific demographic pattern and suggests that something in the physical or culture environment of these people leads to the collection of lipid within the intima of certain high-pressure arteries; many authorities would place at least a portion of the blame on the diet we eat as adults. It is clear from work with experimental animals that dietary elevation of blood lipids, particularly the Beta$_1$ lipoproteins, is mandatory for the development of atherosclerosis. Also, the striking difference in blood lipid levels among people of the world correlates directly with the incidence of atherosclerosis. But, most convincingly, results from longitudinal clinical studies with ACVD-prone groups of American males suggests that a dietary regimen aimed at reducing blood lipids, particularly cholesterol, will reduce the incidence of atherosclerotic arterial disease as well as the recurrence of coronary heart disease in patients who have suffered myocardial infarction.

The third dietary factor in the control of ACVD is one that was discovered quite by accident, which, even now that it has been recognized, seems inexplicable. It appears that the rate of sudden death from coronary heart disease is higher in areas where the water is soft than in areas where its trace metal content is high. Further, the only 2 metals showing negative correlation with the incidence of such death patterns were lithium (for white populations) and vanadium (for non-white). Although these investigations must be continued and greatly expanded, they suggest that the complete absence of these metals in the diet may constitute a serious predilection to sudden death from ACVD. The fact that a "sudden

---

11-24. DIETARY MANAGEMENT OF SERUM LIPIDS

1) LOWER INTAKE OF SATURATED FATS
    restrict use of meat and dairy fats

2) RAISE INTAKE OF POLYUNSATURATED FATS
    increase use of vegetable oils

3) LOWER INTAKE OF CHOLESTEROL
    limit consumption of egg yolk to 2 or 3 per week: restrict intake of organ meats such as liver and shellfish

& high carbohy

11-25. NUTRITION AND DENTAL CARIES

1) INFLUENCE OF DIET PARTICULARLY POTENT DURING DEVELOPMENT AND GROWTH
    fluoride intake
    avoidance of refined carbohydrates

2) FLUORIDATION OF PUBLIC WATER SUPPLIES IS MOST EFFECTIVE MEANS OF *ASSURING A NUTRITIONALLY ADEQUATE INTAKE OF FLUORIDE*

---

death" component can be separated from the rest of the syndrome reinforces the conviction that ACVD results from many interrelated conditions.

2. Dental Caries

Dental caries is a chronic disease of extremely widespread distribution. Indeed, this disease is so common that in some areas of the United States it is known to affect up to 90 per cent of the population. The most frequent serious consequence of dental caries is loss of one or more teeth, a condition which leads to a number of other disabilities such as malocclusion, peridontal disease and the early loss of additional teeth.

Like other chronic disease, dental caries is a problem that is more profitably approached by prevention rather than treatment. Aside from the control of dental plaque through proper oral hygiene, perhaps the most important preventive factor is diet. Again, showing remarkable correspondence with its relationship to other chronic diseases, the influence of diet on dental caries is particularly potent during the early years of life when teeth are undergoing calcification.

As nearly as can be determined, the fluoride ion is the dietary element most critical to the development and maintenance of a caries-free dentition (assuming the general availability of other components of hard tissue). Fluoride works by becoming incorporated into the hydroxyapatite lattice in place of an *occasional* hydroxyl ion. This random distribution of fluoride produces a more compact and less soluble crystal matrix and hence the tooth (or bone) is less subject to dissolution.

The first hint of this role of the fluoride ion was detected in the 1930's when it was discovered that individuals drinking water containing 1 to 2 parts per million (ppm) of this ion had considerably less trouble with tooth decay that those whose water contained less fluoride. It was subsequently demonstrated that the simple adjustment of the fluoride content of a community's water supply to 1.2 ppm could predictably reduce the incidence of dental caries by 60 to 70 per cent among children raised in that area.

Opposition to fluoridation of a public water supply is often based on its being considered a form of mass medication when, in truth, the addition of fluoride ion to public water simply serves to restore its ion concentration to an optimal (and presumably more natural) level.

Additional Reading

Brusis, O. A. and McGandy, R. B. Nutrition and man's heart and bloodvessels. Fed. Proc. 30:1417, 1971

Dietschy, J. M. and Wilson, J. D. Regulation of cholesterol metabolism. N. Engl. J. Med. 282 (3 parts): 1128, 1179, 1241, 1970

Enos, W. F. et al. Pathologenesis of coronary disease in American soldiers killed in Korea. J. Am. Med. Assn. 158:912, 1955

Hodge, H. C. and Smith, F. A. Fluorides and man. Ann. Rev. Pharmacol. 8:395, 1968

McGill, H. C. (ed.) The Geographic Pathology of Atherosclerosis. Williams and Wilkins Co., Baltimore, 1968

McNeil, D. R. The Fight for Fluoridation. Oxford University Press, New York, 1959.

Neri, L. C. et al. Risk of sudden death in soft water areas. Am. J. Epidemiol. 94:101, 1971

Scherp, H. W. Dental caries: prospects for prevention. Science 173:1199, 1971

Spain, D. M. Atherosclerosis. Sci. Amer. 215:49, 1966

Voors, A. W. Minerals in the municipal water and atherosclerotic heart death. Am. J. Epidemiol. 93:259, 1971

chapter 12
DISORDERS OF THE VASCULAR SYSTEM

DIMINISHED CARDIAC OUTPUT (HEART FAILURE)

LEARNING OBJECTIVE

To be able to describe how diseases of each of the following can cause diminution in the output of the heart, citing specific clinical examples of each:

- a) pericardium
- b) myocardium
- c) endocardium
- d) cardiac rhythm (fibrillation)
- e) cardiac development
- f) the lung

12-1. BLOOD: VASCULAR SYSTEM

1) REACTIVE TISSUE
   humoral immunity
   acute inflammation

2) PERFUSION NETWORK
   principal defects include:
       diminished cardiac output (heart failure)
       decompensated heart failure
       disorders of vascular control
       vascular obstruction
       structural vascular defects
       changes in viscosity of the blood

The normal 70-Kg man is made up of about 50 liters of ordinary water. Important as this water is as a chemical constituent of the body it enjoys equal importance as a vehicle for the perfusion of tissues situated too far from a surface to obtain nutrient and discharge waste. In this same 70-Kg man, the heart must propel about 6 liters of blood through miles of vessels during every minute while he rests and even more when he is active. Fully one-fourth of this cardiac output percolates through 2 million renal glomerular filters and trickles down an equal number of tubular systems, where it is resorbed except for a scant 1 ml/minute of waste concentrate called urine.

The task of suffusing the blood with all necessary nutrients, distributing it throughout the body, transferring its metabolites to and from tissue across capillary walls and finally returning it to the heart is truly an enormous one and liable to failure at many critical steps. Illustration 12-1 includes a list of the sources of the more important disorders of this perfusion system. Some idea of the actual importance of these disorders can be gained from the often-repeated fact that diseases of the heart and arteries are the single most prominent cause of death in the United States.

Many different kinds of diseases can lead to the common result of diminished cardiac output (heart failure). In this first learning objective, we will consider those listed in Illustration 12-2 as examples.

1. Diseases of the Pericardium

The pericardium forms a sac in which the heart must be free to move and expand in order to function properly. Anything that obstructs freedom of movement within the pericardial sac interferes with the output of the heart. Two somewhat different diseases will serve to exemplify this category.

Cardiac Tamponade

Cardiac tamponade is a condition in which fluid under pressure accumulates in the pericardial space. Pressure within the pericardial sac prevents heart function by preventing the

12-2. DIMINISHED CARDIAC OUTPUT (HEART FAILURE)

1) PERICARDIUM

2) MYOCARDIUM

3) ENDOCARDIUM (VALVES)

4) CARDIAC RHYTHM

5) CARDIAC DEVELOPMENT

6) LUNG (cor pulmonale)

adequate filling of ventricular chambers. Cardiac tamponade often results from rupture of the heart or aorta, from a penetrating wound or from an inflammatory disease of the pericardium.

Constrictive Pericarditis

Another disease of the pericardium that restricts the action of the heart by limiting its excursion within the pericardial space is constructive pericarditis. This may be caused by either sepsis or by the aseptic effusion associated with rheumatic fever and metabolic disturbances such as uremia. A fibrinous exudate coats the epicardial surface, the organization of which covers the heart with scar. In contracting, this scar constricts the wall of the heart and limits its motion.

2. Diseases of the Myocardium

Almost all diseases of the myocardium will result in some degree of diminished cardiac output. We will use 3 examples of widely varied etiology; bear in mind, however, that this is a very limited sample.

Toxic Myocarditis

Bacterial pathogens that do not invade produce a strong exotoxin. In some diseases, this toxin has a pronounced effect on the heart. This is clearly exemplified in diphtheria where the toxin poisons heart muscle to the extent that fatty degeneration is seen and heart failure is a common cause of death.

Beriberi

A dietary shortage of thiamine which acts as a cofactor in energy metabolism leads to a weakening of myocardial contractions and eventual failure of the heart. This is seen quite vividly in the disease, beriberi, where signs of heart failure are among the first to be recognized.

Myocardial Infarct

The myocardial infarct is the most common cause of diminished cardiac output. If a large area of heart muscle is rendered necrotic and the patient recovers, cardiac output is often diminished to a significant degree.

3. Diseases of the Endocardium

Diseases of the endocardium that are most significant in reducing cardiac output are those which distort the valves. Two kinds of valvular deformities are most prominent in this regard, insufficiency and stenosis.

Valvular Insufficiency

Valvular insufficiency is the failure of proper valve closure. It usually results from the distortion of valve cusps (leaflets) to the extent that their union in a proper seal becomes impossible. Insufficiency results in leakage and the back-flow or regurgitation of blood through the affected valve. A different kind of insufficiency (relative insufficiency) results from the dilatation of the heart to a point where valve cusps fail to meet.

Stenosis

The second form of valvular distortion, stenosis, is the gradual constriction of the valve ring (annulus) by fibrosis to the point where its orifice is critically reduced. Since the valve annulus is the portal of the valve, its gradual closure slows the flow of blood. Both insufficiency and stenosis are seen most often as cardiac lesions in chronic rheumatic fever. In this disease, the valves are affected in a certain order, the one most often damaged being the mitral valve, followed closely by the aortic and, with less frequency, the tricuspid and pulmonic valves. Valvular deterioration in rheumatic fever frequently becomes so severe that the entire valve must be excised and replaced with a prosthesis.

4. Diseases of Cardiac Rhythm

Disturbances of cardiac rhythm are also responsible for slowing or sudden stoppage of the heart. Undoubtedly, the most serious form of arrhythmia is fibrillation in which myocardial fibers contract in an independent and uncoordinated way. This, of course, results in the complete cessation of cardiac output.

The heart may fibrillate because of some defect intrinsic to its conduction system or because of damage to tissue surrounding the conduction network. In the latter form, it is often seen as a complication of a developing myocardial infarct. The main branches of the conduction system course through tissue of the interventricular septum, an area of the heart frequently involved in myocardial infarction.

5. Diseases of Cardiac Development

The embryologic, fetal and even postnatal development of the heart and great vessels takes place in a series of very complex stages. On occasion, 1 or more stages of development will fail and a persisting defect will result. Although certain of these defects are compatible with life, they always result in a poorly functioning heart with inadequate operating potential.

The subject of congenital heart defects will be considered in Chapter 13.

6. Diseases of the Lung

A brief review of cardiopulmonary anatomy shows that the function of the heart is critically dependent upon blood flow through the lungs. Diseases of the lung that interfere with cardiac output are those that impede the passage of blood through the pulmonary vascular system. When restriction of blood flow through the lungs prevents adequate heart function the condition is called *cor pulmonale*. Cor pulmonale can be acute, such as the condition resulting from pulmonary embolism, or chronic, as might result from obstructive or granulomatous lung disease. It is usually associated with an increase in pressure within the pulmonary system and this will occasionally lead to atherosclerosis of the pulmonary artery and its main branches.

DECOMPENSATED (CONGESTIVE) HEART FAILURE

LEARNING OBJECTIVE

To be able to discuss the phenomenon of decompensated heart failure, contrasting right-sided and left-sided failure with regard to:

a) effect on lungs
b) effect on liver and spleen
c) general appearance of the patient
d) the most important causes of each

Any of the conditions mentioned in the previous learning objective can lead to slowing of the output of blood from the heart, or "heart failure." The normal heart adapts well to circulatory needs. This allows an individual to operate comfortably within any reasonable life style without experiencing distress. When a normal person engages in athletics, he does so with reasonable assurance that his heart will keep up with whatever rate of output is needed. However, the failing heart can no longer supply resting circulatory needs without resorting to mechanisms that the normal heart uses only to compensate for increased effort (Illustration 12-3) and so *exercise tolerance is diminished*.

As heart failure progresses, compensating mechanisms are "used up." Ultimately, there is no further way to make up for the worsening performance of the heart and at this point it is said to be *decompensated*; the deterioration of its ability to pump blood has progressed to such an extent that it can no longer be adequately supplemented. The availability of natural compensating mechanisms determines that each normal person has a degree of exercise tolerance. Significantly, as heart failure approaches the point of decompensation exercise tolerance diminishes to 0.

1. Right-sided Heart Failure

Although the cardiovascular-pulmonary system is a closed perfusion circuit and each part is ultimately dependent upon the proper function of all others, there is still the possibility for a selective initial failure of either the right or left chambers of the heart and the emergence of 2 distinct syndromes. In far-advanced heart fail-

---

12-3. DECOMPENSATED HEART FAILURE

---

1) SLOWING OF CARDIAC OUTPUT (HEART FAILURE) IS COMPENSATED BY PHYSIOLOGIC MECHANISMS THAT NORMALLY PERMIT INCREASED EXERTION

　　use of RBC oxygen reserves
　　erythrocytosis
　　diminished exercise tolerance

2) SLOWING OF CARDIAC OUTPUT TO A RATE THAT CAN NO LONGER BE COUNTERBALANCED BY EXERTION MECHANISMS LEADS TO *DECOMPENSATED HEART FAILURE*

　　no exercise tolerance

---

ure, these syndromes merge so that diseases provoking 1 will ultimately include elements of the other (Illustration 12-4).

In right-sided heart failure, blood is not moved at an adequate rate from the venous system and collects under abnormally high pressure on the venous side of the circulation. *The most conspicuous effects of right-sided heart failure are those that result from systemic venous congestion and the ultimate oxygen starvation of congested tissue.*

Effects of Chronic Venous Congestion

All tissues are affected in chronic right-sided heart failure. As blood begins to collect in the venous system, additional capillary vascular space opens and abdominal organs become engorged with slowly circulating, largely depleted blood. Since heart failure is usually part of a chronic and worsening syndrome, visceral congestion grows more severe with time. In the liver, hypoxia is manifested as necrosis of hepatocytes around the central vein of each lobule. This gives rise to a characteristically appearing cut surface termed "nutmeg" liver. In long-standing congestive failure, fibrosis resulting from the death of liver parenchyma leads to a condition known as cardiac cirrhosis.

The chronically congested spleen becomes greatly enlarged and will also undergo fibrosis if the condition persists. The gradual slowing of kidney perfusion leads to engorgement of these organs with exhausted blood and the inadequate elimination of metabolic wastes (prerenal azotemia). In response, the kidney conserves salt which leads to a larger blood volume. In an attempt to compensate for poor circulation, the kidney releases erythropoietin, which stimulates the generation of higher circulating levels of red blood cells (secondary erythrocytosis).

The person suffering from congestive heart failure may appear blue, particularly at the nailbeds and vermillion borders of the lips. This is due to the prominence of congested venules and the generally poor state of oxygenation of the blood. There is also a widening and rounding of the ends of the fingers known as "clubbing" and a swelling of the ankles on standing (dependent edema). The effects of systemic congestion are summarized in Illustration 12-5.

Causes of Right-sided Heart Failure

Right-sided heart failure is seen most clearly in cor pulmonale: however, strong suggestions of right-sided failure are seen in all diseases that cause a primary left heart failure. This is

---

12-4. HEART FAILURE SYNDROMES

---

1) RIGHT-SIDED HEART FAILURE
　　most conspicuous effect is systemic (venous) congestion
　　most clearly seen in cor pulmonale and mitral stenosis

2) LEFT-SIDED HEART FAILURE
　　most conspicuous effect is pulmonary edema
　　most clearly seen in coronary heart disease, hypertension

3) COMBINED
　　elements of both
　　most common syndrome

12-5. EFFECTS OF SYSTEMIC CONGESTION

1) VISCERAL ANOXIA AND FIBROSIS
   "nutmeg" liver leading to "cardiac cirrhosis"
   congestive splenomegaly leading to splenic fibrosis

2) DEPENDENT EDEMA
   ankles when standing
   dorsum when prone

3) "CLUBBING" OF NAILS

4) CYANOSIS IN FAR ADVANCED CASES

12-6. PULMONARY EDEMA

1) FAILURE OF LEFT HEART WITH NORMAL OPERATION OF RIGHT CAUSES BLOOD TO COLLECT IN PULMONARY SYSTEM UNDER ABNORMALLY HIGH PRESSURE

2) CONGESTION OF PULMONARY VESSELS CAUSES INTRA-ALVEOLAR FLUID ACCUMULATION
   usually accompanied by erythrocytes

3) DYSPNEA, ORTHOPNEA RESULT

4) COMPLICATIONS OF CHRONIC PULMONARY EDEMA INCLUDE
   —hypostatic pneumonia
   —"brown induration"

particularly true in severe mitral stenosis, where the constricted mitral annulus prevents transfer of a complete stroke volume to the left heart.

2. Left-sided Heart Failure

When failure of the heart begins with the left chamber, blood collects in the pulmonary system under unusually high pressure. Pulmonary hypertension accounts for the fact that *the most prominent feature of developing left-sided heart failure is pulmonary edema.* Chronic pulmonary edema results in the gradual fibrous thickening of alveolar septae and predisposes an individual to repeated episodes of bronchopneumonia (hypostatic pneumonia). One of the most characteristic signs of pulmonary edema is paroxysmal nocturnal dyspnea with orthopnea (need to sit up to breathe). The effects of pulmonary edema are summarized in Illustration 12-6.

Causes of Left-sided Heart Failure

Left-sided heart failure is most commonly caused by coronary heart disease, hypertension and disorders of the aortic or mitral valves. It rarely occurs without some accompanying manifestations of right heart failure.

Additional Reading

Fishman, A. P. Chronic cor pulmonale. Hosp. Pract. 5: 101, 1971
Gazes, P. C. Cardiac failure in adults. Postgrad. Med. 49:130, 1971

EDEMA AND SHOCK

LEARNING OBJECTIVE

To be able to discuss each of the following 3 vascular disorders and, where applicable, mention cause, pathogenesis, clinical appearance, associated diseases, clinical course, complications and possible outcome:

    a) edema (local and generalized)
    b) serous effusion (ascites, pleural effusion and pericardial effusion)
    c) shock (cardiogenic, hypovolemic, normovolemic)

Major perfusion diseases often take origin in vessels. These are of many kinds, 1 group of which is functional. We will consider the first 2 functional vascular diseases at this point and the remaining 2 in the following learning objectives (Illustration 12-7).

1. Edema and Serous Effusion

Edema is the presence of abnormally large amounts of fluid in intercellular tissue spaces. Serous effusion, a closely related phenomenon, is the emission of this same kind of fluid from the serous lining of body cavities (Illustration 12-8).

Local edema is always seen as part of acute inflammation: however, this same disorder, minus the usual inflammatory cells, results from a variety of conditions which are fundamentally non-inflammatory. In the latter, the fluid is considered a *transudate* (Illustration 12-9) and the effect is either edema or serous effusion or both.

Generalized edema is known as *anasarca*. In generalized edema, the transudate tends to shift to the lowermost areas of the body (ankles while standing). This phenomenon is called dependent edema and is often seen as a sign of congestive heart failure (Illustration 12-10).

2. Shock

In previous learning objectives, we have seen that the gradual slowing of cardiac output and the pooling of large amounts of blood under abnormally high pressure in the venous system are the essential components of the syndrome of congestive heart failure. We must now

---

12-7. DISORDERS OF VASCULAR CONTROL

1) EDEMA AND SEROUS EFFUSION

2) SHOCK

3) VASOSPASM

4) HYPERTENSION

12-8. EDEMA AND SEROUS EFFUSION

EDEMA
    the presence of abnormally large amounts of fluid within the intercellular tissue spaces of the body
        inflammatory
        local, non-inflammatory
        generalized (anasarca)

SEROUS EFFUSION
    abnormal transudate from serous surfaces
        ascites (peritoneal cavity)   #5
        pleural effusion
        pericardial effusion

12-9. TRANSUDATE

1) A MATERIAL THAT CROSSES A MEMBRANE

2) PRACTICALLY DEFINED AS:
    fluid that emits from vessels in abnormal but non-inflammatory conditions

12-10. CAUSES OF EDEMA

1) LOCAL (non-inflammatory)
   venous obstruction
   lymphatic obstruction

2) GENERALIZED (anasarca)
   venous congestion in decompensated heart failure
   hypoproteinemia secondary to protein loss, protein starvation or liver disease
   sodium retention due to renal disease or hormonal imbalance

12-11. SHOCK (CIRCULATORY COLLAPSE)

1) NORMAL CIRCULATION DEPENDS UPON:

   (sudden failure)

   adequate cardiac output

   PROPER PERIPHERAL RESISTANCE

   | sudden failure
   ↓

   VASCULAR SHOCK*
   hypovolemic
   normovolemic

   ↓

   cardiogenic shock

   * All instances of vascular shock begin as a serious disparity between blood volume and vascular space, either blood is lost or there is a large, sudden gain in vascular space

consider a condition in which something like this same congestion occurs with comparative suddenness. Although such a condition can be caused by sudden heart failure (cardiogenic shock), it is more often seen when the heart is perfectly normal. In the latter situation, it is caused by failure of the second requirement for adequate blood circulation, peripheral resistance. The condition itself, whether of cardiogenic or vascular origin, is called *shock* (Illustration 12-11).

Classification of Vascular Shock

Vascular shock is based on the sudden collapse of peripheral resistance. *It always begins as a serious disparity between blood volume and vascular space*, i.e. there is too little blood volume for the vascular space or too much space for a normal blood volume (Illustration 12-11). On the basis of this distinction, we can consider all vascular (non-cardiogenic) shock as being either *hypovolemic* or *normovolemic* shock.

Hypovolemic Shock

Hypovolemic shock is provoked by excessive loss of body fluid and diminished blood volume. It is caused by a number of factors, the most common of which is hemorrhage. The pathogenesis of hypovolemic shock is outlined in Illustration 12-12 and its mechanism will be discussed below.

12-12. HYPOVOLEMIC (HEMORRHAGIC) SHOCK

1) LOSS OF ANY VOLUME OF BLOOD UP TO 1 PINT IS USUALLY NOT SERIOUS

2) LOSS OF 2 to 3 PINTS USUALLY RESULTS IN REVERSIBLE SHOCK

3) LOSS OF MORE THAN 3 PINTS WILL USUALLY LEAD TO IRREVERSIBLE SHOCK UNLESS FLUID VOLUME IS RESTORED

4) HYPOVOLEMIC SHOCK ALSO SEEN IN
   extensive burn
   acute peritonitis
   chronic diarrhea or vomiting
   fluid deprivation

Normovolemic Shock

Normovolemic shock is the kind occurring when a person sustains a sudden, gross increase in vascular space, usually as a result of the loss of peripheral vascular tone. It occurs in 3 principal clinical forms as listed in Illustration 12-13. In each of these, the causative factor interferes with normal vasomotor control, causing the unwarranted opening of capillary beds (particularly those of the viscera) and seriously reducing systemic blood pressure. In effect, they cause a sudden, abnormal increase in available vascular space beyond that which can be filled with the normal blood volume. This causes the pooling of blood within visceral (splanchnic) capillary beds, where it is hidden or sequestered from functioning circulatory routes. This splanchnic sequestration of blood is comparable to its having been lost through hemorrhage.

The Mechanism of Shock

One way of looking at shock is to consider it a result of the malfunction of a mechanism that normally protects an animal (or human) from the effects of blood-loss secondary to serious injury. In the era of prehistory, when sophisticated body machinery was evolving, survival would have been enhanced by a mechanism that would keep an animal alive while recovering from the effects of serious hemorrhage. Blood loss in such times was, no doubt, a rather common experience and, if nothing protected the injured animal from the perfusion difficulties of hypovolemia, life would have been somewhat less feasible. The principal problem in blood-loss hypovolemia is to keep high priority tissues, such as the brain and heart, adequately supplied while blood volume is being restored. To do this, most of the remaining blood is shunted through the "carotid circuit" where it traverses the carotid, cerebral and coronary arteries and their branches, while circulation through viscera, muscles and skin is greatly diminished. In recovery, as tissue fluid leaks into the vascular tree and blood volume approaches normal, more and more of the restricted circulatory routes are re-opened until full circulation is ultimately regained. Having once re-established blood volume, the animal could then set about

---

12-13. NORMOVOLEMIC SHOCK (MECHANISMS OF INITIATION)

1) **NEUROGENIC FAILURE OF VASCULAR TONE**
   simple syncope (fainting)
   prolonged, severe pain
   extremes of fright or emotional insult

2) **ANAPHYLAXIS**
   widespread release of histamine and other materials through generalized IgE reaction
   sudden drop in BP accompanied by dyspnea, vomiting, pruritus, fever and possible loss of consciousness

3) **ENDOTOXEMIA**
   endotoxin-producing
   organisms cause widespread activation of complement, vasodilatation and hypotension

---

to restore formed elements and solutes (Illustration 12-14). The service of this carotid circuit mechanism is probably lifesaving in cases of hemorrhage where volume loss does not exceed 3 pints. However, its operation in those instances where hemorrhage is simulated by the splanchnic sequestration or blood may be the source of trouble in that it may actually prevent sequestered blood from rejoining the circulation (Illustration 12-15).

Stages of Shock

Whatever the cause, the body senses the loss of blood or gain in vascular space as hypotension (it has been said that we can have hypotension without shock but never shock without hypotension). In response to a drop in blood pressure, vasopressive substances are secreted and blood is shunted into the carotid circuit. This reflex-like response is apparently intended to shut down circulation through less

12-14. MECHANISM OF SHOCK

PROBABLY EVOLVED AS A MEANS OF SUSTAINING SERIOUS BLOOD LOSS

HEMORRHAGE ⟶ LOW CAROTID PRESSURE

REMAINING BLOOD IS SHUNTED INTO "CAROTID CIRCUIT" TO ASSURE PERFUSION OF BRAIN AND HEART

VISCERAL (SPLANCHNIC) CAPILLARY BEDS CLOSED

CUTANEOUS CIRCULATION SHUT DOWN

CAROTID PRESSURE RESTORED WHILE BLOOD VOLUME IS BUILT UP

12-15. MECHANISM OF SHOCK

1) SERVICE OF CAROTID CIRCUIT MECHANISM IS PROBABLY LIFE SAVING IN CASES OF MANAGEABLE HEMORRHAGE
    (up to 3 pints)

2) SERVICE OF CAROTID CIRCUIT MECHANISM CAN PROBABLY BE TROUBLESOME IN NORMOVOLEMIC SHOCK
    large proportion of blood volume become shut out of circulation as splanchnic capillary beds are closed

12-16. STAGES OF SHOCK

1) REVERSIBLE
    vasomotor control can be regained

2) IRREVERSIBLE
    vasomotor control cannot be regained because of changes in vessels resulting from anoxia

12-17. EFFECTS OF SHOCK

1) CONFINED LARGELY TO VISCERAL CONGESTION

2) SEEN PRINCIPALLY IN:
    kidney
    liver
    lungs

3) "SHOCK" KIDNEY
    acute tubular necrosis
    glomerular congestion
    rbc casts and hematuria

essential routes, particularly the volumnous visceral and cutaneous capillary beds, so that blood can be conserved for use by more essential tissues. If the shunted volume is adequate the patient will be well sustained until blood volume is restored (hypovolemic shock) or peripheral vasomotor control is re-established (normovolemic shock). In such cases, the shock is said to have been *reversible*. This is undoubtedly the mechanism that accounts for the simple faint (syncope) and recovery. If the blood volume remaining (after loss or splanchnic entrapment) is not adequate for brain and heart perfusion and the carotid circuit pressure remains low, peripheral routes will not be reopened in time to prevent anoxic changes in the tissues denied circulation. When oxygen starvation becomes extreme, visceral tissue begins liberating large amounts of lactic acid and other wastes into circulatory channels. Once such anoxia changes have supervened, neurologic control cannot be regained and the process leads to total vascular collapse and death. The appearance of anoxia changes heralds the onset of *irreversible shock*. In recent years, shock therapy has developed to the degree where some cases demonstrating signs of tissue anoxia may now be rescued (Illustration 12-16).

The Effects of Shock

Tissue changes resulting from shock are largely those to be expected from visceral congestion and anoxia. If normal circulation is restored before extensive tissue damage ensues, all are reversible. Renal anoxia is particularly dangerous because of the propensity of tubular epithelial cells to ischemic necrosis. Recovery from shock is often complicated by the presence of extensive acute tubular necrosis which precludes re-establishing adequate renal function. Renal anoxia also leads to the leakage of erythrocytes through the glomerular filter and some hematuria usually follows any serious shock episode.

Additional Reading

Bill, H. and Thal, A. The peculiar hemodynamis of septic shock. Postgrad. Med. 48:106, 1970

Cherry J. Endotoxin shock. Surg. Clin. N. Amer. 50:403, 1970

Schumer, W. Evolution of the modern therapy of shock: Science *vs.* Empericism. Surg. Clin. N. Amer. 51:3, 1971

Wood, J. E. The venous system. Sci. Amer. 218:86, 1968

VASOSPASM AND HYPERTENSION

LEARNING OBJECTIVE

To be able to discuss each of the following 2 kinds of vascular dysfunction, describing each specific syndrome in some detail:

   a) **vasospasm (Raynaud's phenomenon and ergotism)**

   b) **hypertension (essential, renal and correctable)**

The second kind of vascular dysfunction to be discussed is represented by vasospasm and hypertension. Both of these conditions are characterized by vasoconstriction and *increased* peripheral resistance.

1. Vasospasm

Vasospasm occurs as the unprovoked, sudden constriction of peripheral vessels, usually affecting the extremities. We will employ the 2 conditions listed in Illustration 12-18 as our examples.

Raynaud's Phenomenon

Raynaud's phenomenon (or disease) is a condition in which there is paroxysmal, transient constriction of peripheral arteries, usually those of the most distal extremities. When it occurs as part of another disease (such as scleroderma), it is called Raynaud's phenomenon and, when it occurs as a seemingly primary condition, it is known as Raynaud's disease. Raynaud's disease is usually a rather mild affliction, characteristically seen in young to middle-aged women. An attack is usually provoked by cold or emotional stress and consists of transient blanching of the fingers followed by recovery of normal circulation. Raynaud's phenomenon tends to be more severe and may even lead to gangrene of the extremities.

Ergotism

Ergotism is a vasospastic disease caused by ingestion of foods made from rye contaminated with the fungus, *Claviceps purpurea.* In early times, this disease was seriously prevalent in certain areas of Europe. Because vascular spasms in this condition are strong and painful and because alkaloids of the fungus induce many other signs and symptoms including disturbed behavior, the disease came to be known as "St. Anthony's fire." Vasoconstriction in ergot poisoning is prolonged and severe and often leads to gangrene of the extremities. Extracts of the fungus were later used as an abortifacient and in the treatment of

12-18. VASOSPASM

1) RAYNAUD'S PHENOMENON
   when seen in association with another disease, otherwise known as Raynaud's disease

2) ERGOTISM
   an interesting historical problem with a modern epilog

12-19. HYPERTENSION*

1) ESSENTIAL

2) RENAL (INCLUDING "MALIGNANT")

3) CORRECTABLE

pheochromocytoma (functional tumor of adrenal medulla)

hyperaldosteronism (functional tumor of adrenal cortex)

food idiosyncrasy (cheese, licorice)

* Hypertension is usually defined as systemic pressure exceeding 140/90 or 150/90 but actual value must be arrived at for each patient considering age and other factors

migraine; experiments intended to develop less toxic substituent forms of ergot alkaloids led to the discovery of LSD.

2. Hypertension

Hypertension has been defined as the sustained elevation of a person's systemic blood pressure at a level exceeding that which is normal for his age and sex. We will consider hypertension as occurring in the 3 forms listed in Illustration 12-19.

Essential Hypertension

Essential hypertension is the most common of the 3. The term *essential* refers to the fact that it occurs as a single, idiopathic condition in an otherwise healthy individual and is not part of another disease. It is seen in women more often than in men, is most common in middle life or later and leads to changes in the cardiovascular system such as cardiac hypertrophy, renal vascular deterioration and the acceleration of atherosclerosis. Hypertensive heart disease will be considered in more detail in Chapter 13.

Renal Hypertension

Hypertension from any cause eventually leads to sclerosis of renal arterioles. Also, it can be easily demonstrated that any condition restricting blood flow through the kidneys will give rise to hypertension through the renin-angiotensin mechanism. In any single case of hypertension associated with renal deterioration, there is always the question as to which condition acted as cause and which became the effect. A form of hypertension that originates in the kidney and is associated with grave consequences is malignant hypertension (malignant nephrosclerosis). Malignant hypertension is a drastically serious condition in which the blood pressure continues to rise until the patient dies of some kind of vascular failure, usually an intracranial hemorrhage. Malignant hypertension may be superimposed on essential hypertension or may occur independent of this condition. Pathologic findings in patients dying of malignant hypertension almost always include the appearance of fibrinoid necrosis in the walls of arterioles, most conspicuously those of the renal arterial system.

Correctable Hypertension

In addition to the foregoing patterns of hypertension (which are incurable), there are a variety of similar conditions that are correctable. These include the pheochromocytoma, a functional tumor of the renal medulla, as well as the adrenocortical adenoma producing aldersterone in Conn's syndrome. In addition, one must also include various diet-related conditions such as those associated with idiosyncrasies toward cheese (and other tyramine-containing foods such as beer) and licorice. The therapeutic use of monoamine oxidase inhibitors predisposes an individual to tyramine-provoked hypertension, since both agents occupy the body's monoamine oxidases and prevent them from detoxifying endogenous catecholamines.

Additional Reading

Feagin, O. T. and Oates, J. A. Correctable causes of hypertension. Postgrad. Med. 44:156, 1968

Fraley, E. E. and Feldman, B. H. Renal hypertension. N. Engl. J. Med. 287:550, 1972

Horowitz, D. et al. Monoamine oxidase inhibitors, tyramine and cheese. J. Am. Med. Assn. 188:90, 1964

Koster, M. and David, G. K. Reversible, severe hypertension due to licorice ingestion. N. Engl. J. Med. 278:1381, 1968

Warren, S. and Chute, R. M. Pheochromocytoma. Cancer 29:327, 1972

VASCULAR OBSTRUCTION

LEARNING OBJECTIVE

To be able to discuss the pathogenesis, clinical course, clinical results and morphologic changes associated with the following obstructive vascular conditions:

a) thrombosis (solitary and DIC)
b) embolism (pulmonary thromboembolism, tumor embolism, fat embolism, septic and parasitic emboli, gas embolism)
c) obstructive diseases primary to vessels (atherosclerosis and Buerger's disease)

The many examples of vascular obstruction are an important cause of perfusion difficulties. Obstructive vascular lesions can be divided into the 3 categories listed in Illustration 12-20. Characteristic of these lesions is that they lead to ischemia which, if severe, may cause actual infarction of the area of tissue supplied by a vessel. The clinical manifestations of obstructive vascular lesions, then, are usually more attributable to necrosis of tissue supplied by the obstructed vessel than to the vascular lesion itself.

1. Thrombosis

The Solitary Thrombus

A thrombus is a clot that forms within a blood vessel or the heart. Its exact specifications are detailed in Illustration 12-21. Note that there are 3 essential characteristics to the thrombus: (1) it is located *within* the vessel; (2) in a *living* body; and (3) it *remains attached* to the vessel at the site of its formation. Although many factors contribute to the formation of a thrombus, the 3 principal causes are: (1) endothelial damage, (2) slowing of blood flow and (3) hypercoagulability of the blood. With damage to the endothelial wall, Hageman factor is activated and a platelet patch forms, releasing clot-promoting factors. Given sluggish blood flow, clot formation begins to outstrip the action of factors that normally protect the body from intravascular coagulation, and the thrombus begins to grow (propagate). Since veins of the extremities, particularly those of

---

12-20. OBSTRUCTIVE VASCULAR LESIONS*

1) THROMBOSIS

2) EMBOLISM

3) DISEASES PRIMARY TO VESSELS

— — — — —

* Obstructive lesions characteristically lead to ischemia and may result in an infarct

---

12-21. THROMBOSIS

THROMBUS: Intravascular (or intracardiac) clot within a living body that remains at the site of its formation

1) CAUSATIVE FACTORS
   endothelial damage
   slowing of blood flow (such as might occur when a limb is immobilized)
   hypercoagulability of blood (post-surgery or fracture)

2) FATES
   dislodgement or fragmentation to become embolus
   contraction, organization, recanalization
   calcification

---

the legs, represent the longest, slowest moving column of blood in the body, conditions favoring thrombosis are ideal in these vessels. Most serious examples of thrombosis occur in leg veins and most cases are seen in bed-ridden patients recovering from surgery or serious injury. The propagating thrombus grows by the apposition of alternating layers of conglutinated platelets and fibrin. The result is a solid, rubbery structure consisting of a series of lamina. On microscopic examination, the platelet layers can be distinguished as thin blue-staining lines alternating with bulky deposits of pink fibrin. These platelet lines are called the *lines of Zahn* and are useful in differentiating between an antemortem clot that forms in a moving stream and a postmortem clot that forms in a static mass of blood.

Thrombophlebitis

Venous thrombosis (phlebothrombosis) can be a serious emergency. If the clot becomes large and is located in the main venous channel, the body must contend with significant venous obstruction that will cause blood to accumulate in distal veins under abnormally high pressure. This will invariably lead to gross edema of the affected member. When infection and inflammation become superimposed on phlebothrombosis, the syndrome is known as *thrombophlebitis*.

Fates of the Thrombus

Many clinical courses are possible in thrombophlebitis and the outcome depends largely on the fate of the thrombus. These are listed in Illustration 12-21. One of the most serious developments is the detachment or fragmentation of the thrombus. Under these circumstances, the thrombus becomes an embolus (foreign particulate material in the blood stream) and will invariably lodge in the first capillary network encountered.

Disseminated Intravascular Coagulation (DIC)

Thrombosis occurs in 2 principal clinical patterns (Illustration 12-22). Having described the pathogenesis and fates of the solitary thrombus, we must now consider that in which thrombosis occurs as a generalized disorder, disseminated intravascular coagulation or DIC. Under certain circumstances, endothelial damage may be experienced as a widespread disease. Such generalized endothelial damage is thought to be the basis for DIC. About 50 per cent of patients with DIC are obstetric cases with complications of pregnancy. The balance are

---

12-22. THROMBOSIS (PRINCIPAL CLINICAL PATTERNS)

1) SOLITARY THROMBUS
   usually occurs during recovery from surgery in relatively immobile patient

2) DISSEMINATED INTRAVASCULAR COAGULATION (DIC)
   complication of terminal cancer, generalized vascular disease, or pregnancy
   may lead to "consumption coagulopathy"

---

distributed among various other primary disease, most of which are terminal cancer. In the latter category of patients, the DIC is often called *marantic thrombosis*. The patient manifesting DIC continues to consume platelets and clotting factors and will ultimately suffer a clotting defect. Paradoxically, despite all of the detrimental coagulation manifested, the patient with DIC may be unable to carry out normal hemostasis.

2. Embolism

Any abnormal particulate matter in the blood stream is called an *embolus*. In addition to the thrombus (the most common embolus), an embolus may consist of such diverse materials as fat globules, air bubbles and clusters of tumor cells. Emboli are arrested in the first vessel encountered that is too small to permit passage and usually cause dramatically sudden ischemia of the tissue supplied by the occluded vessel. If the ischemia is severe, the tissue will become necrotic and the resulting lesion is called an *infarct*.

We will consider the embolus under the 5 categories listed in Illustration 12-23.

Pulmonary Thromboembolism

The lodging of an embolus in a branch of the pulmonary artery is perhaps the most common serious example of this phenomenon. It has

12-23. EMBOLISM

EMBOLUS: Abnormal particulate matter in the blood stream

EXAMPLES:
    pulmonary thromboembolism
    tumor embolism
    fat embolism syndrome
    septic and parasitic emboli
    gas embolism

been estimated that up to 47,000 deaths occur each year in the United States from pulmonary embolism. The development of a thrombus in deep leg veins which subsequently dislodges to become impacted in the pulmonary circulation is the sequence of events accounting for the great preponderance of pulmonary embolism. Such a thrombus travels up the inferior vena cava as a single embolus or as an embolic "shower" and, after slipping through the right heart, becomes arrested in a branch of the pulmonary artery. Depending upon its size and location, it may cause a variety of signs and symptoms ranging from sudden death to mild chest pain and dyspnea. Serious pulmonary embolism may lead to the development of a pulmonary infarct, which will appear as a hemorrhagic lesion because of the dual blood supply to the lung. Pulmonary embolism is most often seen in the immobilized patient recovering from surgery or serious injury. Under such circumstances, the blood is usually hypercoagulable and its rate of circulation diminished.

Tumor Embolism

Although the thrombus is the most clinically important embolus and accounts for over 90 per cent of all cases of embolism, other materials are occasionally encountered. A common, but usually asymptomatic, embolus is the cluster of tumor cells. These often find their way into the blood stream by erosion of the wall of the vein and their impaction within the lung may lead to metastasis as well as occlusive phenomena.

Fat Embolism Syndrome

The fat embolism syndrome is a perplexing condition in which globules of fat are found occluding the microvasculature of the lung or brain. In most cases, this fat is released into the blood stream secondary to skeletal or soft tissue trauma. However, this syndrome is not always the result of mechanical injury and may develop in association with a number of different conditions such as diabetes, burns and severe infections. Presumably, the latter group of diseases include some kind of failure in the emulsion stability of fat as it is transported in the blood stream. The disturbance of emulsification allows chylomicra to coalesce into globules of dangerously large dimensions which can occlude smaller vessels. Fat embolism is most common in the third and fourth decades of life when long bone fractures most often occur and again in very advanced age when pathologic fractures are frequent. Fatal cases of this syndrome are usually associated with multiple, severe injuries and are rarely diagnosed *per se* because of the understandable tendency to attribute death under these circumstances to intractable shock. Clinical manifestations of fat embolism depend upon the location of vascular occlusion. If the lung is involved, there may be dyspnea and tachypnea, whereas brain lesions begin as restlessness, confusion, belligerent behavior and, in extreme cases, death. Often a petechial rash develops across the base of the neck, in the axillae and on the conjunctivae, but this is a later sign and unreliable.

Septic and Parasitic Emboli

Colonies of bacteria or single large parasites are often seen as emboli. The former is a common outcome of bacterial endocarditis in which bacteria, growing as fibrin-entrapped colonies (vegetations) on damaged heart valves, become detached and are carried through the arterial system. A common sequel to septic embolization is focal embolic glomerulonephritis, in which bacteria lodge in renal glomeruli causing their suppurative destruction.

Gas Embolism

The gas embolus is probably quite common, if one considers all possibilities for its occurrence: however, in the majority of cases, the embolus is without clinical significance ("silent bubble"). One of the most historically interesting causes for gas embolism is the use of the caisson in underwater construction. Before proper measures for decompression were appreciated, much suffering and several deaths resulted from construction workers' being transported too quickly from the caisson to the surface. Under such circumstances, the nitrogen became dissolved in great quantities in the blood while an individual breathed the hyperbaric environment of the cassion and bubbled out of solution as the person returned to the lower ambient pressure of the atmosphere. These bubbles caused widespread obstruction of capillary blood flow, manifested as severe pain (bends), dyspnea and frequent loss of consciousness. Chronic lesions included bone necrosis and spinal cord injury with paralysis. The syndrome came to be known as *caisson disease*. A similar, but less severe, disorder results from rapid assent to high altitudes. This condition is known as *dysbarism*. Gas embolism can also occur from the accidental injection of air or from a gas-forming infection (Illustration 12-24).

3. Obstructive Diseases Primary to Vessels

Many examples of vascular obstruction result as a complication of a disease primary to the

---

12-24. GAS EMBOLISM

COMPOSITION OF AIR:
    NITROGEN: 75.51 parts by weight
    OXYGEN: 23.15 parts by weight

---

1) ACCIDENTAL INJECTION OF AIR

2) GAS FORMING INFECTION

3) DYSBARISM
    rapid ascent to high altitude

4) DECOMPRESSION SICKNESS (CAISSON DISEASE) (BENDS)
    rapid ascent to earth's surface

12-25. OBSTRUCTIVE DISEASES PRIMARY TO VESSELS

1) ARTERIOSCLEROSIS
    most common example is atherosclerosis

2) ARTERIAL INFLAMMATORY DISEASES
    Buerger's disease (thromboangiitis obliterans)
    immune arteritis
        polyarteritis nodosa
        giant cell arteritis
        temporal arteritis

---

vessel wall. These may be arbitrarily considered as either *arteriosclerosis* or *arterial inflammatory disease* (Illustration 12-25). The former is a large group of diseases all of which lead to the hardening of arteries. By far the most common example of this category is atherosclerosis, which is discussed in detail elsewhere. Arterial inflammatory diseases are a widely diverse group of disorders, each of which is based on in inflammatory change in the vessel wall. Although not the most common, an example that serves as an excellent illustration is Buerger's disease.

Buerger's disease or thromboangiitis obliterans is an obliterating, segmental, inflammatory disease primarily affecting blood vessels of the extremities and beginning in medium and small-sized arteries. The age of onset is usually between 20 and 40, males are affected at a ratio of 75:1 and approximately half of all cases occur in those of Jewish extraction. Lesions occur in episodes producing complete and usually permanent vascular obstruction and often the need for amputation. Acute attacks are provoked or at least aggravated by smoking and, in some patients, abstinence from tobacco results in complete remission.

Additional Reading

Behnke, A. R. Decompression sickness: advances and interpretations. Aerospace Med. 42:255, 1971

Cabezas-Moya, R. and Dragstedt, L. R. An extreme example of Buerger's disease. Arch. Surg. 101:632, 1970

Deykin, D. The clinical challenge of disseminated intravascular coagulation. N. Engl. J. Med. 283:636, 1970

Dines, D. E. et al. Fat embolism syndrome. Mayo Clin. Proc. 47:237, 1972

Fitts, W. T. Jr. Thromboembolism: The clinical picture. J. Trauma 9:661, 1969

Harland, W. A. The problem of atherosclerosis. Practitioner 206:321, 1971

Jarcho, S. Alphonse Jaminet. Am. J. Cardiol. 21:258, 1968

Sartwell, P. E. Oral contraceptives and thromboembolism: A further report. Am. J. Epidemiol. 94:192, 1971

Scully, N. M. A new look at pulmonary embolism. Surg. Clin. N. Amer. 50:343, Apr, 1970

de Takats, G. and Vaithianathan, T. Bodily defenses against thrombosis. Am. J. Surg. 120:73, 1970

Wessler, S. Buerger's disease revisited. Surg. Clin. N. Amer. 49:703, 1969

STRUCTURAL VASCULAR DEFECTS

LEARNING OBJECTIVE

To be able to discuss the cause, pathogenesis and clinical course of the following vascular lesions:
  a) **aneurysm (congenital saccular, atherosclerotic, mycotic, syphilitic)**
  b) **varix (superficial, hemorrhoidal, esophageal)**
  c) **telangiectasia**
  d) **arteriovenous fistula**

On many occasions, disturbance of perfusion is traceable to a structural defect of a vessel. These most often take the form of an abnormal dilatation or outpouching and may be seen in arteries and veins of all caliber. We will consider each of the 4 kinds of structural defects listed in Illustration 12-26.

1. Aneurysm

An aneurysm is a sac-like, fusiform lesion formed by the abnormal dilatation of an artery (or vein). It most often results from structural weakness of the wall which may be congenital or acquired (Illustration 12-27).

> **12-26. STRUCTURAL VASCULAR DEFECTS**
>
> 1) ANEURYSM
>
> 2) VARIX
>
> 3) TELANGIECTASIA
>
> 4) ARTERIOVENOUS FISTULA

> **12-27. ANEURYSM**
>
> 1) CONGENITAL
>   congenital saccular ("berry") aneurysm
>
> 2) ACQUIRED
>   atherosclerotic
>   syphilitic
>   mycotic
>   dissecting

Congenital Saccular Aneurysm (Berry Aneurysm)

The congenital saccular aneurysm is found in a cerebral artery, usually at a bifurcation within the circle of Willis. It may develop slowly, throughout a person's early life, and usually becomes manifest in adulthood when it bursts or begins to leak. It is the most common cause of uncomplicated subarachnoid hemorrhage and the usual explanation for a cerebrovascular accident or "stroke" in the young adult.

Atherosclerotic Aneurysm

An atherosclerotic aneurysm is one that occurs secondary to the weakening of a vessel wall by atherosclerosis. It is seen quite often in the aorta where it occurs within the *abdominal* segment, at the iliac bifurcation.

Syphilitic Aneurysm

The syphilic aneurysm is a lesion occurring as a result of the weakening of the aortic wall in tertiary syphilis. It is found within the *thoracic* segment of the aorta, usually in the proximal portion of the arch.

Mycotic Aneurysm

The mycotic aneurysm is one that results from infection of a vessel wall. Bacterial enzymes digest and weaken the vessel, causing relatively sudden outpouching into an aneurysm.

2. Varix

The varix is a tortuous, abnormally dilated vein. It differs from an aneurysm in that the vessel is affected throughout a significant segment of its length. It may be caused by constitutional weakness in the adventitial layers or by the experiencing of sustained, unusual pressure within a vein or venous network. Some people appear to be unusually susceptible to the formation of varices, whereas others appear to form them only under abnormal provocation.

Three examples of varices are listed in Illustration 12-28. The first of these is the very common "varicose veins," actually varices of superficial (hence readily observable) veins. These are extremely common and are seen with great frequency in the legs of multiparous woman over the age of 30.

12-28. VARIX

VARIX: a tortuous, abnormally dilated vein

EXAMPLES:
1) VARICOSE VEINS
      superficial

2) HEMORRHOIDS

3) ESOPHAGEAL VARICES
      secondary to portal venous obstruction

The common hemorrhoid is a lesion which begins as a varix of a hemorrhoidal vein. This leads to stasis, thrombophlebitis and the usual complaint of tenderness.

The final example of the varix that we will use is the occurrence of esophageal varices secondary to obstruction of the portal venous network. The portal venous system is one of the few in the entire body that begins and ends in a capillary bed. It is the first system to intercept blood from the intestine and the major route for the return of splanchnic blood to the heart. Obstruction of the portal venous system usually occurs secondary to the hepatic fibrosis of chronic liver disease. With diffuse scarring of the liver and portal obstruction, the large volume of splanchic blood must find other routes for return to the central venous system. One of these is the thin-walled veins that are located within the esophageal wall just under the mucosa. In being forced to convey such an abnormally large volume of blood these veins dilate and become varicose, protruding into the lumen. An ever-present hazard in this condition is erosion of the mucosa and vein wall with resulting serious, and usually fatal, blood loss. Hemorrhage from esophageal varices is second only to hepatic failure as a cause of death in hepatic fibrosis (cirrhosis).

3. Telangiectasia

Telangiectasia is a lesion resulting from the permanent dilatation and abnormal prominence of capillaries, venules and arterioles. In the acquired form these are usually seen on the upper parts of the body of pregnant women or patients with chronic liver disease.

4. Arteriovenous Fistula

The arteriovenous fistula is an abnormal communication between the arterial and venous components of the circulatory system. It is an endothelial-lined tract of major caliber that bypasses a microvascular network and permits the direct, uncontrolled transfer of blood from the arterial to the venous system. It often results from the faulty healing of traumatic wounds and, if large enough, may impose a significant extra load on the heart.

Certain diseases are associated with widespread formation of arteriovenous fistulas. Most notable among these is osteitis deformans in which arteriovenous fistulae are found in bone.

HYPERVISCOSITY OF THE BLOOD

LEARNING OBJECTIVE

To be able to outline the effect of the following on the viscosity of the blood:
   a) hyperproteinemia (as exemplified by increased fibrinogen and paraproteinemia)
   b) polycythemia
   c) sclerocythemia (as exemplified in spherocytosis and sickle cell disease)

The final category of perfusion difficulties to be mentioned is that of blood vicosity changes. Since perfusion failures are more often seen with hyperviscosity, we will confine our attention to conditions in which viscosity is increased (Illustration 12-29).

Perhaps the most common factor causing an increase in the viscosity of blood is hyperproteinemia. This is seen as a normal concomitant of acute inflammation in which the circulating concentration of fibrinogen increases, and also as dysproteinemia (paraproteinemia) of the monoclonal gammopathy. As mentioned in an earlier discussion, either situation will be manifested as an increase in erythrocyte aggregation (rouleaux formation) and as an increase in the erythrocyte sedimentation rate.

It has been repeatedly demonstrated that there is also a close, direct relationship between hematocrit and whole blood viscosity. The greater the concentration of circulating erythrocytes, the more viscid will be the blood. This becomes particularly important in conditions such as polycythemia vera, in which erythrocyte concentration is grossly increased.

Our final example of conditions causing hyperviscosity are those in which red cells become overly rigid (sclerocythemia). An example of this phenomenon is seen in sickle cell disease where it may contribute significantly to the failure of deformed cells to traverse capillary beds.

Additional Reading

Litwin, M. S. Physical factors affecting human blood viscosity. J. Surg. Res. 10:433, 1970

Wells, R. Syndromes of hyperviscosity. N. Engl. J. Med. 283:183, 1970

12-29. HYPERVISCOSITY OF THE BLOOD

1) HYPERPROTEINEMIA
       increased fibrinogen, paraproteinemia
       causes increase in erythrocyte aggregation with increased ESR and rouleaux

2) POLYCYTHEMIA

3) SCLEROCYTHEMIA
       (conditions in which red cells become rigid)
           sickle cell disease
           spherocytosis

part 4

systems review — a

chapter 13
THE HEART

CONGENITAL HEART DISEASE

LEARNING OBJECTIVE

To be able to discuss the phenomenon of congenital heart disease and contrast cyanotic and acyanotic types, using the following as examples:
   a) **the tetralogy of Fallot**
   b) **septal defects**
   c) **the patent ductus arteriosus**

Major diseases of the heart can be considered as occurring in 9 categories (Illustration 13-1): however, only the first 5 will receive attention in this discussion. These 9 categories by no means exhaust the possibilities for heart disease. We have considered several others previously and this final summing up will only serve

---

13-1. MAJOR CATEGORIES OF HEART DISEASE

1) CONGENITAL HEART DISEASE

2) ISCHEMIC HEART DISEASE

3) HYPERTENSIVE HEART DISEASE

4) RHEUMATIC HEART DISEASE

5) INFECTIVE ENDOCARDITIS

- - -

6) SYPHILITIC HEART DISEASE

7) PULMONARY HEART DISEASE

8) PERICARDITIS

9) CARDIOMYOPATHIES

---

to lend some degree of completeness to our perspective.

In its embryonic development the heart, like many other organs of the human body, roughly recapitulates the stages of the evolution of this organ. It begins as a simple bulge in the dorsal aorta, becoming first a primitive 2-chambered pump and finally the complex 4-chambered organ of higher life forms. The process of cardiac development is amazingly intricate. The success of each stage depends upon completion of the 1 preceding it and the whole sequence is absolutely dependent on precisely correct differential rates of cell proliferation and the proper laying down of interstitial material such as collagen.

Congenital heart disease is based on developmental error. Such an error results in a structural defect in the heart or great vessels. All such defects are present from birth, although many are not recognized until later when some outward manifestation such as a heart murmur, low exercise tolerance or increased incidence of respiratory infection is noticed.

Congenital heart disease is a reasonably common occurrence, reports varying from 1.2 to 7.2 such lesions per 1,000 live births. The etiology of the developmental error is essentially unknown; however, hereditary factors are thought to play a great part. Teratogens such as thalidomide and rubella are also known to cause congenital heart defects. An enormous variety of congenital heart defects is possible, many of which are incompatible with life. We will consider 2 large categories, cyanotic defects and acyanotic defects (Illustration 13-2).

1. Cyanotic Congenital Heart Defects

If a congenital defect is compatible with life, its severity will depend upon its effect on circulatory kinetics. Cyanotic defects are those that have the most disastrous effect because they permit the direct mingling of venous and arterial blood (right-to-left-shunt). Almost all cyanotic defects are incompatible with life. Even if a cyanotic defect is mild enough to

---

13-2. CONGENITAL HEART DISEASE

1) CYANOTIC DEFECTS
　　right-to-left (venous-to-arterial)
　　blood shunt

2) ACYANOTIC DEFECTS
　　no shunt or left-to-right (arterial
　　to venous) blood shunt

13-3. CYANOTIC CONGENITAL DEFECTS

1) USUALLY INCOMPATIBLE WITH EX-
　　TRA-UTERINE LIFE OR FATAL WITHIN
　　A YEAR AFTER BIRTH

2) TETRALOGY OF FALLOT IS THE ONE
　　SEEN MOST COMMONLY IN CHIL-
　　DREN SURVIVING BEYOND 2 YEARS
　　large ventricular septal defect
　　aorta overrides right ventricle (ei-
　　　ther fully or partially)
　　stenosis of pulmonary outflow
　　　tract
　　right ventricular hypertrophy

---

sustain life, the patient will demonstrate a gradually worsening cyanosis with time.

Cyanosis (dusky, bluish skin color) requires the mixture of large quantities of venous with arterial blood. Cutaneous blood is usually rich in oxyhemoglobin, hence the color of normal caucasian skin is usually pink. The appearance of cyanosis suggests serious failing of the circulatory system.

The most common cyanotic defect in children surviving past the age of 2 years is the tetralogy of Fallot. This lesion is called a tetralogy because it includes the 4 abnormalities listed in Illustration 13-3. Cyanosis is usually not apparent at birth, but appears within the first few months of independent life. Complete surgical repair of this lesion is possible but is generally delayed until 6 to 8 years of age.

2. Acyanotic Congenital Heart Defects

Acyanotic congenital heart defects are those in which there is either no shunt or left-to-right shunt. They are not as severe as cyanotic defects and almost all are amenable to surgical treatment.

Over 90 per cent of congenital heart defects in living patients are of the acyanotic type. The most common are listed in order of their incidence in Illustration 13-4. We will consider the first 2 of these as our examples.

Septal defects are openings in either the atrial or ventricular septa that persist. The *foramen ovale,* an embryonic opening between the atria, may remain patent or an opening may persist between the ventricles (usually small and located in the membranous portion of the septum). All degrees of severity are possible and cyanosis is usually absent in long-standing

---

**13-4. EXAMPLES OF ACYANOTIC CON-
GENITAL HEART DEFECTS**

(in order of frequency)

1) SEPTAL DEFECTS

2) PATENT DUCTUS ARTERIOSUS

3) COARCTATION OF THE AORTA

---

untreated cases. *The interventricular septal defect is the most common of all congenital heart defects.*

Patent ductus arteriosus is thought to be the second most common form of congenital heart defect. Although, like other congenital heart defects, its etiology is essentially unknown, factors of heredity are operative in its occurrence. It is also seen in association with other congenital deformities when rubella is contracted by the mother during the first trimester of pregnancy.

Clinical manifestations of the patent ductus will vary with the size of the blood channel it provides. In every case, the shunt begins as left-to-right transfer because of the greater strength of the left ventricle: however, a large patent ductus may lead to right ventricular

13-5. PATENT DUCTUS ARTERIOSUS

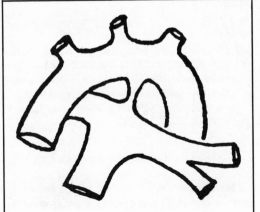

1) DUCTUS IS NORMAL FETAL STRUC-TURE, ALLOWS BLOOD TO BY-PASS LUNGS BY SHUNTING IT DI-RECTLY FROM PULMONARY ARTERY TO THE AORTA (see above)
2) SHOULD CLOSE WITHIN A FEW WEEKS AFTER BIRTH
3) PERSISTENT PATENCY BEGINS AS L-R SHUNT BUT MAY BECOME R-L AS RIGHT VENTRICLE HYPERTRO-PHIES

hypertrophy, severe pulmonary hypertension and even the equalization of pressures between the pulmonary and systemic circulatory systems. Thus, the patent ductus may become a right-to-left shunt if not corrected.

Total surgical correction of the patent ductus arteriosus is a relatively simple procedure with a low mortality rate. Since the risk of contracting infective endocarditis during later life is slightly greater in untreated cases, surgical correction is almost always recommended (Illustration 13-5).

Additional Reading

Hay, S. Incidence of selected congenital malformations in Iowa. Am. J. Epidemiol. 94:572, 1971
Jackson, B. T. The pathogenesis of congenital cardiovascular anomalies. N. Engl. J. Med. 279:25, 1968
Wegner, N. K. Stop and look—before you listen: Non-cardiac clues to the diagnosis of cardiovascular disease. Mt. Sinai J. Med. XXXVII:331, 1970

ISCHEMIC HEART DISEASE

LEARNING OBJECTIVE

To review information about atherosclerosis presented in Chapters 3, 11 and 12 and to be able to compare and contrast the 2 forms of ischemic heart disease manifested in angina pectoris and the myocardial infarct or "heart attack," including the following:

a) atherosclerosis as an antecedent condition
b) factors that provoke myocardial ischemia in both angina pectoris and the myocardial infarct
c) pathogenesis of the myocardial infarct
d) usual course of both conditions
e) complications and emergency situations presented by both

Ischemic heart disease is the term used for myocardial disorders based on insufficiency of the coronary circulation. This kind of heart disease is, far and away, the most prominent, accounting for approximately 50 per cent of all heart disorders now prevailing in living patients. The 2 most important clinical syndromes of cardiac ischemia are angina pectoris and myocardial infarction (Illustration 13-6). Both are almost always a result or complication of atherosclerotic narrowing of coronary arteries, and so *one should first review discussions of atherosclerosis presented in Chapters 3, 11 and 12.*

1. Angina Pectoris

Angina pectoris (literally "chest pain") is a disease in which the patient experiences paroxysms of a characteristic, constricting pain in the thorax. The condition most often giving rise to angina pectoris is gradual narrowing of coronary arteries to the point where circulation to the heart becomes marginally sufficient. With coronary circulation compromised, sudden demands for cardiac activity precipitate episodes of relative myocardial ischemia and result in the onset of a very characteristic,

---

13-6. ISCHEMIC HEART DISEASE

1) ANGINA PECTORIS
    usually caused by gradual athero-
    sclerotic narrowing of coronary
    arteries to the point where circula-
    tion is insufficient

2) MYOCARDIAL INFARCT (heart attack)
    usually caused by sudden occlu-
    sion of a coronary arterial branch
    resulting in complete ischemia of
    the area of heart muscle supplied
    by that branch

13-7. EXAMPLES OF FACTORS THAT MAY PRECIPITATE ANGINA PECTORIS

1) EXERTION

2) EMOTIONAL STRESS

3) A HEAVY MEAL

---

severe, crushing pain in the chest, usually described as radiating into the arms or neck. Examples of factors precipitating an attack of angina pectoris are listed in Illustration 13-7. The person who will experience angina pectoris is balanced on the very edge of cardiac circulatory adequacy; anything representing a demand for more cardiac output may result in an attack.

An episode of angina pectoris is quickly relieved by some kind of potent coronary vasodilator such as nitroglycerine. As a matter of fact, the response of such a condition to nitroglycerine is a very reliable confirmatory sign of angina pectoris and substantiates its being based on circulatory inadequacy.

The significance of angina pectoris is not so much the pain (although this may be excruciating), but rather that each attack may result in the diffuse necrosis of a number of myocardial fibers. The necrosis is neither as severe nor as concentrated as seen in the myocardial infarct, but each attack probably takes its toll of heart muscle.

Although most angina pectoris is brought about by atherosclerotic narrowing of coronary arteries, there are other factors that can cause it. Indeed, any of a number of factors that interfere with circulation through the coronary arteries are at least potential antecedents of angina pectoris. Some of these are listed in Illustration 13-8.

2. Myocardial Infarction

Myocardial infarction, like angina pectoris, is almost always a complication of atherosclerosis. Since the epidemiology of myocardial infarction will follow that of atherosclerosis very closely, the student is again urged to review information about the latter presented in earlier Chapters.

The myocardial infarct results from the sudden and more or less complete occlusion of a branch of the coronary arterial system. This leads to coagulation necrosis of a single, well defined area of heart wall and, if the patient survives, its subsequent replacement by scar.

We will trace the stages of the myocardial infarct from its inception as acute ischemia to its outcome as scar formation, mentioning the clinical picture, the histopathology and some of the complications that arise at each of the 5 stages listed in Illustration 13-9.

13-8. UNCOMMON CAUSES OF ANGINA PECTORIS

1) SYPHILITIC AORTITIS
    occlusion of coronary ostia by
    chronic inflammatory process

2) AORTIC VALVULAR INSUFFICIENCY
    low diastolic pressure

3) ANEMIA
    when superimposed on coronary
    atherosclerosis

13-9. PATHOGENESIS OF THE MYO-CARDIAL INFARCT

1) CORONARY OCCLUSION
no morphologic changes are ob-servable until at least 4 hours fol-lowing complete occlusion

2) FIRST DAY
first degenerative changes in heart muscle can be observed, also opening stages of acute inflamma-tory response

3) FIRST WEEK
inflammation peaks and begins to subside, ingress of macrophages, beginning repair, infarcted area becoming soft, serum enzyme changes detectable

4) SECOND AND THIRD WEEKS
necrotic tissue completely removed, fibrosis quite evident

5) FOUR WEEKS AND BEYOND
repair is complete and collagen maturation well under way

Coronary Occlusion

As a result of coronary atherosclerosis, the intimal lining of the coronary arterial system is bulged into the lumen of the vessel. Damage to this area of the endothelium (perhaps due to constant buffeting by erythrocytes) can result in the formation of a thrombus which may propagate to completely occlude an already impaired coronary artery. Another mechanism for occlusion is the possibility of sudden hemorrhage into an atheroma from the vasa vasorum. This latter mechanism is probably less important, but often mentioned. Although both are feasible means of completely occlud-ing a branch of the coronary system, in many cases neither can be demonstrated. In effect, then, the cause of many "heart attacks" cannot

be established with certainty. Where no occlu-sive lesion can be found, the cause is often ascribed to fibrillation or an intractable spasm of a coronary artery. But even in those heart attacks known to be based on coronary thrombosis, when death ensues quickly, no infarct will be evident because insufficient time will have elapsed for the ischemic area to undergo detectable degeneration. The descrip-tion of the following pathogenetic stages, then, applies only to those infarcts which are based on occlusion and in which the patient survives long enough for ischemic degenerative changes to become evident.

First Day

With sudden ischemia, the deprived area of the heart wall begins to degenerate. The myocardium is always in critical need of oxygen and will survive only a short time without adequate circulation. As seen in angina pectoris, myocardial ischemia is extremely painful; the heart attack is often described as a constricting or crushing chest pain that radiates into the arms, neck or abdomen. The patient may lose consciousness because of shock and, if the infarct is impinging on the interventricular system, may experience a disturbance of im-pulse conduction, fibrillation, total cessation of cardiac output and death. If death ensues within 4 hours, there will be no morphologic evidence of the patient's having sustained a myocardial infarct, unless an occluding lesion is discovered in the coronary system. Since death was so sudden, the affected muscle will appear normal even though it may have entered the first stages of necrosis. After 5 to 6 hours the first degenerative changes may be noticed in both the cytoplasm and nuclei of dying muscle. Also, within the first 24 hours, one may notice the opening stages of the acute inflammatory response that will develop to wall off the infarct. Complications and hazards in the first day include sudden death from fibrillation, and the development of stagnant, intractable shock which may also lead to death.

First Week

In the first week, from the second to the fourth day, a neutrophil exudate gradually forms so that by the end of the fourth day a strong acute inflammatory response is seen surrounding the infarct. This begins to subside on the fifth and sixth days and, as neutrophils disappear, their place is taken by macrophages. Also observable in the first week is the beginning of fibrous scar formation at the periphery of the infarct. With the wholesale disruption of cells now well along in its progress, intracellular enzymes begin to appear in the blood. Certain of these are helpful as confirmatory signs in the diagnosis of the myocardial infarct, since they are particularly well represented in cardiac muscle (although not found exclusively there). One of these, SGOT (serum glutamic-oxalacetic transaminase), which becomes elevated between 8 and 12 hours following infarction, reaches a peak between 24 and 48 hours and falls to normal within 3 to 8 days. Another is LDH (lactic dehydrogenase). This becomes elevated between 24 and 48 hours, reaches a peak between 48 and 72 hours and slowly falls to normal between 5 and 10 days. The first week, of course, also presents many new hazards. Since the area of the infarct is becoming soft, the patient is liable to rupture of the wall of the heart and to the development of cardiac tamponade. Damage to the endocardium overlying the infarcted area may result in the formation of a thrombus on the wall of the heart (mural thrombus) which can undergo fragmentation resulting in thromboemboli.

Second and Third Weeks

By the beginning of the second week a zone of necrotic muscle has been removed at the periphery of the infarct; by the end of this week the entire area of necrosis will be gone. Fibrosis, of course, will be well underway and quite evident. Here, again, new hazards appear. As healing progresses the wall of the heart may become distended, creating a non-functioning pouch which interferes with its operation (cardiac aneurysm). Also a hazard during the second and third weeks is the post-myocardial infarction syndrome (Dressler's syndrome), presumably the result of the mounting immunologic response to tissue debris released from the infarct. This includes fever, pericarditis, pleuritis and pneumonia. A similar clinical picture may be observed following cardiac surgery or trauma; hence, a more appropriate term, *post-cardiac injury syndrome,* has been suggested.

Signs of this condition are probably brought about by immune complex injury.

Four Weeks and Beyond

With the advent of the fourth week, collagen has now all but replaced the infarcted muscle. Assuming no other complication, the patient must now face the possibility that he has lost too much cardiac muscle to continue his normal life style. At this stage, the principal hazard is cardiac insufficiency which, in turn, could be so severe so as to lead to decompensated heart failure. Paradoxically, an infarct occurring in the young man is usually more serious than one occurring in an older man. This is because the young man, although he has experienced atherosclerotic degeneration of his coronary arteries, has not done so to the extent that numerous collateral circulatory routes have developed. When a coronary artery becomes occluded in a young man it usually leads to the damage of a large area of heart muscle, whereas, in the older individual, extensive collateral routes will be available to make up some of the deficit.

Additional Reading

Edwards, J. E. What is Myocardial Infarction? Circulation XXXIV (Suppl. 4) 5, 1969

Friedberg, C. K. Angina pectoris. Geriatrics 22:144, 1967

Jenkins, C. D. Psychologic and social precursors of coronary disease. N. Engl. J. Med. 284:244 and 301 (two parts) 1971

Kannel, W. B. Lipid profile and the potential coronary victim. Am. J. Clin. Nutrit. 24:1074, 1971

Roberts, W. C. The pathology of acute myocardial infarction. Hosp. Pract. 12:88, 1971

Rosenblatt, M. B. et al. Causes of death in 1000 consecutive autopsies. N.J. State J. Med. 71:2189, 1971

Russek, H. L. and Russek, L. G. Etiologic factors in ischemic heart disease. Geriatrics 27:81, 1972

Thompson, J. G. Production of severe atheroma in a transplanted heart. Lancet, Nov. 26, 1088, 1969.

HYPERTENSIVE HEART DISEASE

LEARNING OBJECTIVE

To review information about hypertension presented in Chapter 12 and be able to discuss this entire subject emphasizing its effect on the heart and including the following:
   a) definition of hypertension
   b) epidemiology of essential or primary hypertension
   c) effects of longstanding hypertension

Hypertension is the condition of sustained, abnormally high *systemic* blood pressure. We will see in later subjects that there is the possibility for developing hypertension in both the pulmonary and portal circulatory systems: however, these are different and usually unrelated conditions. Systemic blood pressures tend to be higher in older individuals and so an accurate definition of hypertension depends upon the age group in which it is being considered. Generally speaking, in men and women between the ages of 20 and 60, hypertension is defined as systolic pressures higher than 140 to 150 and diastolic pressures higher than 90.

By far, the most common kind of hypertension is the "essential" or primary type although hypertension secondary to a variety of other disorders is often seen (see Chapter 12). Essential hypertension is approximately twice as common in women as in men and it tends to be seen with greater frequency in the obese and in members of the black race. Its etiology is unknown, although it is clearly related to an increase in the peripheral vascular resistance to blood flow. Its effects on the heart, major vessels, brain and kidneys shorten life and lead to a variety of distinguishing morphologic changes.

The effect of hypertension on the heart (Illustration 13-10) depends upon its duration and severity. In early stages, hypertension causes simple hypertrophy of the left ventricular wall, increasing the weight of the heart but not its size. This condition is called "concentric" hypertrophy, because the heart wall grows at the expense of the chamber's area and the normal outward shape of the heart is retained. In later stages, the heart dilates and for a time the increased thickness may be obscured by the stretching of the heart wall. Hypertrophy continues, however, and soon the heart appears both enlarged and more muscular.

In the latest stages of severe cases, hypertensive heart disease may progress to heart failure, systemic congestion and death.

RHEUMATIC HEART DISEASE

LEARNING OBJECTIVE

To be able to discuss the entire phenomenon of rheumatic fever and rheumatic heart disease, including the following:
   a) its relationship to streptococcal infection
   b) epidemiology
   c) the Jones criteria
   d) heart lesions
   e) clinical course and systemic effects of rheumatic heart disease
   f) potential for emergency situations in the rheumatic heart patient

---

13-10. THE EFFECT OF HYPERTENSION ON THE HEART

1) CONCENTRIC HYPERTROPHY

2) DILATATION AND CONTINUED HYPERTROPHY
   cardiac enlargement

3) ULTIMATE HEART FAILURE

Rheumatic fever is a delayed complication of infection with Group A beta hemolytic streptococcus. It occurs in only 3 per cent of individuals sustaining such infections: however, this is thought to result in approximately 100,000 new cases of rheumatic fever per year in the U.S. It is clearly a disease of the very young with most first attacks occurring in the decade between 5 and 15.

Rheumatic fever is undoubtedly based on an

13-11. RHEUMATIC FEVER

1) POST-STREPTOCOCCAL PHENOMENON

   follows infection with beta hemolytic, group A strep

2) IDIOPATHIC INFLAMMATION OF HEART, JOINTS AND OTHER TISSUES

   carditis is only manifestation that can cause life-threatening complications

3) RECURRENT ATTACKS CAUSE PROGRESSIVE DEFORMATION OF HEART VALVES

   particularly mitral valve
   fibrous thickening
   verrucous outgrowths
   stenosis

4) A SINGLE, WELL-DOCUMENTED ATTACK IS INDICATION FOR THE LIFELONG USE OF PROPHYLACTIC ANTIBIOTICS

13-12. JONES CRITERIA (MODIFIED*)

1) MAJOR MANIFESTATIONS
   carditis
   polyarthritis
   chorea

2) MINOR MANIFESTATIONS
   fever
   previous attack
   positive acute phase reactants (such as increased ESR)
   prolonged P-R interval

3) SUPPORTING EVIDENCE OF STREPTOCOCCAL INFECTION
   recent scarlet fever
   positive throat culture
   increased titer of anti-streptococcal Ab.

— — —

* Originally proposed by T. Duckett Jones in 1944. Revised by AHA Council on Rheumatic Fever and Congenital Heart Disease. Postgrad. Med. 44:73, 1968

---

immunologic reaction to some product of the infecting bacteria. Like acute glomerulonephritis (see Chapter 18), it is a poststreptococcal inflammatory disease, but unlike the kidney disease it has not yet been shown to be based on the accumulation of immune complexes in affected tissue (Illustration 13-11).

A single attack of rheumatic fever may occur in a range of clinical severity from acute and fulminant to chronic and subclinical. There is no specific symptom or sign pathognomonic of rheumatic fever: however, certain clinical standards called the "Jones criteria" have been established to be used as guidelines in diagnosis. These are outlined in Illustration 13-12.

Inflammation of the heart (carditis) occurs in about one-half the patients during the initial attack of rheumatic fever. It most often affects all 3 layers of the heart (pancarditis). Carditis is the only manifestation of rheumatic fever that can lead to chronic disease and death. Recurrent attacks of rheumatic fever cause progressive distortion of heart valves (Illustration

---

13-13. RHEUMATIC HEART DISEASE

1) FIBROUS THICKENING OF VALVE LEAFLETS

2) VERRUCOUS (WART-LIKE) GROWTHS ALONG LINE OF CLOSURE

3) STENOSIS

4) THICKENING OF CHORDAE TENDINAE FIBROSIS OF PAPILLARY MUSCULATURE

13-13), which in turn may lead to severe congestive heart failure and its consequences. The valve most commonly affected is the mitral: however, the aortic valve is often involved either alone or in combination with the mitral.

Valve distortion in chronic, recurrent rheumatic fever takes 2 forms: 1) fibrous thickening of the leaflets with verrucous thickening along the line of closure and 2) stenosis of the valve annulus. The heart deformity most characteristic of chronic rheumatic fever is mitral insufficiency and stenosis. In far advanced cases heart lesions become manifested clinically as failure of both the left and right sides of the heart, leading to severe systemic and pulmonary congestion.

Like other diseases that give rise to irreversible degenerative changes, the most effective treatment of rheumatic fever is its prevention. Given a proven incident of rheumatic fever, authorities now recommend that the patient be treated prophylactically with antibiotics for the rest of his life.

Additional Reading

Quie, P. G. and Ayoub, E. M. Rheumatic fever. Postgrad. Med. 44:73, 1968

INFECTIVE ENDOCARDITIS

LEARNING OBJECTIVE

To be able to discuss the entire phenomenon of infective endocarditis including the following:
   a) **predisposing factors**
   b) **pathogenesis**
   c) **causative agents and clinical varieties**
   d) **prevention**

Infective endocarditis is a disease in which endocardial surfaces, (principally heart valves) are damaged by a parasitic microorganism. Agents responsible for infective endocarditis find their way into the blood stream, become attached to valve leaflets or some other area of the endocardium and either destroy tissue or grow out in soft friable masses known as *vegetations.* Vegetations consist of the infecting microorganisms trapped in fibrin.

In addition to causing direct damage to the valve leaflet, the vegetations of infective endocarditis shed septic material into the blood stream which becomes arrested in other organs to establish new sites of infection. Both brain and kidney are often affected in this way.

At one time it was thought that infective endocarditis could be clearly divided into acute and subacute forms, depending upon the virulence of the infecting organism. Today there is more of a tendency to consider this disease a single entity, the clinical course of which will depend upon a number of additional factors such as the defense status of the host and the treatment regimen employed.

One characteristic of the disease that does seem dependent upon the virulence of the infecting organism is the nature of the heart lesion. Less virulent organisms such as non-hemolytic streptococci produce vegetative lesions, with attendant embolic complications while virulent organisms such as hemolytic streptococci and staphylococci produce the more destructive, ulcerating lesions that often result in valvular insufficiency.

The widespread use of antibiotics has caused a change in the relative frequency of causative organisms. Today, most cases of this disease are caused by either Streptococcus, viridans or staphylococcus, the latter being associated with more severe ulcerating infections occurring in essentially normal hearts. Although other infectious agents are comparatively rare as a cause of infective endocarditis, almost any pathogen has this potential. In fact, there now appears to be an increase in the incidence of endocarditis caused by antibiotic-resistant gram-negative bacteria and even fungi (Illustration 13-14). The significant incidence of monilial endocarditis has rendered the older term "bacterial endocarditis" inaccurate.

Eighty percent of cases of infective endocarditis occur in patients with rheumatic heart lesions and about 10% in patients with congenital heart deformities. The remaining 10% occur in patients with seemingly normal hearts and are usually the ulcerative form caused by more virulent organisms such as staphylococci.

Given either rheumatic or congenital heart disease, a normally innocuous bacteremia can result in the implantation of organisms on the endocardial surface and the development of a

13-14. INFECTIVE ENDOCARDITIS*

1) BACTERIAL (OR FUNGAL) INFECTION OF ENDOCARDIAL SURFACE
   usually valves

2) 80% OCCURS ON RHEUMATICALLY DEFORMED ENDOCARDIUM, 10% ON CONGENITALLY DEFORMED AND 10% ON SEEMINGLY NORMAL HEARTS

3) VEGETATIVE OR ULCERATIVE
   depending upon character of causative organism

4) EXTREMELY SERIOUS INFECTION, DIFFICULT TO TREAT
   many cases now caused by anti-biotic-resistant, gram-negative organisms and fungi

— — —

* The older term "bacterial endocarditis," although still widely used, is now considered inadequate in view of the frequency of fungal cases

severe infection. It must be remembered, therefore, that *before rendering any treatment that may result in even the slightest release of bacteria into the blood stream one is obliged to make absolutely sure that the patient is not affected with any kind of heart deformity.* If such treatment must be performed and the patient is known (or suspected) to have a deformity of the heart, it is absolutely necessary to use prophylactic antibiotics.

Additional Reading

Quinn, E. L. Bacterial endocarditis. Postgrad. Med. 44:82, 1968

chapter 14

HEMATOPOIETIC AND LYMPHORETICULAR SYSTEMS

NORMAL HEMOSTASIS

LEARNING OBJECTIVE

To be able to describe the process of hemostasis and briefly outline the contributions and interactions of:
- a) vessels
- b) platelets
- c) the intrinsic coagulation mechanism

Higher and more complex animals use circulatory systems that operate at pressures considerably greater than lower organisms of more simple construction. With the evolutionary emergence of increased blood pressure came the risk of sudden, serious hemorrhage, an intolerable selective hazard that dictated the parallel development of improved means of stopping the flow of blood from damaged vessels. In man, we see both the high perfusion pressure and the elaborate staunching mechanisms of far advanced species.

The sequence of events leading to the arresting of blood loss from an injured vessel is called hemostasis. Effective hemostasis depends upon contributions from 3 sources (Illustration 14-1). Because of their critical importance in all clinical disciplines, we will spend some time discussing each of these components of normal hemostasis.

1. Vessels

The major role of vessel integrity in successful hemostasis is apparent. The vessels conduct the blood and any lasting hemostatic device must be based first of all on intact, serviceable vessels. In a disease such as scurvy, in which intracellular cement substance of the endothelial membrane is deficient, one sees a profound tendency to spontaneous hemorrhage. Also, the neurologically mediated contraction of vessels that follows local injury undoubtedly facilitates

---

14.1 THREE COMPONENTS OF NORMAL HEMOSTASIS

1) **VESSELS**
   contain the blood
   constrict following injury to allow formation of platelet patch

2) **PLATELETS**
   adhere to exposed collagen and conglutinate to form temporary patch aggregate platelets release clot-promoting factors (PF-3)

3) **COAGULATION MECHANISM**
   allows replacement of platelet patch with fibrin
   fibrin is later replaced with scar if injury has been extensive

---

succeeding steps and represents another contribution of vessels to the over-all scheme of hemostasis.

2. Platelets

The second important factor in hemostasis is the platelet or thrombocyte. The platelet is a small (2 to 5 micron) fragment of cytoplasm. They are given off by the megakaryocyte, a large cell residing in hematopoietic marrow. Healthy platelets are disc-shaped, possess mitochondria, ribosomes, lysosome-like electron-dense granules, a cytocavitary network and a unit plasma membrane. They do not contain rough endoplasmic reticulum or a nucleus. They are slightly phagocytic and have a life span in the circulation of approximately 3 to 15 days. The normal circulating concentration of platelets is 150,000 to 350,000 per cu. mm. The level is elevated in response to emotional stress, trauma, surgery, and in particular, following removal of the spleen.

The principal function of the platelet is its role as an agent of hemostasis. In this respect, its contribution differs considerably from that of the clotting mechanism, as can be seen in a closer look at the actual sequence of events following injury to a blood vessel:

1. The vessel is damaged and immediately contracts. (This vascular contribution to hemostasis is usually insufficient to stop hemorrhage.)
2. Within seconds platelets adhere to the site of damage and the defect is occluded by a platelet mass known as the "hemostatic plug."
3. The intrinsic coagulation mechanism is activated.
4. As a clot is formed the hemostatic plug disintegrates and is replaced by a more durable fibrin mass. Complete replacement occurs within a matter of hours or, at most, a few days, depending on the extent of the injury.
5. The clot is ultimately replaced by a regenerated endothelial membrane or scar or both.

It is important to note that conglutinated platelets comprise a primary, but transient, patching material for damaged vessels. The initial platelet layer does not attach to damaged endothelial cells, but rather to newly exposed collagen fibers. Thus, it is the exposure of collagen that starts platelet activity, just as it sets off the normal activation of Hageman factor.

Illustration 14-2 is an outline of the interrelationship between the platelet and solute systems mediated by Hageman factor.

3. The Coagulation Mechanism

The third important factor in hemostasis is the coagulation mechanism. We have encountered this system earlier in Chapter 2, but we must now outline its operation in some detail.

The whole strategy of the coagulation mechanism is directed toward causing an insoluble protein clot to form suddenly from soluble, blood-borne percursors. This tough protein matrix of the clot is called fibrin. A more or less complete list of factors involved in coagulation is provided in Illustration 14-3.

Although it is recognized as a gross oversimplification, it is convenient to organize the operation of the coagulation mechanism into 3 stages (Illustration 14-4).

Whereas this simplified concept of coagulation should be recognized as scientifically incomplete, it is still very useful as a means of roughly classifying defects of coagulation.

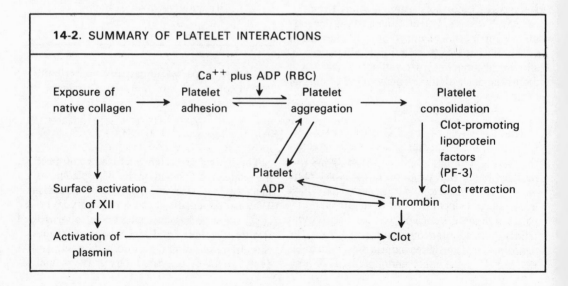

14-2. SUMMARY OF PLATELET INTERACTIONS

14-3. CLOTTING FACTORS

I	FIBRINOGEN
II	PROTHROMBIN
III	THROMBOPLASTIN
IV	CALCIUM
V	LABILE FACTOR
VI	(none)*
VII	STABLE FACTOR
VIII	ANTIHEMOPHILIC FACTOR
IX	CHRISTMAS FACTOR
X	STUART-PROWER FACTOR
XI	PLASMA THROMBOPLASTIN ANTECEDENT (PTA)
XII	HAGEMAN FACTOR
XIII	FIBRIN STABILIZING FACTOR

- - - - - - - - - -

* This numeral was once used to designate what was thought to be an active form of factor V

14-4. "CLASSICAL" SEQUENCE OF COAGULATION STAGES

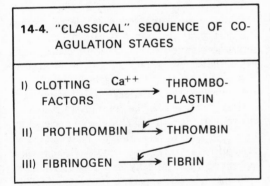

I) CLOTTING FACTORS $\xrightarrow{Ca^{++}}$ THROMBO-PLASTIN

II) PROTHROMBIN $\longrightarrow$ THROMBIN

III) FIBRINOGEN $\longrightarrow$ FIBRIN

Note that at Stage I the process gives rise to a substance called thromboplastin. Thromboplastin is not a single, well characterized material but a group of activated antecedent factors which (by acting on prothrombin) give rise to thrombin. This distinction is important because another kind of thromboplastin is released by tissue damage and provides a completely separate pathway for the initiation of a clot. We see, therefore, that there are actually 2 alternative ways to accomplish Stage

I: 1) an intrinsic pathway (so-called because all factors are contained within circulating blood) and 2) an extrinsic pathway in which thromboplastin is provided from outside the blood-vascular system.

Illustration 14-5 is a highly simplified diagram of the relationship between the intrinsic and extrinsic coagulation mechanisms.

Note that the intrinsic system operates through the activation of 4 coagulation factors in sequence. Factor XII (Hageman factor), when activated, activates factor XI which activates factor VIII. At each stage there is a geometric increment in the number of participating molecules. For example, 10 molecules of activated Hageman factor may each activate 10 molecules of factor XI, each of which may activate 10 of factor IX, etc. This geometric increase in the number of participating molecules is called "biologic amplification," the "gain" depending upon the number of molecules and the number of stages. The effect has been likened to a cascade or avalanche in which a few events occurring at the beginning of a sequence can be expanded to a countless number of similar events at the end.

It is important to realize that the more primitive extrinsic system proceeds more or less directly from tissue disruption to fibrin formation and is comparatively inefficient. The intrinsic system, however, using the principle of amplification, is capable of generating copious amounts of fibrin and responding very suddenly. That such a sensitive and efficient system is needed to maintain a high-pressure blood system can be seen from the fact that defects of the intrinsic coagulation mechanism frequently lead to fatal hemorrhage.

The very efficiency of the intrinsic coagulation system would endanger the life of an individual unless some means of controlling its activation was also available. Consider, for example, that, if clotting factors were activated and then allowed to remain intact while they diffused throughout the body, the obvious result would be general solidification of the blood. To prevent such catastrophe, the coagulation mechanism is coupled to other intrinsic molecular systems which provide a check and balance on its operation. Look back for one moment to Illustration 14-5. Note that factor XII (Hageman factor) is situated at the very threshold of the intrinsic coagulation mechanism. It is the activation of Hageman factor

14-5. SIMPLIFIED DIAGRAM OF THE RELATIONSHIP BETWEEN INTRINSIC AND EX-
TRINSIC COAGULATION MECHANISMS

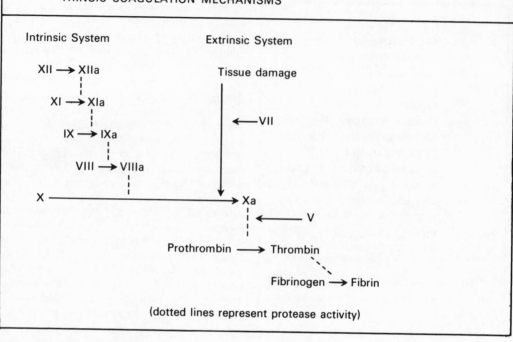

(dotted lines represent protease activity)

14-6. CENTRAL   ROLE   OF   HAGEMAN
FACTOR

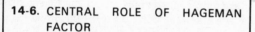
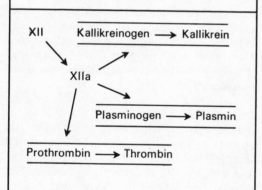

that starts the entire sequence. Bear in mind, however, that this same Hagemen factor also serves to couple the coagulation mechanism to other molecular systems. Figure 14-6 depects this coordinating role of Hageman factor. Note that through Hageman factor the coagulation system is coupled to the fibrinolysin system so that clot formation and clot digestion can enter into a balanced relationship. Note also that Hageman factor couples the kallikrein-kinin system to the 2 already mentioned. The need for this is less apparent, but it might be speculated that it assures the focusing of activated coagulation factors at the site of hemorrhage or inflammation and prevents their dissemination throughout the body.

Additional Reading

Bleyer, W. et al. The development of hemostasis in the human fetus and newborn infant. J. Pediat. 79:838, 1971
Gaston, L. W. Blood clotting factors. N. Engl. J. Med. 270:236, 1964
Rodman, N. F. and Mason, R. G. Platelet-platelet interaction: relationship to hemostasis and thrombosis. Fed. Proc. 26:95, 1967

DISORDERS OF HEMOSTASIS

LEARNING OBJECTIVE

To be able to compare and contrast the two principal categories of hemostatic disorders, discussing the causes, clerical signs and hazards of:

- a) thrombocytopenic purpura
- b) non-thrombocytopenic purpura
- c) hemophilia A (as an example of the Stage I coagulation disorder)
- d) varieties of the Stage II coagulation disorder

Disorders of hemostasis are usually divided into the 2 principal kinds, *purpura* and *coagulation disorders*. In Illustration 14-7, we see that purpura is generally caused by a disturbance of vessels or platelets, whereas coagulation disorders are always traceable to some deficiency in the intrinsic coagulation mechanism.

1. Purpura

Purpura is a rather inexact term usually taken to mean a condition characterized by episodes of spontaneous bleeding. These hemorrhages often occur into skin or mucous membranes resulting in areas of deep, purplish pigmentation, hence the term, purpura. Skin discoloration in purpura can vary from petechial hemorrhages to large patches of ecchymosis. By tradition, purpura itself is further subdivided into 2 types, *thrombocytopenic purpura* (Illustration 14-8) and *non-thrombocytopenic purpura* (Illustration 14-9). In the former, the concentration of circulating platelets will be lowered by any of a variety of systemic disorders, whereas the latter is most often traceable to some kind of vessel defect.

14-8. THROMBOCYTOPENIC PURPURA (LOW PLATELET CONCENTRATION)

1) SHORTENED PLATELET LIFESPAN
   - drug reactions
   - infections
   - ITP (primary autoimmune)
   - TTP (widespread thrombosis)
   - hypersplenism

2) FAILURE OF PLATELET PRODUCTION
   - idiopathic marrow failure
   - chemical suppression
   - irradiation
   - myelophthisic conditions
     - leukemia
     - myelofibrosis
     - multiple myeloma
     - histiocytosis
   - metabolic disorders
   - infections

14-7. DISORDERS OF HEMOSTASIS

1) PURPURA
   tendency toward spontaneous hemorrhage caused by a number of disorders of either vessels or platelets

2) COAGULATION DISORDERS
   tendency toward spontaneous and prolonged bleeding caused by a deficiency of one or more clotting factors

---

14-9. NON-THROMBOCYTOPENIC PURPURA

1) VESSEL DEFECTS
   - scurvy
   - certain infections
     - diphtheria
     - rickettsial disease
     - typhoid fever
     - scarlet fever

2) PLATELET DEFECTS
   (very rare)

The clinical picture of purpura varies from the innocuous to the very severe. Depression of the platelet count below 50,000 cu mm of blood will usually result in clinically apparent purpura as outlined in Illustration 14-10. The patient complains of "bruising easily" and demonstrates frequent spontaneous hemorrhage into skin or mucous membrane, from around the necks of the teeth or into hollow viscera.

The condition of purpura greatly increases the risk of fatal intracranial hemorrhage (cerebrovascular accident) and for this reason is particularly dangerous.

2. Coagulation Disorders

Coagulation disorders, the second major class hemostatic disorders, occur in a variety of heritable and acquired forms. The common effect of all such disorders is failure to form fibrin.

Coagulation disorders result in the clinical phenomenon known as "rebleeding." If a patient with a defect of the intrinsic coagulation mechanism sustains a mild injury, bleeding will soon be arrested by the formation of the hemostatic plug: however, as the plug disintegrates, fibrin will not be generated to take its place and bleeding resumes. This phenomenon of the resumption of bleeding after its having stopped is one hallmark of the coagulation disorder.

Most coagulation disorders are based on the deficiency of factors operating in Stages I and II of the coagulation scheme. We will use an example of a disorder originating in each of the 3 stages to establish a more complete picture (Illustration 14-11).

14-10. SIGNS OF PURPURA

1) SPONTANEOUS HEMORRHAGE INTO SKIN OR MUCOUS MEMBRANES

2) "EASILY BRUISED"

3) EPISTAXIS, HEMATURIA, MELENA, HEMATEMESIS

4) RISK OF CVA

5) HEMORRHAGE AROUND TEETH

14-11. COAGULATION DISORDERS

1) HEMOPHILIA (Stage I Defect)
   hemophilia A is most common example: accounts for approximately 80 per cent of all cases

2) PROTHROMBIN DEFICIENCY (Stage II Defect)
   hemorrhagic disease of newborn
   chronic liver disease
   diseases leading to steatorrhea
   anticoagulant therapy using warfarin drugs

3) FIBRINOGEN DEFICIENCY (Stage III Defect)
   congenital (very rare)
   chronic liver disease

14-12. HEMOPHILIA-A (STAGE I COAGULATION DEFECT)

1) CONGENITAL ABSENCE OF CLOTTING FACTOR VIII

2) INHERITED AS SEX-LINKED RECESSIVE CHARACTER

3) HEMARTHROSIS IS COMMON

4) REBLEEDING: PROLONGED HEMORRHAGE: LETHAL POTENTIAL IN INJURY OR SURGERY

Hemophilia-A

Hemophilia-A, an inherited deficiency of clotting factor VIII, is the most common of the congenital coagulation disorders (Illustration 14-12). It is inherited as a sex-linked recessive trait and its occurrence is practically confined to the male. It accounts for approximately 80 per cent of the cases of "pure" Stage I coagulation defects.

14-13. PROTHROMBIN DEFICIENCY (STAGE II COAGULATION DEFECT)

1) PROTHROMBIN IS PRODUCED BY THE LIVER: VITAMIN K (FAT SOLUBLE) IS NEEDED

2) HEMORRHAGIC DISEASE OF THE NEWBORN IS COMMON EXAMPLE

3) ADULT FORMS INCLUDE:
    chronic liver disease
    diseases causing steatorrhea
    anticoagulant therapy

14-14. FIBRINOGEN DEFICIENCY (STAGE III COAGULATION DEFECT)

1) OCCURS IN CONGENITAL AND ACQUIRED FORMS
    (congenital form very rare)

2) ACQUIRED FORMS ASSOCIATED WITH:
    obstetrical disorders
    chronic liver disease

The most outstanding clinical feature of hemophilia-A is hemarthrosis (bleeding into joint spaces). Also conspicuous is the risk of serious or even fatal hemorrhage from minor trauma or surgery. Continued bleeding beyond 24 hours following any surgical procedure should arouse mild suspicion of a coagulation defect of this type. If bleeding persists beyond 48 hours grave suspicion is warranted.

Prothrombin Deficiency

Prothrombin deficiency occurs in a variety of circumstances, perhaps the most common being the neonatal deficiency of prothrombin based on the lack of intestinal bacteria as a source of vitamin K.

The possibility for prothrombin deficiency in the adult arises with chronic liver disease, absorptive defects and anticoagulant therapy with warfarin-type drugs that act as competetive inhibitors of vitamin K (Illustration 14-13).

Fibrinogen Deficiency

Fibrinogen deficiency occurs in both congenital and acquired forms: however, the former is very rare.

Since fibrinogen is produced by the liver anything that destroys liver parenchyma or interferes with its normal function can give rise to some degree of acquired fibrinogen deficiency. This is most often seen in associations with disorders of pregnancy and chronic liver diseases (Illustration 14-14).

Additional Reading

Craig, J. W. Vitamin K deficiency in adults. Nutrit. Rev. 26:165, 1968

Crowell, E. B. et al. The effect of oral contraceptives on factor VIII levels. J. Lab. Clin. Med. 77:551, 1971

Deykin, D. Warfarin therapy. N. Engl. J. Med. 283:691, 1970

Edson, J. R. Hemophilia; von Willebrand's disease and related conditions. Human Path. 1:387, 1970

Girolami, A. Report of a case of congenital afibrinogenemia. Blut 24:23, 1972

Hathaway, W. E. Bleeding disorders in children due to platelet dysfunction. Am. J. Dis. Child. 121:127, 1971

Karapatkin, S. Drug-induced thrombocytopenia. Am. J. Med. Sci. 262:68, 1971

Stormorken, H. Physiopathology of hemostasis. Sem. in Hematol. 8:3, 1971

Wesler, S. and Alexander, B. A guide to anticoagulant therapy. Am. Heart Assn., 1970

DEFICIENCIES OF THE FORMED ELEMENTS OF BLOOD

LEARNING OBJECTIVE

To be able to outline the location, functions and products of hematopoietic marrow and compare the following 3 causes of anemia, listing prominent clinical examples of each:

    a) acute and chronic hemorrhage
    b) excess hemolysis
    c) marrow failure

Hematopoietic marrow is the tissue that supplies most of the formed elements of blood (cells and platelets). It is found in practically all bones of the child and in all except long bones in the adult. In the fetus, one finds hematopoietic activity in the spleen and liver as well, but such extramedullary activity ceases before or shortly after birth (Illustration 14-15).

Diseases affecting the formed elements of blood are conveniently classified as either *deficiency disorders* or *proliferative disorders* (Illustration 14-16). They may affect a single element or all cell series. Having already discussed the platelet, we will consider the very complex picture of anemia as our second example of deficiency disorders of the formed elements of blood. Proliferative disorders will be considered as a separate subject in the following learning objective.

14-15. DISTRIBUTION OF HEMATOPOIETIC MARROW

1) CHILD:
    all bones

2) ADULT:
    all bones except long bones

  – – – – – – – – –

  Hematopoietic activity in the spleen ceases before birth
  Small foci of liver activity may persist at the time of birth

---

14-16. DISEASES AFFECTING THE FORMED ELEMENTS OF BLOOD

1) DEFICIENCY DISORDERS
    red cell: anemia
    white cell: leukopenia
    platelet: thrombocytopenia
    all series: pancytopenia

2) PROLIFERATIVE DISORDERS
    red cell: polycythemia
    white cell: leukemia
    platelet: thrombocythemia
    all series: leukoerythroblastosis

14-17. ANEMIA (DEFICIENCY OF CIRCULATING ERYTHROCYTES)

1) THE ANEMIA OF HEMORRHAGE

2) THE ANEMIA OF EXCESS HEMOLYSIS (hemolytic anemia)

3) THE ANEMIA OF MARROW FAILURE
    nutritional deficiency
    marrow suppression

  – – – – – – –

Above classification adapted from: Ward, F. A. A Primer of Hematology. New York, Appleton-Century-Crofts, 1971.

1. Anemia (Erythrocyte Deficiency)

Anemia is a deficiency of circulating red cells. *It is not a disease in itself, but rather a sign of disease.* It is caused by one of 3 basic kinds of underlying disturbances (Illustration 14-17).

The Anemia of Hemorrhage

Hemorrhage is the condition in which blood elements are found outside the vascular space (endothelium-lined channels). Of course, the most easily detected blood cell is the erythrocyte and so one usually accepts the definition of hemorrhage as meaning the presence of erythrocytes outside the vascular space.

Hemorrhage can result from angiorrhexis (the rupture of a vessel) or by diapedesis (the escape of blood through abnormally permeable capillaries).

Unless hemorrhage results in the loss of considerable amounts of blood, its effects are negligible: however, given serious blood loss, 2 syndromes are possible (Illustration 14-18).

In *acute, serious hemorrhage,* the body is deprived of whole blood so that the blood picture immediately following acute hemorrhage shows no change. In the first stage of recovery, tissue fluid will find its way into the blood stream and dilute the remaining cellular elements and the picture begins to appear as if the person were anemic. Since the cells are normal, this kind of anemia is described as normocytic. Because most acute hemorrhages result from trauma, the person will most often have a healthy marrow and be fully capable of producing adequate amounts of normal erythrocytes. He will set about immediately to restore the normal circulating concentration of cells. Circulating immature erythrocytes (reticulocytosis) may be seen for a short time as the marrow responds, but eventually the blood picture returns to normal.

In *serious chronic hemorrhage* the body is deprived of a significant amount of blood each day, week or month over a protracted period of time. Aside from normal menstrual bleeding, the most common reason for this is a lesion of the gastrointestinal tract. It is particularly important in chronic hemorrhage that this loss is to the *outside* of the body, because such a loss will ultimately lead to a significant deficiency of iron. Since iron is very slowly absorbed, transported and processed in the manufacture of blood cells, one of the very first changes that is noticed in chronic serious hemorrhage will be an iron deficiency (hypochromic, microcytic) anemia.

14-18. THE ANEMIA OF HEMORRHAGE

---

1) IN ACUTE SERIOUS HEMORRHAGE THE BLOOD PICTURE WILL DEPEND UPON THE TIME ELAPSED

2) IN CHRONIC HEMORRHAGE THE ANEMIA WILL BE OF THE IRON DEFICIENCY TYPE

14-19. THE ANEMIA OF EXCESS HEMOLYSIS (HEMOLYTIC ANEMIA)

---

1) EXTRACORPUSCULAR DEFECT
   disease is extrinsic to the erythrocyte

2) INTRACORPUSCULAR DEFECT
   disease is based on an inherited defect intrinsic to the erythrocyte
   membrane defect
   hemoglobinopathy

The Anemia of Excess Hemolysis

When erythrocytes are destroyed at a rate in excess of the ability of marrow to replace them the result is *hemolytic anemia.* Hemolytic anemia can result from 2 different kinds of diseases, the *extracorpuscular defect* and the *intracorpuscular defect* (Illustration 14-19).

In the *extracorpuscular defect,* the disease itself is extrinsic to the erythrocyte, but results in the red cell's actually being damaged or at least being abnormally fragile and having a greatly shortened lifespan. Erythrocyte fragility is manifested as spherocytosis, a condition in which circulating erythrocytes assume the shape of a sphere and become unusually liable to normal mechanisms of attrition. Extrinsic factors cause erythrocyte damage and fragility, either directly such as the parasite of malaria or through immunologic mechanisms such as is seen in acquired hemolytic anemia. They are listed in Illustration 14-20.

In the *intracorpuscular defect,* the disease is inherited as a fault intrinsic to the erythrocyte itself. These faults are seen as 2 principal kinds, the membrane defect and the hemoglobin defect or hemoglobinopathy (Illustration 14-21). Again, regardless of the cause, affected erythrocytes are fragile and have a short lifespan. As our example of hemolytic anemia

---

14-20. THE EXTRACORPUSCULAR DEFECT AS A CAUSE OF EXCESS HEMOLYSIS

1) DIRECT HEMOLYSIS
    malaria (over-all most common cause of hemolytic anemia)
    toxemia
    snake venom
    phenylhydrazine

2) IMMUNOLOGIC HEMOLYSIS
    acquired hemolytic anemia (an autoimmune phenomenon)
    erythroblastosis fetalis (Rh incompatibility between mother and fetus)

14-21. THE INTRACORPUSCULAR DEFECT AS A CAUSE OF EXCESS HEMOLYSIS

1) MEMBRANE DEFECT
    congenital hemolytic anemia (hereditary spherocytosis)

2) HEMOGLOBIN DEFECT (HEMOGLOBINOPATHY)
    sickle cell disease will be used as example

14-22. SICKLE CELL DISEASE

1) HEMOGLOBIN-S IS INHERITED (AUTOSOMAL CODOMINANT)
    homozygote = disease
    heterozygote = trait
    (virtually confined to black race)

2) DIMINISHED SOLUBILITY IN DEOXYGENATED FORM CAUSES SICKLING
    anemia (sickle cells are more fragile, have shorter lifespan)
    capillary obstruction
    micro-infarction
    fibrosis

---

based on an intracorpuscular defect, we will use the very common *sickle cell disease.*

Sickle cell disease and its accompanying anemia is based on the inheritance of a form of hemoglobin known as hemoglobin-S (Illustration 14-22). Hemoglobin-S is inherited according to an autosomal co-dominant pattern. The homozygous condition results in 100 per cent hemoglobin-S, whereas the heterozygote has only 50 per cent or less. The gene for hemoglobin-S originated in Africa and its distribution is virtually confined to the black race. Heterozygosity is a relatively innocuous condition and is even thought to confer some degree of resistance to malaria. In the case of the homozygote, however, the prognosis is very poor and most patients die before the age of 30. Hemoglobin-S differs form normal adult hemoglobin (hemoglobin-A) by only a single amino acid at 1 position in the globin portion of the molecule. Yet this slight difference is enough to render hemoglobin-S less soluble in its deoxygenated form.

Because of its diminished solubility, hemoglobin-S tends to form crystalline aggregates when it has given up its oxygen. The formation of these aggregates causes distortion of the erythrocyte, drawing it into a thin, elongate form resembling a sickle. Cells that have formed sickles cannot traverse capillary beds normally and tend to obstruct the microcirculation causing tiny areas of infarction and fibrosis. Poorly healing leg ulcers are a common complication, because of circulatory obstruction. Visceral fibrosis, cor pulmonale and recurrent thrombosis are also seen.

The syndrome of hemolytic anemia (Illustration 14-23) is fairly consistent, regardless of the cause.

The Anemia of Marrow Failure

Marrow failure is the third and perhaps the most complicated of all causes of anemia. The marrow, because of intense mitotic activity and

---

14-23. THE SYNDROME OF HEMOLYTIC ANEMIA

1) PALE, ATROPHIC SKIN AND MUCOSA

2) JAUNDICE (ICTERUS)

3) TENDENCY TO GALLSTONE FORMATION

4) HEPATOSPLENOMEGALY

5) SHORT RBC LIFESPAN

6) SPHEROCYTOSIS

7) FATIGUE, WEAKNESS, ANGINA PECTORIS

14-24. THE ANEMIA OF MARROW FAILURE

1) NUTRITIONAL DEFICIENCY
   iron (most common)
   B (pernicious anemia) discussed in Chapter 11
   folic acid (similar to B_{12} deficiency in clinical appearance)

2) MARROW SUPPRESSION
   drugs and chemicals
   radiation
   myelophthisic (marrow-displacing) conditions
   infections and metabolic disorders

---

its diversity of specialized cells is **extremely** sensitive to a number of adverse conditions which, for purposes of convenience we are dividing into: 1) nutritional deficiencies and 2) marrow suppression (Illustration 14-24). Again we will be considering only anemia: however, other cell series can also be affected.

Anemia resulting from nutritional deficiency is usually traceable to shortage of 1 of 3 agents: iron, vitamin B_{12} or folic acid. A discussion of *pernicious anemia* (B_{12} deficiency) is presented in Chapter 11. *Folic acid deficiency* bears a strong resemblance to pernicious anemia, but it is based on a dietary shortage of this agent rather than the inability to absorb vitamin B_{12}.

Iron deficiency anemia is by far the most common of the 3 causes of nutritional deficiency anemia. It is particularly common among women of child-bearing age, because of their iron loss in menstruation: however, it can come about in a number of different ways (Illustration 14-25).

In the evaluation of a patient with iron deficiency who demonstrates no apparent cause, one must always consider the possibility of chronic blood loss, particularly into the gastrointestinal tract.

Iron deficiency anemia is often associated with the atrophy of lingual epithelium (atrophic

---

14-25. IRON DEFICIENCY ANEMIA

1) MOST COMMON OF THE NUTRITIONAL DEFICIENCY ANEMIAS
   hypochromic, microcytic cells

2) RESULTS FROM:
   low intake
   decreased absorption
   increased loss
   competitive inhibition (as in heavy metal poisoning)

3) PARTICULARLY COMMON IN THE WOMAN OF CHILD BEARING AGE

4) IN MALES AND POST-MENOPAUSAL FEMALES IT MOST OFTEN POINTS TO CHRONIC BLOOD LOSS

5) OFTEN ASSOCIATED WITH ATROPHIC GLOSSITIS

glossitis) which results in a sore, beefy, red tongue. Erythrocytes will be hypochromic (pale red) and microcytic (smaller than normal). Death due to uncomplicated iron deficiency is rare and the condition responds readily to dietary iron.

Additional Reading

Bell, R. M. S. and Gelfand, M. Sickle cell disease in Rhodesia. J. Trop. Med. Hygiene. 74:148, 1971

Bowe, E. T. Immunization against Rh. Postgrad. Med. 45:110, 1969

Goldwein, M. Autoimmune hemolytic anemias: A review. Am. J. Clin. Path. 56:293, 1971

Jonxis, J. H. P. The development of hemoglobin. Ped. Clin. N. Amer. 12:64, 1965

Klieger, J. A. The Rh factor: Past, present and future. Med. Clin. N. Amer. 53:1063, 1969

Koepke, J. A. Iron-deficiency anemia. Postgrad. Med. 51:163, 1972

Linman, J. W. Physiologic and pathophysiologic effects of anemia. N. Engl. J. Med. 279:812, 1968

Poynton, H. G. and Davey, K. W. Thalassemia. Oral Surg., Oral Med., Oral Path. 25:564, 1968

Reich, C. The cellular elements of the blood. Clinical Symposia, Summit, N.J., Ciba Pharmaceutical Div., Ciba Corp., 1962

Streiff, R. R. Folic acid deficiency anemia. Sem. In Hematol. 7:23, 1970

Sullivan, L. W. Vitamin B_{12} metabolism and megaloblastic anemia. Sem. in Hematol. 7:6, 1970

Wiesenfeld, S. L. Sickle cell trait in biological and cultural evolution. Science 157:1134, 1967

PROLIFERATIVE DISORDERS OF THE FORMED ELEMENTS OF BLOOD

LEARNING OBJECTIVE

To be able to describe proliferative disorders of the formed elements of blood discussing polycythemia vera and leukemia as examples. Where applicable mention:

  a) etiology and pathogenesis
  b) clinical signs
  c) clinical varieties
  d) complications
  e) usual course of the disease

Proliferative disorders of the formed elements of blood are those conditions in which 1 or more of the products of normal marrow are manufactured in excess and without regard for need. Recognized clinical patterns of this kind of disorder are listed in Illustration 14-26. All of these are neoplastic or quasi-neoplastic conditions. We will use polycythemia vera and leukemia as examples here and discuss multiple myeloma under diseases of the lymphoreticular system.

Polycythemia Vera

Polycycthemia vera or primary polycythemia is a condition in which there is the uncontrolled production of erythrocytes (Illustration 14-27). These erythrocytes are usually normochromic, normocytic and fully functional, but because of the enormous increase in their number the blood becomes hyperviscous and difficult to circulate. Hemoglobin values of

---

14-26. PROLIFERATIVE DISORDERS OF THE FORMED ELEMENTS OF BLOOD

1) POLYCYTHEMIA VERA
   uncontrolled production of erythrocytes

2) LEUKEMIA
   uncontrolled production of white cells

3) ERYTHROLEUKEMIA
   exaggerated production of all cell series

4) MYELOFIBROSIS
   overgrowth of marrow by indigenous fibrous tissue

5) MULTIPLE MYELOMA
   multicentric malignancy of marrow plasma cells

6) PRIMARY THROMBOCYTHEMIA
   idiopathic overproduction of platelets

14-27. POLYCYTHEMIA VERA (PRIMARY POLYCYTHEMIA)
1) OVERPRODUCTION OF ERYTHRO-CYTES
2) HYPERVISCOSITY congestion cyanosis
3) THROMBOSIS AND HEMORRHAGE ARE COMMON COMPLICATIONS
4) OFTEN TERMINATES IN ANOTHER NEOPLASTIC MARROW DISEASE chronic myelogenous leukemia myelofibrosis

14-28. LEUKEMIA
1) MYELOGENOUS acute—any age chronic—usually middle age
2) LYMPHOGENOUS acute—childhood chronic—old age
3) STEM CELL acute and fulminating anaplastic cells older age groups

more than 20 gm per 100 cc are often encountered.

Polycythemia vera (primary polycythemia) must be differentiated from the secondary or compensatory erythrocytosis seen in response to heart disease, lung disease, methemoglobinemia and occult malignant tumors producing erythropoietin. True polycythemia, in contrast to reactive erythrocytosis, is a neoplasm-like proliferation of red cells. It is essentially incurable: however, the patient may survive in relative comfort for 10 to 15 years. Thrombosis and hemorrhage are common complications and may be the cause of death. Consistent with its neoplastic character, polycythemia vera often terminates as chronic myelogenous leukemia or less frequently as myelofibrosis.

2. Leukemia

Leukemia is a term meaning literally white blood. Actually the blood never really becomes white: however, there often (but not necessarily) is a dramatic increase in the number of circulating white cells. Leukemia cells originate in either the marrow or in lymphoid tissue.

Myelogenous (marrow-originating) leukemia, like polycythemia, is a neoplasm or perhaps, more accurately, the *result* of a neoplasm of marrow. The white cells produced in leukemia are tumor cells and, like other tumor cells, are unable to respond to normal homeostatic controls or carry out normal functions. Thus a patient suffering from leukemia of cells resembling granulocytes does not enjoy enhanced protection from infection nor does a patient suffering from lymphocytic leukemia exhibit a stronger immunologic response.

Leukemia is actually many diseases, the categories of which correspond to the particular cell type involved in the neoplastic process and the duration of the disease process. The usually recognized types of leukemia are listed in Illustration 14-28. Their occurrence within fairly specific age groups supports the hypothesis of multiple etiologies.

Additional Reading

Mathe, G. Immunotherapy in the treatment of acute lymphoid leukemia. Hosp. Pract. 12:43, 1971
Silverstein, M. N. Polycythemia vera, 1935-1969: An epidemiologic survey in Rochester, Minnesota. Mayo Clin. Proc. 46:751, 1971

LYMPHORETICULAR INFECTIONS

LEARNING OBJECTIVE

To review Chapter 4 and be able to compare
and contrast simple, reactive lymphadenopathy
and infectious mononucleosis mentioning:
  a) etiology and pathogenesis
  b) clinical signs
  c) clinical varieties
  d) complications
  e) usual course of the disease

The lymphoreticular system (Illustration 14-
29) is the source of the immunologic and other
defense faculties of the body. Its normal
function has been discussed in some detail in
Chapter 1, and a group of its diseases in
Chapter 4.

The stock-in-trade of the lymphoreticular
system is its ability to react to the appearance
of foreign material within the body. In every
instance, this reaction includes cellular proliferation, and so proliferation is an integral
part of the *normal* activity of this system.
Replication of cells is the means of amplifying
the reaction in this case, just as the use of

**14-29. COMPONENTS OF THE LYMPHO-
RETICULAR SYSTEM**

1) ORGANIZED LYMPHOID TISSUE
   central
   peripheral

2) LYMPHATIC VESSELS

3) PHAGOCYTIC RETICULAR CELLS

4) PHAGOCYTIC SINUSOIDAL LINING
   CELLS
   liver
   spleen
   lung
   lymph nodes
   bone marrow

**14-30. DISEASES OF THE LYMPHORE-
TICULAR SYSTEM**

1) IMMUNOLOGIC DEFICIENCY
   (see Chapter 4)

2) ALLERGY
   (see Chapter 4)

3) AUTOIMMUNITY
   (see Chapter 4)

4) IMMUNOPROLIFERATIVE DISEASE
   (to be discussed in this Chapter)

---

multiple molecular factors is in the clotting
mechanism. This proliferative activity may be
well controlled and local as seen in the case of a
single regional lymph node reacting to the
presence of foreign material (review Chapter 1
for a summary of humoral and cellular reactions within a single lymph node) or it may
involve the entire lymphoreticular system as
seen in the the very interesting disease, infectious mononucleosis.

Infectious mononucleosis is a benign, self-
limiting disease of viral etiology that has its
most conspicuous effect on lymphoid cells
(Illustration 14-31).

Although many other tissues are involved,
the reaction of the lymphoreticular system is
unusual in that there is generalized lymphadenopathy and atypical lymphocytosis (the
appearance in circulating blood of a large,
rather primitive-appearing lymphocyte). Another unexplained manifestation of infectious
mononucleosis is the appearance of the "heterophile antibody" in the patient's serum. This is
an antibody that is detected by its ability to
agglutinate sheep red blood cells in a diagnostic
assay known as the Paul-Bunnel test. This
heterophile antibody is transient and does not
persist beyond the clinically apparent course of
the disease. It is a convenient means of
differentiating this disease from viral hepatitis,
to which it bears a strong resemblance in many
ways.

Interestingly, antigens of the Epstein-Barr

IMMUNOPROLIFERATIVE DISEASE

14-31. INFECTIOUS MONONUCLEOSIS

1) BENIGN, SELF-LIMITING VIRAL INFECTION

2) 2 to 4 WEEK ACUTE PHASE
   chills, fever, sore throat, fatigue, palatal petechiae

3) ATYPICAL LYMPHOCYTOSIS

4) HETEROPHILE ANTIBODY

5) SOFT SPLENOMEGALY
   predisposed to rupture

6) LIVER INVOLVEMENT RESEMBLES HEPATITIS

7) ASSOCIATED WITH E.B. VIRUS
   causative relationship not established

LEARNING OBJECTIVE

To be able to outline the general phenomenon of neoplastic proliferation of cells that mediate immunologic defenses and discuss multiple myeloma, lymphoma and Hodgkin's disease with regard to the following:
   a) etiology and pathogenesis
   b) clinical signs
   c) clinical varieties
   d) complications
   e) usual course of the disease

Immunoproliferative diseases are those that result from the neoplastic proliferation of cells that carry out immunologic defense. Like other examples of neoplastic disorders, these are characterized by uncontrolled proliferation of genetically altered cells and a variety of untoward effects on the host. In this case, however, the picture is complicated by the fact that the disease takes origin in the system that is normally responsible for the protection of other tissues. Also complicating the picture of immunoproliferative disease is the diffuse distribution of normal lymphoreticular cells, their propensity for wandering throughout the body, their normally aggressive character, the extreme heterogeneity of cell types that make up

virus can be detected in all heterophile-positive cases of infectious mononucleosis. This unusual relationship between a tumor-associated virus and a benign, self-limiting infection has been pointed out in Chapter 7 and should be reviewed at this time.

Additional Reading

Burnet, M. A modern basis for pathology. Lancet 1:1383, 1968
Evans, A. S. Infectious mononucleosis: Recent development. GP XI:127, 1969
Zacharski, L. R. Lymphocytopenia: Its causes and significance. Mayo Clin. Proc. 46:168, 1971.

14-32. IMMUNOPROLIFERATIVE DISEASE

1) REACTIVE IMMUNOPROLIFERATION
   local lymphadenitis
   generalized lymphadenitis (as seen in infectious mononucleosis)

2) NEOPLASTIC IMMUNOPROLIFERATION
   monoclonal gammopathy
   lymphoma
   Hodgkin's disease

lymphoreticular tissue and the fact that some of these manufacture immunoglobulins.

The three types of neoplastic immunoproliferative diseases that will be discussed are the monoclonal gammopathies, the lymphomas and Hodgkin's disease. These are listed in Illustration 14-33. Listed also is the category of disease known as malignant histiocytosis: however, diseases in this group will not be discussed.

3. Monoclonal Gammopathy

According to the clonal selection theory, reaction of the immunologic systems to the appearance of an antigen is based on the selection (by the antigen) of a clone of immunocompetent cells that first proliferates and then goes on to carry out either the synthesis of a specific antibody or the aggressive functions of a sensitized lymphocyte (see Chapter 1). In monoclonal gammopathy, we are witnessing the neoplastic transformation of 1 of these clones of the type that is able to produce antibody. While proliferating, cells of this kind

---

14-33. NEOPLASTIC IMMUNOPROLIFERATION

1) THE MONOCLONAL GAMMOPATHIES (AND OTHER PLASMACYTIC TUMORS)
   diffuse myelomatosis
   multiple myeloma
   plasma cell leukemia
   solitary plasmacytoma
   solitary myeloma

2) THE LYMPHOMAS
   lymphocytic lymphoma
   stem cell lymphoma
   histiocytic lymphoma

3) HODGKIN'S DISEASE
   lymphocytic predominance
   nodular sclerosis
   mixed cellularity
   lymphocytic depletion

4) MALIGNANT HISTIOCYTOSIS

14-34. MULTIPLE MYELOMA (AS AN EXAMPLE OF MONOCLONAL GAMMAOPATHY)

1) MULTICENTRIC MALIGNANCY OF CELLS RESEMBLING PLASMA CELLS
   starts as single nodule
   causes resorption

2) MOST MANUFACTURE LARGE AMOUNTS OF FUNCTIONLESS IMMUNOGLOBULIN
   paraprotein or myeloma protein

3) ABUNDANCE OF ABNORMAL PROTEIN CAUSES A VARIETY OF DIAGNOSTIC SIGNS:
   intravascular rouleau
   amyloidosis
   renal atrophy
   Bence-Jones proteinuria (actually light chains from disrupted paraprotein)

---

produce an abundance of an essentially functionless immunoglobin (paraprotein).

The specific kind of monoclonal gammopathy that we will use as our example is the *multiple myeloma* (Illustration 14-34). Multiple myeloma is a multicentric malignancy of cells that strongly resemble plasma cells. It is thought to begin in bone marrow as a single nodule and its spread is associated with sharply demarcated areas of bone resorption giving the radiographic appearance of multiple "punched out" lesions.

Myeloma cells, as expected, manufacture hugh quantities of immunoglobin which is released into the bloodstream to circulate throughout the body. This abnormal globin is called *paraprotein* or *myeloma protein* and is almost always of a single isotype. Myelomas producing all 5 isotypes (IgG, IgA, IgM, IgD, IgE) have been described and the ratio of their frequency of occurrence corresponds roughly to the prevalence of each immunoglobulin in the body.

The principal morphologic changes associated with multiple myeloma are caused by the rapid, widespread erosion of bone and the presence of large amounts of paraprotein. The former leads to pathologic fractures and possible neurologic deficit if the spine is involved; the latter gives rise to a variety of abnormal changes including intravascular rouleaux, amyloidosis, renal atrophy and the presence in the urine of a peculiar type of protein (Bence-Jones protein) which has recently been shown to be the light chain components of disrupted paraproteins.

Multiple myeloma is always ultimately fatal, although the course of the disease in many cases is slow and protracted.

2. Lymphoma

Lymphomas are tumors of lymphoid tissue. Although the term might suggests that they are benign, almost all tumors primary to peripheral lymphoid tissue are malignant. There are a number of histologic varieties of lymphoma, the appearance and clinical behavior of which depend upon the site, lymphoid cell of origin and degree of malignancy.

Most examples of lymphoma originate in lymph nodes: however, some are extranodal in both origin and distribution. Perhaps the most closely studied of the latter is *Burkitt's lymphoma,* mentioned earlier, which takes origin in lymphoid tissue of facial bones and viscera. Another example of an extranodal lymphoma is a disease of the skin known as *mycosis fungoides.* This form of lymphoma is always fatal, originates in lymphoid tissue of the skin and often terminates with widespread visceral involvement.

In general, lymphomas arising in lymph nodes are classified, first of all, according to whether they exhibit nodular or diffuse architecture (the former are less aggressive), and secondly, according to the predominant cell type. This classification is outlined in Illustration 14-35. If malignant cells from a lymphoma are regularly or periodically released into the blood stream causing an enormous increase in the number of circulating white cells (greater than 50,000 cell per cu mm) the tumor is more correctly termed a lymphocytic leukemia.

Evidence is conclusive that lymphocytic leukemias and lymphomas of lower animals are

---

14-35. LYMPHOMA (EXCLUDING HODGKIN'S DISEASE)

Although most examples of lymphoma originate in lymph nodes, some are extranodal in both origin and distribution

1) NODULAR
    lymphocytic lymphoma
        well-differentiated
        moderately well differentiated
        poorly differentiated
    stem cell lymphoma (mixed cell type)
    histiocytic lymphoma (reticulum cell sarcoma)

2) DIFFUSE
    (same subclassfications as above)

---

caused by oncogenic viruses (usually RNA viruses). But despite morphologic similarity of these diseases to human lymphoma, the infectious etiology of the latter has not yet been demonstrated. Certain factors are known to predispose to human lymphoma; these include immunosuppressive therapy, anticonvulsant therapy (with hydantoin derivatives) and certain primary immunologic deficiencies (ataxia telangiectasia and the Wiscott-Aldrich syndrome).

Unfortunately, systems of classification of lymphoma take little cognizance of the most recent ideas about lymphocyte populations. Although the subject needs a great deal more clarification, it would appear at this stage that most non-Hodgkin's lymphomas are disorders of the B-cell system, whereas Hodgkin's disease (discussed below) appears to be a T-cell neoplasm.

3. Hodgkin's Disease

Hodgkin's disease is a progressive neoplastic disease of peripheral lymphoid tissue. It was once invariably fatal: however, new methods for the treatment of cases intercepted very early are beginning to produce encouraging

14-36. HODGKIN'S DISEASE: HISTO-
LOGIC CLASSIFICATION

1) LYMPHOCYTIC PREDOMINANCE
lymphocytes/histiocytes predominate: Reed-Sternberg cells are
rare

2) NODULAR SCLEROSIS
nodules of abnormal lymphoid tissue surrounded by bands of collagen: few Reed-Sternberg cells:
necrosis, lymphocytes, plasma
cells and granulocytes in varying
amounts

3) MIXED CELLULARITY
more Reed-Sternberg cells: less
lymphocytes: some necrosis,
plasma cells, granulocytes and
histiocytes: diffuse fibrosis: no collagen bands

4) LYMPHOCYTIC DEPLETION
lymphocytes are scarce: diffuse,
non-collagenous fibrosis: Reed-
Sternberg cells are very common

to the number of Reed-Sternberg cells seen in a microscopic section of affected lymphoid tissue and inversely proportional to the predominance of lymphocytes.

The progress of Hodgkin's disease is reckoned in stages which correspond to the extent of its spread from the point of origin. The more malignant types spread quickly and reach advanced stages soon after the disease begins, whereas the more benign varieties tend to remain localized longer. Success of treatment is strongly dependent on intercepting the disease while it is still in one of the early stages.

Additional Reading

Franssila, K. O. et al. Histologic classification of Hodgkin's disease. Cancer 20:1594, 1967

results. Considered as a single disease, it is seen 2 to 3 times more frequently in men than women. It may develop at any time of life, but occurs most frequently between the ages of 20 and 40.

Hodgkin's disease is thought to start at a single focus and spread throughtout the lymphoid tissue of the body. A common site of origin is lymph nodes of the cervical chain.

The disease is seen as 4 morphologic variants, each of which can be assigned a different prognosis. Some authorities favor the interpretation that there are actually 2 separate diseases represented in the 4 variants of Hodgkin's disease: however, they are conventionally considered as only 1. The most modern and widely accepted system for subclassifying Hodgkin's disease on the basis of histologic characteristics is outlined in Illustration 14-36. The malignant character of the disease is directly proportional

chapter 15
MUSCULOSKELETAL AND NERVOUS SYSTEMS

DISEASES OF SKELETAL MUSCLE

LEARNING OBJECTIVE

To be able to discuss the liability of skeletal muscle to various kinds of diseases and describe the following:

 a) atrophy of skeletal muscle
 b) muscular dystrophy
 c) myasthenia gravis
 d) neoplasms of skeletal muscle

Skeletal or voluntary muscle is a comparatively hardy tissue, remarkably free of primary infections, and rarely involved in either primary or metastatic tumor growth. We will consider diseases of skeletal muscle under four categories (Illustration 15-1).

1. Muscular Atrophy

Atrophy of skeletal muscle is seen in a variety of disorders (Illustration 15-2), all of which are *extrinsic* to affected muscle tissue. The muscle mass undergoing atrophy shows uniform change, all muscle fibers responding to approximately the same degree. In far-advanced atrophy, muscle cells may actually undergo necrosis and be replaced with fibrous tissue.

2. Muscular Dystrophy

In contrast to atrophy, muscular dystrophy is a group of muscle-wasting diseases that are *intrinsic* to the affected muscle. Individual fibers are affected on a random basis and the histologic picture is one of healthy-appearing cells alternating with others undergoing degeneration.

Muscular dystrophy is actually a group of diseases, *all of which are inherited*. Individual diseases making up this group can be distinguished only on the basis of their characteristic inheritance pattern.

The clinical course of the disease is variable, however, it can lead to death through its effect on the muscles of respiration.

15-1. DISEASES OF SKELETAL MUSCLE

1) ATROPHY

2) MUSCULAR DYSTROPHY

3) MYASTHENIA GRAVIS

4) NEOPLASMS

15-2. ATROPHY OF MUSCLE

1) PROLONGED DISUSE OR INTERFERENCE WITH INNERVATION

2) STARVATION

3) ADVANCED AGE

4) PANHYPOPITUITARISM

5) MESENCHYMAL AUTOIMMUNE DISEASE
   dermatomyositis
   SLE

---

3. Myasthenia Gravis

Myasthenia Gravis is a neuro-muscular disease in which the basic defect has been traced to a disturbance of impulse transmission at the myoneural junction (Illustration 15-3). It is characterized by episodes of weakness, most often affecting the facial, oculomotor, laryngeal, pharyngeal and respiratory muscles.

An episode may be precipitated by infection or emotional upset and usually consists of weakness, accompanied by drooping eyelids, diplopia, and slurring of speech. A variety of other, less constant signs may also be present. Most signs and symptoms are relieved by rest or the administration of anticholinesterase drugs.

There appears to be a strong correlation between the myoneural transmission defect of myasthenia gravis and overactivity of the thymus. The great majority of patients with myasthenia gravis show either hyperplasia or neoplasia or the thymus while 75% of thymoma patients manifest myasthenia gravis. Neither the exact nature of the defect nor its association with the thymus have been thoroughly elucidated.

4. Neoplasms of Muscle

Tumors of muscle are exceedingly rare, the only significant malignancy being the rhabdo-

myosarcoma. These are often quite aggressive and the five-year survival rate is discouraging low. Although some tumors do metastasize to muscle, particularly in the terminal stages of malignant disease, skeletal muscle is an exceedingly rare site for the metastatic growth of malignant tumors originating elsewhere in the body.

Additional Reading

Alpert, L. I. A histologic reappraisal of the thymus in myasthenia gravis. Arch. Path. 91:55, 1971
Goldstein, G. and Manganaro, A. Thymin: A thymic polypeptide causing the neuromuscular block of myasthenia gravis. Ann. N.Y. Acad. Sci. 183:230, 1971
Zacks, S. I. Recent contribution to the diagnosis of muscle disease. Human Path. 1:465, 1970
Zundel, W. S. and Tyler, F. H. The muscular dystrophies. N. Engl. J. Med. 273:537 and 596 (two parts), 1965

TRAUMATIC, INFLAMMATORY AND NECROTIZING LESIONS OF BONE

LEARNING OBJECTIVE

To review information on fractures presented in Chapter 3 and discuss the following:
  a) classification of fractures and clinical stages of the process of fracture healing.
  b) cause, pathogenesis and clinical varieties of suppurative osteomyelitis
  c) a brief description of other forms of osteomyelitis
  d) a brief description of osteoradionecrosis

Bone is such a highly complex, diversified tissue that it is difficult to assemble its disorders into some kind of reasonably simple organization. We will be using the system of classification outlined in Illustration 15-4.

Types of lesions to be included in the first of these categories are listed in Illustration 15-5.

15-3. MYASTHENIA GRAVIS

1) WEAKNESS DUE TO INTERFERENCE WITH TRANSMISSION AT MYONEURAL JUNCTION

2) CORRECTED BY NEOSTIGMINE (PROSTIGMINE): SIMULATED BY CURARE

3) ASSOCIATED WITH HYPERACTIVITY OF THE THYMUS
    70% of patients with myasthenia gravis show hyperplasia of the thymus
    15 to 30% have thymoma
    75% of thymoma patients have myasthenia gravis

15-4. DISEASES OF BONE

1) TRAUMATIC, INFLAMMATORY AND NECROTIZING LESIONS

2) DYSTROPHY, DYSPLASIA AND DYS-OSTOSIS

3) NEOPLASMS

15-5. TRAUMATIC, INFLAMMATORY AND NECROTIZING LESIONS OF BONE

(Examples)

1) FRACTURE
   (review information in Chapter 3)

2) OSTEOMYELITIS
   suppurative
      hematogenous and secondary
      to compound fracture
   tubercular
   symphilitic

3) OSTEORADIONECROSIS

1. Fractures

Fractures have been discussed in Chapter 3 and should be reviewed at this time.

2. Osteomyelitis

Osteomyelitis is an inflammatory lesion based on a bacterial infection of bone marrow. Although any pathogen can infect bone marrow, most cases are caused by hemolytic staphylococci. The infecting organism usually gains access to bone marrow either directly through a compound fracture or indirectly via the bloodstream. The latter type of staphylo-coccal osteomyelitis is seen most often in children, possibly because of the unusual circulation extant in rapidly growing bones. In most cases the source of the infecting organism is not apparent.

Tubercular osteomyelitis is the result of the seeding of bone marrow with blood-borne tubercle bacilli from a pulmonary infection. Quite in contrast to pyogenic staphylococcal infections of marrow, tubercular osteomyelitis is insidious in onset and very destructive of hard tissue.

Syphilitic osteomyelitis is not common, but can occur in association with either the congenital or acquired disease. Osteochondritis, periostitis and gumma formation are seen.

Additional Reading

Waldvogel, F. A. et al. Osteomyelitis. N. Engl. J. Med. 282:260, 1970

DYSTROPHY, DYSPLASIA AND DYSOSTOSIS

LEARNING OBJECTIVES

To develop a comparison among the 3 kinds of bone diseases classified as dystrophy, dysplasia and dysostosis using the following diseases as examples:
   a) osteoporosis
   b) osteitis deformans
   c) osteogenesis imperfecta

Without a comprehensive system of classification, the rich variety of bone lesions could amount to a discouraging challenge for student and practitioner alike. Those that are clearly traumatic, inflammatory, necrotizing or neoplastic present no ambiguity: however, there is a large group that are none of these. For this group we will adopt the classification system outlined in Illustration 15-6.

Osteitis deformans = Paget's disease (handwritten)

15-6. DYSTROPHY, DYSPLASIA AND DYSOTOSIS (RUBIN CLASSIFICATION)

1) DYSTROPHY
disorder of bone resulting from a disturbance in nutrition or metabolism *extrinsic* to the affected bone

2) DYSPLASIA
disorder of bone resulting from an acquired disturbance of growth or metabolism *intrinsic* to the affected bone

3) DYSOSTOSIS
disorder of bone based on an *inherited* defect of developmental or mesenchymal tissues

---

1. Dystrophy

The osteodystrophies are generalized bone lesions in which the underlying cause is traceable to a disturbance of metabolism or nutrition *extrinsic* to bone. A list of examples are presented in Illustration 15-7.

Osteodystrophies, although extremely diverse in cause, are usually manifested as either osteoporosis or a rachitiform disease as indicated in Illustration 15-7.

Osteoporosis is generalized rarefaction of bone. Like other bone changes secondary to systemic disease, it affects the entire skeleton and results in diminution of bone density. Since the most convenient means of detecting osteoporosis is by radiography, one usually comes to think of this condition as a decrease in radiodensity. The composition of bone in osteoporosis is normal: however, there is less calcified substance per unit volume of tissue than would be expected in healthy bone. Stated in another way, the bone substance is of normal composition but abnormally delicate in construction. Osteoporosis like anemia is a sign of disease rather than a disease in itself. Osteoporosis signals the existence of an underlying osteodystrophy which must be treated if bone changes are to be reversed. The most common causes of osteoporosis are those dystrophies resulting from advance age, menopause or prolonged steroid therapy.

Rachitiform diseases are those which bear morphologic resemblance to rickets. The latter has been discussed in some detail in Chapter 1 and should be reviewed.

2. Dysplasia

Dysplasias of bone are those conditions that appear to originate as acquired diseases *intrinsic* to affected skeletal tissue. They are usually characterized by either undergrowth or overgrowth of bone (Illustration 15-8). We will consider only 1 of these, osteitis deformans or Paget's disease.

Osteitis deformans is a acquired disease intrinsic to bone. Its etiology is completely unknown: however, it is manifested as the unprovoked resorption of normal bone and its replacement by poorly calcified, irregular bony matrix (Illustration 15-9). Certain bones are affected more often than others; they increase in size, but are soft and may be deformed if involved in weight bearing. The process may be monostotic, i.e. affect only a single bone, or it may involve a number of bones or even the

---

15-7. OSTEODYSTROPHY

(Examples)

1) HORMONAL (OSTEOPOROSIS)
hyper- and hypofunction of
    thyroid
    parathyroid
    adrenal
    pituitary
advanced age
menopause
prolonged steroid therapy

2) RACHITIFORM
deficiency of Vitamin D
deficiency of calcium
renal disease
heavy metal poisoning

3. Dysostosis

Dysostosis is a condition in which skeletal deformities are based on an inherited defect of developmental or mesenchymal tissues. Examples of this kind of bone disease are presented in Illustration 15-10. We will consider only the second of these.

Osteogenesis imperfecta is a rare inherited disease thought to be based on a constitutional abnormality of all connective tissue (Illustration 15-11). It is seen in at least 3 distinct clinical forms differing in the time of onset of major signs. All appear to be based on a similar connective tissue defect and become manifest

---

15-8. DYSPLASIA OF BONE

(Examples)

1) HYPOPLASIA
   hypophosphatasia
   chondroepithelial dyspl.

2) HYPERPLASIA
   osteitis deformans (Paget's disease)

15-9. OSTEITIS DEFORMANS (PAGET'S DISEASE)

1) RESORPTION AND SIMULTANEOUS OVERGROWTH OF POORLY CALCIFIED, IRREGULAR BONE

2) BONES INCREASE IN SIZE BUT ARE SOFT

3) EXTREME ELEVATION OF BLOOD ALKALINE PHOSPHATASE

4) IRREGULAR OSTEOID LINES IMPART MOSAIC APPEARANCE TO SPICULES

5) PATIENT OUTGROWS HATS: TEETH SPREAD: BOWING OF LONG BONES

6) USUALLY OCCURS AFTER 50: MAY TERMINATE IN OSTEOSARCOMA

15-10. DYSOSTOSIS

(Examples)

1) CLEIDOCRANIAL DYSOSTOSIS

2) OSTEOGENESIS IMPERFECTA

15-11. OSTEOGENESIS IMPERFECTA

1) UNDERLYING DEFECT IS ABNORMALITY OF CONNECTIVE TISSUE

2) MOST CASES INHERITED AS AUTOSOMAL DOMINANT: MOST ALSO CONGENITAL

3) EXTREME FRAGILITY OF BONES, MULTIPLE SPONTANEOUS FRACTURES

4) BLUE SCLERAE, LAX LIGAMENTS, DEAFNESS

5) FREQUENTLY ACCOMPANIED BY DENTINOGENESIS IMPERFECTA

6) AT LEAST THREE CLINICAL FORMS

---

entire skeleton. The more generalized forms of this disease may be manifested as an enlarged skull, bowed lower extremities and the opening of spaces between maxillary teeth. Serum alkaline phosphatase levels are usually very high, presumably owing to intense, generalized osteoblastic activity. A frequent complication of this condition is the development of osteogenic sarcoma.

very early in life. The afflicted child has brittle bones that fracture easily. Ligaments are usually lax and the sclerae may be blue. Osteogenesis imperfecta is often accompanied by an analogous defect of teeth (dentinogenesis imperfecta) in which pulp chambers and nerve canals are obliterated by an overgrowth of poorly formed dentin.

Additional Reading

Harris, W. H. and Heany, R. P. Skeletal renewal and metabolic bone disease. N. Engl. J. Med. 280:193, 253 and 303 (three parts), 1969
Donaldson, C. L. Effect of prolonged bed rest on mineral metabolism. Metabolism 19:1071, 1970

NEOPLASMS OF BONE

LEARNING OBJECTIVE

To discuss the over-all picture of bone tumors and compare osteogenic sarcoma and the giant cell lesions of bone mentioning the following:
   a) clinical varieties of each
   b) epidemiology and location within skeleton
   c) clinical course
   d) complications

Neoplasms of bone occur in a variety of histologic types, both benign and malignant. From this wide selection we will be using only the 2 examples listed in Illustration 15-12.

The most common malignant tumor found in bone is one that has metastasized from some other site; the most common malignant tumor originating in bone is the multiple myeloma, discussed in Chapter 14. The latter actually arises from lymphoid cells of the marrow and hence shares more of the qualities of lymphoid tissue than bone.

Sarcomas primary to bone are not common: however, their usually aggressive nature and their tendency to occur in young adults render them different from most other malignancies and worthy of special consideration.

15-12. NEOPLASMS OF BONE

(Examples)

1) OSTEOGENIC SARCOMA

2) GIANT CELL TUMORS

15-13. OSTEOGENIC SARCOMA

1) MOST COMMON MALIGNANT TUMOR PRIMARY TO BONE
   (exclusive of multiple myeloma)

2) GREATEST INCIDENCE 10 to 25 years

3) ABOUT 50 PER CENT IN FEMUR OR TIBIA AT KNEE

4) OSTEOLYTIC OR OSTEOPLASTIC

5) WIDE SURGICAL EXCISION NECESSARY
   15–20% 5 year cure rate

---

1. Osteogenic Sarcoma

Osteogenic sarcoma (Illustration 15-13) is a comparatively rare but highly dangerous malignancy of mesenchymal cells. It originates in bone and usually exhibits some degree of osteoblastic activity, hence the term "osteogenic." Excluding multiple myeloma, osteogenic sarcoma is the most common malignant tumor primary to bone. Its peak incidence is seen in the age group between 10 and 25 years. Most cases of osteogenic sarcoma originate in seemingly normal bone: however, about 15 per cent are seen as complications of another bone disease such as osteitis deformans. In the majority of cases involving normal bone the tumor will arise at the knee joint in either the femur or tibia. Osteogenic sarcoma metastasizes early and widely. Preferred sites are the lungs and liver, but any location is possible. Treat-

---

15-14. GIANT CELL LESIONS OF BONE

1) SOME ARE INFLAMMATORY OR RE-
   PARATIVE, OTHERS ARE TRUE NEO-
   PLASMS
   > benign and malignant

2) CLINICAL COURSE DEPENDS ON BI-
   OLOGIC QUALITIES
   > most aggressive forms may actually
   > be osteogenic sarcomas with giant
   > cell differentiation

DISEASES OF JOINTS

LEARNING OBJECTIVE

To be able to compare rheumatoid arthritis and osteoarthritis (neoplasms of joints will not be considered) mentioning epidemiology, suspected cause, pathogenesis, clinical course, complications and associated extra-articular lesions where applicable.

---

ment includes wide excision but the 5-year survival rate is only about 10 to 20 per cent.

2. Giant Cell Lesions of Bone

Somewhat typical of the ambiguous quality of bone tumors is the giant cell series of lesions (Illustration 15-14). Some of these do not fulfil the requirements of a true neoplasm and are looked upon more as inflammatory or repara- tive lesions ("brown tumors" of hyperparathy- roidism, reparative granuloma of jaws, giant cell lesions of synovia and tendon sheath). Others qualify as true tumors, about half of these behaving as frankly malignant neoplasms.

Like osteogenic sarcoma, true giant cell tumors are quite rare and usually found at the knee joint within the lower femur or upper tibia. Unlike osteogenic sarcoma, however, these tumors are seen with greater frequency among older patients.

The clinical course of a giant cell tumor will depend largely on its biologic qualities. Some are cured by simple excision; others tend to recur and behave aggressively, whereas still others invade and metastasize widely.

Joints, like other highly specialized struc- tures of the body, are subject to an almost unique group of diseases. Foremost among these are the inflammatory disorders (anthri- tides) and tumors of synovial tissue (Illustration 15-15). Only the former is common enough to warrant discussion here.

Arthritis is inflammation of a joint. It is seen in a number of diseases (Illustration 15-16):

15-15. DISEASES OF JOINTS

1) ARTHRITIS

2) TUMORS

15-16. ARTHRITIS

1) RHEUMATOID ARTHRITIS

2) OSTEOARTHRITIS

3) SPECIFIC INFECTIOUS ARTHRITIS

4) ARTHRITIS OF GOUT

– – – – – – – – – – – –

In addition to the above arthritis may also be caused by trauma and is often seen as part of another syndrome such as acute rheumatic fever psoriasis, ulcerative colitis, etc.

Additional Reading

Kadin, M. and Binsch, K. On the origin of Ewing's tumor. Cancer 27:257, 1971

however, from the standpoint of public health significance the 2 most important are rheumatoid arthritis and osteoarthritis. We will use these as our examples.

1. Rheumatoid Arthritis

Rheumatoid arthritis is a very common systemic disease in which arthritis is the most prominent and disabling component (Illustration 15-17). It afflicts women approximately 3 times as frequently as men and usually has its onset at a young age during the childbearing years. Although its etiology is unknown it is thought to be based on immunologic injury and shares many features in common with SLE, scleroderma, dermatomyositis and other so-called collagen diseases. It may begin as a acute episode, but will usually follow a chronic course.

Small joints such as those of the fingers are affected first. Initial changes are confined to the synovial membrane which becomes severely inflamed and thickened. Inflammatory changes spread to joint cartilage and ultimately granulation tissue may extend across the joint space forming a fibrous and later bony ankylosis.

Other lesions seen in this disease include granulomatous lesions of the endocardium, heart valves, myocardium, pericardum and pleura. Subcutaneous nodules are often seen, particularly over bony prominences and other areas where the skin is subject to pressure.

2. Osteoarthritis

Osteoarthritis is a disease which appears to be more completely localized to joints than rheumatoid arthritis. It begins as degenerative lesions of articular cartilage which in turn cause slight inflammation and slowly progressive changes in adjacent bone. Quite in contrast to rheumatoid arthritis, osteoarthritis is evenly distributed between the sexes and begins in later rather than early life. Although there is some deformity, this disease does not cause the degree of crippling seen in rheumatoid arthritis.

DISEASES OF THE CENTRAL NERVOUS SYSTEM ASSOCIATED WITH INFECTIOUS AGENTS

LEARNING OBJECTIVE

To be able to outline the entire range of CNS diseases that are known to be associated with infectious agents discussing the following as examples:
    a) viral meningitis and encephalitis
    b) postinfectious encephalomyelitis
    c) rabies
    d) suppurative diseases of the CNS (using meningococcal meningitis and the brain abscess as examples)

The central nervous system is the great coordinator of higher functions of the human body. Although no aspect of life could be said to be simple, one cannot help but single out the human brain and its extensions as the most complex. The brain, like other organs, is a collection of highly differentiated cells supported by a comparatively simple stroma. But it is also the seat of that immeasurably complicated archive of attitudes and experience we call the mind. Up to this point we have

---

15-17. RHEUMATOID ARTHRITIS
1) A SYSTEMIC DISEASE IN WHICH ARTHRITIS IS THE MOST DISABLING COMPONENT
2) INCIDENCE IS HIGHEST IN YOUNG WOMEN
3) LONG, CHRONIC COURSE
4) SMALL JOINTS AFFECTED FIRST inflammatory changes may lead to bony ankylosis

approached each organ or system as if a disease was always to be somehow attached to a structural or chemical derangement within its tissue. In studying the human nervous system, however, we must introduce the novel concept of the purely functional disorder as distinct from those which are traceable to some kind of lesion. As we develop the present subject bear in mind that we will be considering only the latter. Functional disorders of the mind will be treated as a separate topic in the very last chapter of this book.

The central nervous system is liable to invasion by most if not all agents that infect other tissues (Illustration 15-18): however, a number of factors render such infections worthy of special consideration. Some of these, such as the confinement of the brain within the skull, have already been mentioned.

Most pathogens are carried to the central nervous system via the bloodstream; some such as rabies spread along nerve channels, whereas comparatively few extend into the brain by crossing the olfactory mucosa or penetrating the cranial vault. Distinction must be made between inflammation of the meninges (meningitis) and that of the cerebral parenchyma (encephalitis), while a third category (encephalomyelitis) is usually invoked for inflammatory diseases that result in demyelination.

1. Virus-Associated Neurologic Disease

Virus-associated neurologic disease can be conveniently partitioned into 3 categories listed in Illustration 15-19.

Viral meningitis, also called "aseptic" meningitis, is usually a benign, self-limiting acute

---

15-18. DISEASES OF THE CNS ASSOCIATED WITH INFECTIOUS AGENTS

1) VIRUS-ASSOCIATED DISEASE

2) SUPPURATIVE DISEASE

3) MISCELLANEOUS INFECTIOUS DISEASES

15-19. VIRUS-ASSOCIATED NEUROLOGIC DISEASE

1) MENINGITIS (ASEPTIC)
　　enterovirus
　　mumps
　　herpes simplex
　　arborviruses

2) ENCEPHALITIS
　　rabies
　　enterovirus
　　mumps
　　herpes simplex
　　arborviruses
　　slow virus infections

3) ENCEPHALOMYELITIS
　　postinfectious complication of measles vaccination and other infections

---

disease caused by any one of the number of viruses listed. It is characterized by fever, headache and nuchal rigidity (stiff neck). Treatment includes relief of symptoms and rest.

Viral encephalitis, as can be imagined is, in most *acute* cases, an extension and complication of viral meningitis. In addition to signs and symptoms listed for the latter, those of acute viral encephalitis may include loss of consciousness, seizures or focal neurologic deficit. Although the foregoing description would undoubtedly summarize most cases of viral encephalitis, there are a few which differ so profoundly that they deserve special mention; the first of these is *rabies*.

Rabies is a comparatively rare human disease in which a viral infection spreads from an animal bite through nerve sheaths to ultimately involve the brain. The usual victim is a child and the usual animal vector is the domestic dog (although the skunk, fox and bat are now challenging the dog as a source of contagion). Treatment is designed to prevent encephalitis. Killed virus grown in duck embryo culture is used to induce active immunity whereas interim passive protection is provided with human anti-rabies gamma globulin.

Other viral encephalitides that differ radically from the usual acute disease are those of the slow, latent and chronic varieties. These have been described in Chapter 7 and should be reviewed at this point.

2. Suppurative Diseases of the Central Nervous System

Suppurative diseases of the central nervous system are rather common and almost invariably associated with the presence of pus-eliciting bacteria within either the meninges or brain substance. We will use only 2 such diseases as examples (Illustration 15-20).

Meningococcal meningitis is a purulent infection of the leptomeninges caused by the gram-negative organism, *Neisseria meningitides.* Access to the cranial vault is thought to be gained through the olfactory mucosa or bloodstream. Although its clinical manifestations are severe, this infection is treatable. Fulminating cases are still common but usually seen either in children or as the result of late interception.

The *brain abscess* is a lesion usually caused either by direct penetration of pyogenic bacteria into the brain parenchyma or by their metastatic spread from another focus of purulent infection. The most common of the causative organisms are the staphylococci but others such as streptococci are often implicated. The lesion may be single or multiple, the latter being more common if hematogenous spread is involved.

3. Miscellaneous Infectious Diseases

A number of other very important infections of the central nervous system are often seen, but for the sake of brevity we must consider them beyond the scope of this discussion. These include syphilis, tuberculosis, various mycoses and toxoplasmosis.

Additional Reading

Johnson, R. T. Neurologic diseases associated with viral infections. Postgrad. Med. 50:85, 1971

CEREBROVASCULAR ACCIDENT

LEARNING OBJECTIVE

To be able to describe the pathogenesis and results of the cerebrovascular accident, using the following as examples.

a) the congenital saccular aneurysm
b) CVA secondary to cerebral atherosclerosis

The brain, a highly critical tissue, situated as it is within the unyielding cranial vault, is strongly dependent on a continuous supply of blood and highly intolerant of lesions that occupy space or interrupt its perfusion. One very prominent example of the former is hemorrhage into the brain; an example of the latter would be thrombosis of a cerebral artery or its branch. The former is almost always traceable to the rupturing of a bloodvessel whereas the latter usually appears as a complication of atherosclerosis. The resulting clinical syndrome, regardless of its cause, is called a *cerebrovascular accident, CVA,* or simply *stroke.*

Several conditions predispose to the occurrence of the cerebrovascular accident, some of which have been mentioned in discussions of previous chapters. We will discuss the first 2 of those listed in Illustration 15-21.

15-20. SUPPURATIVE DISEASES OF THE CNS

1) MENINGITIS
    caused by a number of pyogenic organisms, the most important being the meningococcus

2) ENCEPHALITIS
    seen as a complication of meningitis or as the brain abscess

15-21. CEREBROVASCULAR ACCIDENT (CVA, STROKE)

1) CONGENITAL SACCULAR ANEURYSM (BERRY ANEURYSM)

2) CEREBRAL ATHEROSCLEROSIS

3) HYPERTENSION

4) HEMOSTATIC DISORDERS

15-22. CEREBRAL ATHEROSCLEROSIS

1) ATHEROSCLEROSIS OF CEREBRAL ARTERIES PARALLELS THAT OF OTHER ARTERIES OF COMPARABLE SIZE

2) COMPLICATIONS INCLUDE
aneurysm, with or without rupture
thrombosis with cerebral infarct

1. Congenital Saccular Aneurysm (Berry Aneurysm)

The congenital saccular aneurysm is an outpouching of the wall of a cerebral artery (located at the base of the brain) resulting from a developmental defect in the media. Little or no effect is noted until the aneurysm bursts, an event that usually occurs in early to middle adult life.

The sudden release of arterial pressure into the subarachnoid space and cerebral tissue often results in sudden death: however, many patients survive with varying degrees of neurologic deficit.

2. Cerebral Atherosclerosis

Arteries at the base of the brain are liable to the same degree of atherosclerotic degeneration as other arteries of comparable size. Indeed the degree of atherosclerotic change in cerebral

arteries, particularly those in or near the circle of Willis, corresponds quite closely to that found in similar vessels of the heart and kidney.

As would be expected severe atherosclerosis may be complicated by two developments of very serious nature, the aneurysm and thrombosis (Illustration 15-22). Both the ruptured aneurysm and the infarct give rise to the clinical appearance of the cerebrovascular accident or stroke.

The CVA based on atherosclerosis characteristically happens in later life after the process of atherosclerosis has had time to advance. That based on the congenital saccular aneurysm, you will remember, usually occurs in young adulthood.

Additional Reading

Bailey, W. L. Intracranial aneurysms. J. Am. Med. Assn. 216:1993, 1971

INTRACRANIAL TUMORS

LEARNING OBJECTIVE

To be able to discuss the entire picture of intracranial tumors mentioning
   a) tissues of origin and relative frequency
   b) epidemiology
   c) clinical course of the glioma
   d) liability of the brain to metastatic tumor

Tumors of the brain are said to cause approximately 2 per cent of all deaths in the United States. They are listed roughly in order of incidence in Illustration 15-23. Like tumors of other organs, brain tumors can originate in any of a number of different cells and will exhibit the usual spectrum of biologic qualities. Unlike other tumors, however, neoplasms primary to the brain rarely, if ever, metastasize

---

15-23. INTRACRANIAL TUMORS

(in order of incidence)

1) GLIOMA

2) METASTATIC TUMOR

3) MENINGIOMA

4) A VARIETY OF OTHERS
   embryonal tumors
   miscellaneous   pituitary   tumors
   sarcoma

---

regardless of their degree of malignancy: yet even the most benign have lethal potential because of the strict confinement of the brain in the cranial vault.

We will examine only the first 2 listed in Illustration 15-23.

1. Glioma

Gliomas are tumors of the supportive tissues of the brain. They are always the most common intracranial tumor regardless of country or group studied. In general, they arise from the astrocyte, the oligodendroglia or ependyma. They all have lethal potential and virtually none ever metastasize extracranially regardless of the degree of malignancy.

The most malignant-appearing glioma is also the most common. It is known as the glioblastoma multiforme, a tumor that usually occurs after middle age. Its onset is usually sudden, its progress surprisingly rapid and its prognosis exceedingly poor.

2. Metastatic Tumors

Any malignant neoplasm has the potential to metastasize to the brain or its meninges. The 2 that do this with greatest frequency are carcinoma of the lung and carcinoma of the breast. A metastatic focus of either of these tumors may be detectable in the brain long before its primary site has been discovered, because even the smallest cerebral metastases usually gives rise to disproportionately severe edema and a sudden increase in intracranial pressure.

Pulmonary carcinoma tends to metastasize to brain substance, whereas carcinoma of the breast frequently involves the dura.

DEMYELINATING DISEASES AND IDIOPATHIC EPILEPSY

LEARNING OBJECTIVE

To be able to compare and contrast the pathogenesis and clinical courses of demyelinating diseases (using multiple sclerosis as an example) and idiopathic epilepsy mentioning:
   a) suspected causes
   b) age at onset
   c) clinical course
   d) complications

Myelin is a fatty material produced by cells of the nerve sheath (Schwann cells). It surrounds the axon, nourishing it and allowing it to conduct nerve impulses over long distances without fading or confusion. Diseases which appear to be based on deterioration of this myelin sheath are called demyelinating diseases. In this learning objective, we will be concerned with comparing demyelinating diseases with another group in which the neurologic effect is prominent but the lesions causing it are obscure.

1. Demyelinating Diseases

Demyelinating diseases are actually a very large, poorly defined group most of which are of unknown etiology (Illustration 15-24). In some of these diseases the process of demyelination occurs in a focal pattern as discrete plaques, whereas in others it is seen as a diffuse condition affecting all tissues within a certain area of the central nervous system. We will

15-24. DEMYELINATING DISEASES

1) MULTIPLE SCLEROSIS

2) LEUKOENCEPHALOPATHY

3) SUBACUTE COMBINED DEGENERA-
   TION

4) POSTINFECTIOUS ENCEPHALOMYE-
   LITIS

- - - - - - - - -

Most of the above are not single diseases but large and poorly defined groups, all of which exhibit demyelination

examine the disease, multiple sclerosis, as an example of demyelinating diseases.

Multiple sclerosis is a demyelinating disease in which the brain and cord are affected in a focal pattern. Plaques are most prominently seen in the long tracts of the spinal cord, hence lower limb motor deficit is a conspicuous sign. Others include intentional tremor, nystagmus and the slurring of speech.

The etiology of multiple sclerosis is unknown. Its onset usually occurs between the ages of 20 and 40 and the patient usually experiences alternating periods of remission and relapse over many years as his condition worsens.

Little more is known about multiple sclerosis today than when it was first described more than 100 years ago. Since it is reasonably common, affects young adults and is refractory to treatment, a great deal of research is now directed toward its understanding.

2. Idiopathic Epilepsy

Whereas the neurologic disorder associated with demyelinating diseases is clearly a functional deficit caused by *demonstrable* lesions of the central nervous system, there is another kind of CNS disease in which the causative lesion is not so obvious and, indeed, in many cases never seen.

Epilepsy or, more correctly, idiopathic epilepsy, is the term used for a kind of disease in which the patient experiences recurrent seizures or episodes of convulsions for which no cause can be demonstrated. Many such episodes, of course, are not epileptic and can be traced to congenital malformations, anoxia, trauma, infection, tumors, poisons or metabolic defects. Epilepsy reaches its peak incidence at around 10 years of age and is usually outgrown by early adult life. Epilepsy occurs with greater frequency in certain families, suggesting that factors which predispose an individual to seizures are inherited at least as a polygenic quality.

True epileptic seizures occur in 3 clinical patterns (Illustration 15-25). We will consider each in turn.

The Petit Mal Seizure

The petit mal seizure is characteristically one of brief duration usually presenting as an abrupt, momentary lapse of consciousness and activity. The patient suddenly stops whatever he is doing and stares, just as suddenly resuming his activity with no awareness of having sustained an attack. All clinical variations are possible, however, and the petit mal seizure

---

15-25. CLINICAL PATTERNS OF EPILEPSY (IDIOPATHIC EPILEPSY)

1) PETIT MAL
   - usually not provoked
   - brief (5 to 30 sec)
   - convulsion minor or absent

2) GRAND MAL
   - usually provoked by emotional disturbance and preceded by an unusual sensory experience or "aura"
   - longer duration
   - strong convulsion
   - patient loses conciousness

3) FOCAL (JACKSONIAN)
   - resembles grand mal but confined to one side of body

may well include a number of other pycho-motor phenomena such as mild convulsions, blinking or lip smacking.

The Grand Mal Seizure

The grand mal seizure is one characterized by a serious convulsive episode. Its onset is often signalled by an unusual sensory experience or "aura" and the patient is unconscious during the seizure. Most patients who have other kinds of seizures will have grand mal seizures at some time.

The Focal (Jacksonian) Seizure

The focal or jacksonian seizure resembles the grand mal in clinical appearance, but is confined to only one side of the body. In some cases there will be a aura: however, the patient may remain conscious but be unable to speak. Focal seizures occur most often during sleep usually in the hours just after retiring or before rising. They are most often seen in the middle years of childhood.

Additional Reading

Soll, R. W. The enigma of multiple sclerosis. Postgrad Med. 52:113, 1972

Dean, G. The multiple sclerosis problem. Sci. Amer 223:40, 1970

Metcalf, C. W. Amyotrophic lateral sclerosis. Arch Neurol. 24:518, 1971

chapter 16
RESPIRATORY SYSTEM

ACUTE RESPIRATORY INFECTIONS

LEARNING OBJECTIVE

To be able to discuss acute bacterial laryngotrachiobronchitis, influenza and the 4 principal forms of pneumonia as examples of acute respiratory infections, mentioning the following:

a) protective faculties of the respiratory system
b) causative agents
c) predisposing factors where applicable
d) usual clinical course
e) complications

The respiratory passages are a common portal of entry for viral and bacterial pathogens as well as a variety of non-living irritants.

In the normal tracheobronchial tree a number of defense mechanisms serve to protect the individual from most of these agents (Illustration 16-1). But despite this formidable array of protective devices, irritation of the respiratory tract is a frequent occurrence and respiratory infections are more common than those of any other major organ system. Most are acute and transient and, despite their common occurrence, rarely lead to irreversible changes in the lung or air passages. We will consider 2 as examples (Illustration 16-2).

1. Laryngotracheobronchitis

Acute laryngotracheobronchitis is an extremely common form of acute respiratory disease and may be caused by a variety of agents. Any inhaled irritant or respiratory pathogen that is not flushed out by the ciliary mucin elevator or neutralized by secretory antibody can cause irritation and inflammation of the larynx or air passages. Aside from inhaled irritants the most frequent causes of

---

16-1. PROTECTIVE FACILITIES OF THE RESPIRATORY SYSTEM

1) MUCIN SECRETION

2) CILIARY ELEVATION OF MUCIN TOWARD THE MOUTH

3) THE COUGH

----

the above are intended to trap and expel all foreign material before or shortly after it enters the bronchial system—deeper protective facilities include:

4) SECRETORY IMMUNOGLOBULINS

5) ACUTE INFLAMMATION

6) THE ALVEOLAR MACROPHAGE

16-2. ACUTE INFECTIONS OF THE RESPIRATORY SYSTEM

1) LARYNGOTRACHEOBRONCHITIS
   most (infective) cases are caused by bacterial pathogens
   an important example of viral etiology is influenza

2) PNEUMONIA (pneumonitis)
   a variety of clinical patterns

this condition are *Staphylococcus aureus* and various streptococci as well as a large group of viruses. Viral infections of the respiratory tract are often secondarily invaded by bacterial pathogens and so many such infections end up as predominantly pyogenic.

2. Pneumonia

Pneumonia or pneumonitis is inflammation of the pulmonary parenchyma. It occurs in 4 principal clinical patterns (Illustration 16-3).

Regional Pneumonia

Regional pneumonia is inflammation localized to a rather well circumscribed area of the lung. It is usually caused by aspiration of an irritant substance, a septic object or in a rather unusual form as lipid aspiration pneumonia. None of these will concern us here.

Lobar Pneumonia

Lobar pneumonia is a form in which whole lobes are involved in the inflammatory process. The microscopic architecture of lung paren-

---

16-3. PRINCIPAL CLINICAL PATTERNS OF PNEUMONIA

1) REGIONAL
   pulmonary abscess
   lipid aspiration

2) LOBAR
   one or more entire lobes are consolidated

3) LOBULAR (BRONCHO-)
   consolidation is distributed lobule by lobule

4) PRIMARY ATYPICAL (PAP)
   totally diffuse involvement of both lungs
   no typical consolidation
   alveolar septae are thick and cellular

---

chyma differs from that of all other organs because it is intended to hold air. Normally, then, pulmonary parenchyma is mostly air space.

When inflamed it changes dramatically. The air cavities (alveoli) rapidly fill with exudate which promptly clots, transforming the vacant, sponge-like lung into a solid-appearing fleshy tissue resembling liver. This process is called *consolidation* and is the most conspicuous change in most bacterial pneumonias. In lobar pneumonia, consolidation characteristically affects one or more entire lobes.

Lobar pneumonia can be caused by a number of respiratory pathogens, all of which are able to evoke a strong inflammatory response; however, over 90 per cent of cases are actually caused by the pneumococcus (*Diplococcus pneumoniae*). An inoculum of this organism is inhaled and finds its way into the normally sterile terminal bronchi and alveolar sacs. Because it is strongly provocative of inflammation, an immediate response ensues. Subsequent changes in the lung are usually considered in 4 stages (Illustration 16-4). In the first stage (*congestion*), the early vascular changes of the acute inflammatory process can be found occurring throughout the affected lobe. Vessels become dilated and engorged with blood preparatory to the release of copious exudate.

In the next stage, exudate pours out of the congested vessels rapidly filling the alveolar spaces. Consolidation follows quickly and the air spaces become obliterated with exudate and hemorrhage. This is called the stage of *red hepatization*, a term used because of the abundance of hemorrhage and the similarity in consistency between the consolidated lung and liver.

As the inflammatory reaction proceeds to later stages, macrophages clear the extravasated blood cells and the consolidated lung takes on a lighter color. With the elimination of blood pigment, the process is said to be in the stage of *gray hepatization*. Finally, the clot undergoes lysis and the process enters the stage of *resolution* which proceeds to recovery, usually without leaving permanent traces.

On very rare occasions the exudate organizes instead of resolving, a phenomenon mentioned in Chapter 3 as an example of aberrant repair. This, of course, has disastrous consequences and may render the affected lobe nonfunctional.

16-4. STAGES OF LOBAR PENUMONIA
1) CONGESTION
2) RED HEPATIZATION
3) GRAY HEPATIZATION
4) RESOLUTION

16-5. AGENTS WHICH CAUSE PRIMARY ATYPICAL PENUMONIA
1) MYCOPLASMA PNEUMONIAE (Eaton Agent) poorly understood, intracellular pathogen
2) VIRUS myxovirus influenza respiratory syncytial virus (RSV) others
3) CHLAMYDIAE AND RICKETTSIAE most prominent example is ornithosis

Lobular Pneumonia

Lobular pneumonia is a pattern in which consolidation is distributed, lobule by lobule. It begins in the airway and spreads into lung parenchyma. Because of its origin in the bronchial tree, it is often called *bronchopneumonia*. Lobular pneumonia is most commonly caused by staphylococci and streptococci but many other organisms have also been implicated.

Although it is seen under a variety of conditions, the lobular pattern of pneumonia is almost always seen among patients with immunologic deficiency, particularly that of the humoral system (see Chapter 4). It is also seen as a complication of measles and other viral infections, pertussis (whooping cough), immunosuppression and any of a number of debilitating conditions. It is a common incidental finding at autopsy regardless of the cause of death.

The clinical course of lobular pneumonia is extremely variable because of its usual association with some other disease.

Primary Atypical Pneumonia

Primary atypical pneumonia, also called *interstitial pneumonia*, is characterized by generalized (not lobar or lobular) distribution and the fact that it takes origin within the walls of the pulmonary alveoli. In cases where the etiology has been identified, the most common causative organism is *Mycoplasma pneumoniae* (also known as the *Eaton agent*), a poorly understood intracellular pathogen. This pattern of pneumonia also results from viral infection of the lung parenchyma (Illustration 16-5), as well as rare cases of rickettsial pneumonitis.

Consolidation does not occur in uncomplicated cases and most of the reaction goes on within the fibrous walls (septae) of the alveoli. These become thickened and cellular-appearing but comparatively little exudate collects within the alveolar space.

The clinical course is variable and probably depends largely on the nature of the causative agent and the defense status of the patient. It can be suddenly and dramatically fatal such as the attacks described in the influenza epidemic of 1914-1918 or so benign as to cause only the most mild discomfort.

Additional Reading

Carruthus, M. M. Practical therapeutics: Diagnosis and management of flu. Am. Fam. Phys. (GP) 2:119, 1970

Foy, H. M. et al. *Mycoplasma pneumoniae* pneumonia in an urban area. J. Am. Med. Assn. 214:1666, 1970

Hinson, K. F. W. Diffuse pulmonary fibrosis. Human Path. 1:275, 1970

Kilbourne, E. D. Influenza 1970: Unquestioned answers and unanswered questions. Arch. Environm. Health 21:284, 1970

Kylstra, J. Experiments in water-breathing. Sci. Amer. 219:66, 1967

Marks, A. Diffuse interstitial pulmonary fibrosis. Med. Clin. N. Amer. 51:439, 1967

Rosenow, E. C. Foreign body aspiration. Postgrad. Med. 49:164, 1971

Smith, C. A. The first breath. Sci. Amer. 209:27, 1963

Thurlbeck, W. M. Physiological considerations in restrictive lung disease. Human Path. 1:259, 1970

BRONCHIAL ASTHMA

LEARNING OBJECTIVE

To be able to discuss bronchial asthma with regard to:
   a) probable cause
   b) predisposing factors
   c) age distribution
   d) associated morphologic changes in the respiratory system

---

Bronchial asthma is a condition in which there are succeeding episodes of bronchial constriction, usually of poorly defined etiology. These bronchospastic attacks are manifested by the acute onset of dyspnea, lasting from one to several hours and are usually interspersed with longer intervals of normal respiratory function. An allergen is sometimes clearly involved: however, more often the relationship of each attack with a precipitating factor is ambiguous. Emotional stress, fatigue and endocrine changes are often described as predisposing, but usually not provoking, influences.

The IgE system almost certainly mediates an attack of acute asthma, since most patients show additional atopic afflictions, but the basic difference between the asthmatic and normal individual may be more reliably attributable to an exaggerated reactivity to chemical mediators of IgE reactions such as histamine, kinins and SRS-A.

Bronchial asthma is most prominent among school-age children where it is usually more clearly associated with inhaled allergens.

16-6. VARIETIES OF ASTHMA (PAROXYSMAL DYSPNEA)

---

1) BRONCHIAL ASTHMA
   usually seen in the young

2) CARDIAC ASTHMA
   associated with heart failure

3) ASTHMA-LIKE SYNDROMES ASSOCIATED WITH PULMONARY INFECTIONS AND TUMORS

Asthma in middle age and beyond is often seen as a complication of infections. Asthma-like signs and symptoms may be associated with heart failure (cardiac asthma) and pulmonary tumors (Illustration 16-6).

Additional Reading

Cohen, S. I. Psychological factors in asthma. Postgrad. Med. J. 47:533, 1971

SECONDARY LUNG DISEASE

LEARNING OBJECTIVE

To review the interaction of the heart and lungs as presented in Chapter 12 and be able to discuss secondary lung disease using the following as examples:
   a) pulmonary edema as an effect of heart failure
   b) pulmonary embolism and infarction leading to acute cor pulmonale

---

Since respiration is so intimately involved with blood circulation, many disorders of the latter ultimately affect the respiratory system, particularly the lung. We will use this opportunity to take a second look at 2 of the most prominent examples of this relationship (Illustration 16-7).

1. Pulmonary Edema

Pulmonary edema has been described in Chapter 12 and is mentioned here only to reinforce the concept of heart-lung interdependency. It should be thoroughly reviewed at this point.

2. Pulmonary Embolism and Infarction

Pulmonary embolism is so common among hospitalized patients it is also deserving of review at this point.

16-7. SECONDARY LUNG DISEASE

1) PULMONARY EDEMA

   primary concomitant of left-sided heart failure
   Review Chapter 12

2) PULMONARY EMBOLISM AND IN-FARCTION

   most common form of acute cor pulmonale

Because the great preponderance of pulmonary emboli begin as thrombi of the veins of the lower torso and extremities and because blood stasis is so potent a predisposing factor in phlebothrombosis, there is a tendency now to get patients out of bed and ambulatory as soon as possible after surgery.

Additional Reading

Divertie, M. B. Lung involvement in the connective tissue disorders. Med. Clin. N. Amer. 48:1015, 1964

Fisher, M. S. Pulmonary embolism. Med. Radiogr. Photogr. 46:54, 1970

Gee, J. B. L. The alveolar macrophage: pulmonary frontiersman. Am. J. Med. Sci. 260:195, 1970

Staub, N. C. The pathophysiology of pulmonary edema. Human Path. 1:419, 1970

Weiss, E. B. Goodpasture's syndrome. Am. Rev. Resp. Dis. 97:444, 1968

CHRONIC OBSTRUCTIVE AIRWAY DISEASE

LEARNING OBJECTIVE

To be able to discuss chronic obstructive airway disease as 2 separate syndromes, chronic bronchitis leading to emphysema and primary emphysema mentioning the following:
   a) 3 principal forms of emphysema
   b) pathogenesis of chronic bronchitis
   c) acquisition and significance of α_1, antitrypsin deficiency
   d) pathogenesis of primary emphysema

With continued irritation of the respiratory system, there is the possibility for the development of irreversible structural defects within the tracheobronchial tree or pulmonary parenchyma. These structural defects interfere with normal protective cleansing of the air passages and lead to their obstruction. Once obstructed, the condition enters a kind of degenerative spiral in which the irritation resulting from obstruction leads to further irritation and obstruction. The syndrome is called chronic obstructive airway disease and the spiral often ends in pulmonary failure and death. Two forms of chronic obstructive airway disease must be differentiated in this discussion (Illustration 16-8).

16-8. CHRONIC OBSTRUCTIVE AIRWAY DISEASE

1) CHRONIC BRONCHITIS AND EMPHY-SEMA

   usually centrilobular—may progress to panlobular if patient survives to advanced age

2) PRIMARY EMPHYSEMA

   panlobular form is seen, even in relatively young—
   α^1 antitrypsin deficiency or other inherited predisposition

---

1. Chronic Bronchitis and Emphysema

The first form of chronic obstructive airway disease to be considered is chronic bronchitis leading to emphysema. Chronic irritation of the bronchi such as results from the excessive inhalation of cigarette smoke or other irritant material will result in chronic inflammation. Given adequate duration, this will inevitably lead to structural changes within bronchial walls. Hyperplasia or even metaplasia of the epithelium, an increase in the dimension of the sub-epithelial layers and the failure of ciliary action occur first causing the accumulation of secretion and chronic cough. This cough is paroxysmal in onset and most severe on rising.

In the next stage, there is repeated and lingering deep respiratory infection which, if severe, will weaken bronchial walls leading to abnormal dilatation and outpouching. This is called bronchiectasis, a condition that irreversibly inhibits the normal airway cleansing action by providing sequestered areas for bacterial growth.

In the final stages, terminal airway structures and alveolar septae begin to dilate and even rupture. This change, irreversible and highly significant for a number of reasons, is called *emphysema*. Emphysema is usually divided into 3 types, depending upon its localization and severity (Illustration 16-9). Since lung parenchyma is actually supporting and anchoring the bronchiolar-size air passages, distortion by emphysema leads to bronchial collapse and further airway obstruction. Also anchored in the pulmonary parenchyma are small vessels of the pulmonary vascular tree. With the onset of emphysema there is distortion of pulmonary arterioles and the gradual development of cor pulmonale. Stages in the pathogenesis of chronic bronchitis and emphysema are reviewed in Illustration 16-10.

The clinical course of chronic bronchitis is variable and depends upon the rate of deterioration of pulmonary function. There is usually a persistent cough productive of purulence, after years of which gradual failure of ventilation usually occurs. Death may be caused by acute respiratory failure precipitated by infection or by complications of cor pulmonale. The pattern of emphysema that results is usually of the centrilobular type.

16.9. EMPHYSEMA (Classification Based on Structural Alterations)

Emphysema is the condition of dilatation (with or without rupture) of terminal bronchioles and alveoli

- - - - -

REGIONAL

not distributed generally, associated with obstructing bronchial lesion or seen as patchy change in senescence

CENTRILOBULAR

generalized distribution primarily affecting only the respiratory bronchioles of all pulmonary lobules

PANLOBULAR

generalized distribution affecting respiratory bronchioles, alveolar ducts and alveoli of all pulmonary lobules

---

2. Primary Emphysema (Alpha₁ Antitrypsin Deficiency)

The second form of chronic obstructive airway disease differs considerably from the first in that it is based on an inherited susceptibility to emphysema. We have seen that emphysema is often encountered as a complication of advanced chronic bronchitis, but that in this situation it is most often in the centrilobular pattern. On occasion this condition worsens to take on a panlobular distribution, in which case the patient begins to demonstrate severe ventilatory distress, including pronounced cyanosis.

In primary emphysema, quite in contrast, severe panlobular emphysema appears to develop without antecedent chronic bronchitis. In other words, the emphysema is seen not as a complication of another disease but as a disease entity in itself.

Primary emphysema has for many years been thought to represent an underlying constitutional predisposition to the breakdown of lung parenchyma. Recently one such predisposition was shown to be associated with the lack or absence of a globulin found in the α_1 electrophoretic fraction of serum and called α_1 antitrypsin.

The possession of an adequate amount of α_1 antitrypsin is controlled by a single gene which acts as an autosomal dominant. Thus, homozygous individuals have an abundance, heterozygotes an intermediate amount, and recessive homozygotes none. The last of these 3 genotypes is clearly predisposed to severe panlobular emphysema, as well as a kind of liver disease that evolves to cirrhosis. Apparently α_1 anti-

---

16-11. PRIMARY EMPHYSEMA (FAMILIAL EMPHYSEMA)

(OCCURS SECONDARY TO α_1 ANTITRYPSIN DEFICIENCY OR OTHER INHERITED PREDISPOSING FACTOR)

1) **CHRONIC BRONCHITIS OR MINIMAL BRONCHIAL IRRITATION**
   comparatively rapid dilatation and rupture of terminal structures of the respiratory lobule

2) **PANLOBULAR EMPHYSEMA**
   significant impairment of respiration and gas exchange-cor pulmonale
   severe dyspnea and cyanosis

16-10. PATHOGENESIS OF CHRONIC BRONCHITIS AND EMPHYSEMA

1) **SUSTAINED IRRITATION OF AIR PASSAGES**
   thickening of bronchial walls
   ciliary arrest
   accumulation of secretions
   chronic cough

2) **IRREVERSIBLE CHANGES IN WALLS OF AIRWAY**
   frequent deep chest infections
   possible bronchiectasis

3) **CENTRILOBULAR EMPHYSEMA**
   further obstruction of airways
   aggravation of all changes noted above

4) **MAY PROGRESS TO PANLOBULAR EMPHYSEMA IF PATIENT SURVIVES TO ADVANCED AGE**

---

trypsin protects the delicate alveolar septae from damage by lysosomal enzymes that are released as cells break down in normal body function. Depending upon the availability of α_1 antitrypsin, a person is more or less protected from emphysema. The picture is clear in the case of its complete absence, but what is not clear is the amount needed to constitute adequate protection.

It is quite likely that some individuals manifesting panlobular emphysema as a complication of chronic bronchitis are suffering from an intermediate but insufficient amount of this globulin and, indeed, some authorities believe that in such cases it might be emphysema that actually precipitates the bronchitis. The pathogenesis of primary emphysema is reviewed in Illustration 16-11.

Additional Reading

Burrows, B. and Earle, R. H. Course and prognosis of chronic obstructive lung disease. N. Engl. J. Med. 280:397, 1969

Guenter, C. A. et al. Alpha₁ antitrypsin deficiency and pulmonary emphysema. Ann. Rev. Med. 22:283, 1971

Lieberman, J. et al. Screening for heterozygous alpha₁ antitrypsin deficiency. J. Am. Med. Assn. 217:1198, 1971

Pratt, P. C. and Kilburn, K. H. A modern concept of the emphysemas based on correlations of structure and function. Human Path. 1:443, 1970

Pump, K. K. The aged lung. Chest 60:571, 1971

CHRONIC GRANULOMA-TOUS LUNG DISEASE

LEARNING OBJECTIVE

To review information on the granuloma presented in Chapter 2 and on tuberculosis and the deep mycoses presented in Chapter 8. To be able to discuss the entire picture of chronic granulomatous lung disease mentioning the cause, pathogenesis, clinical course and complications of the following:

  a) primary and secondary tuberculosis
  b) the deep mycoses (histoplasmosis, coccidioidomycosis and blastomycosis as examples)
  c) pneumoconiosis (coal workers disease, silicosis and berylliosis as examples)

Whereas most foreign material within the lung precipitates an acute inflammatory response, the inhalation of certain kinds of pathogens and non-living material gives rise to the formation of widespread granuloma formation and fibrosis. This is the basis for a category of diseases called *chronic granulomatous lung disease*. It is convenient to separate chronic granulomatous lung diseases into 2 categories (Illustration 16-12), those caused by dust inhalation and those resulting from infection by living organisms.

1. Pneumoconiosis

Chronic granulomatous lung disease caused by non-living foreign material is called *pneumoconiosis*. Both mineral and organic dusts can cause pneumoconiosis; however, since the disease-causing potential of such material is dependent upon *long exposure to high concentra-*

16-12. CHRONIC GRANULOMATOUS LUNG DISEASE

1) PNEUMOCONIOSIS
   widespread pulmonary fibrosis caused by dust inhalation

2) GRANULOMATOUS INFECTIONS
   usually caused by higher (more complex) pathogens
   tuberculosis
   deep mycoses

16-13. DETERMINANTS OF PNEUMOCONIOSIS

1) NATURE OF DUST
   certain materials have unusual antigenic effect

2) PARTICLE SIZE
   $< 3\ \mu$ is most dangerous

3) CONCENTRATION
   heavy concentration is usually required to overcome flushing action of ciliary mucin elevator

4) LENGTH OF EXPOSURE
   long exposure usually needed

5) COEXISTENCE OF OTHER LUNG DISEASE
   particularly any condition impairing ciliary elevation of mucin

---

tions of finely divided particles (Illustration 16-13), most examples are seen as occupational diseases. We will look briefly at those listed in Illustration 16-14.

Silicosis

Without a doubt the model for all pneumoconiosis has been silicosis. This disease has

16-14. EXAMPLES OF PNEUMOCONIO-SIS
1) SILICOSIS
2) COAL WORKERS' PNEUMOCONIOSIS
3) ASBESTOSIS
4) BERYLLIOSIS
5) BYSSINOSIS

that, although very similar to silicosis, differs in certain significant respects. This disease has come to be known as *coal workers pneumoconiosis* or *black lung disease*. It is not restricted to miners and in fact was first described among coal "trimmers," who are responsible for leveling a load of coal as it is placed aboard ships for transport.

The clinical course of black lung disease varies among individuals and is influenced by the same factors that determine severity in other pneumoconiosis. Its importance as a public hazard is based on its occurrence among miners, since this group is the largest of those affected.

Asbestosis

Laborers engaged in the manufacture of insulation and fireproofing materials are exposed to asbestos dust and may contract a form of pneumoconiosis known as *asbestosis*. This disease is similar to silicosis in many respects except that it tends to progress more rapidly and predispose an affected individual to bronchogenic carcinoma and pleural mesothelioma, the latter being a malignant tumor occurring with extreme rarity among persons not exposed to asbestos.

Berylliosis

With industrial use of beryllium, particularly as a coating for fluorescent light tubes, came the delayed realization that this metal could also give rise to a kind of pneumoconiosis. Berylliosis differs from either silicosis or asbestosis in that it exhibits wide variation in individual susceptibility and is not confined to the lungs.

Byssinosis

Byssinosis, a kind of pneumoconiosis contracted through the inhalation of cotton dust, is added here as an example of those caused by the inhalation of vegetable fiber.

2. Granulomatous Infections

Most major examples of infectious granulomatous diseases of the respiratory system have been mentioned in Chapter 8 and should be reviewed at this point.

been described in ancient Egyptian mummies and is common today among a variety of occupations. It can be generated at will in an experimental animal and is even seen as a complication of some forms of drug abuse. Silica (silicon dioxide) is the most prominent constituent of the earth's outer mantle. Not surprisingly, exposure to this material under a variety of circumstances is a common occupational hazard.

Particularly liable to such exposure are underground miners working in an atmosphere heavy with rock dust. But, more recently, it is seen among individuals in various occupations in which silica is used as an abrasive. This includes metal grinders, sandblasters and others.

The onset of symptoms in silicosis is characteristically insidious. Nodular fibrosis associated with granuloma formation occurs slowly over a number of years, leading to the gradual onset of dyspnea with exertion. Complications include chronic bronchitis, emphysema, cor pulmonale and a pronounced predisposition to tuberculosis.

Coal Workers Pneumoconiosis

All kinds of deep mining are potentially hazardous as a lifelong occupation, because the air space within most mines is usually heavily ladened with dust, if not constantly, at least at frequent intervals. We have seen that when this dust has a significant silica content there is great danger of contracting silicosis.

In recent years, it has become apparent that coal dust, regardless of its silica content, can cause a kind of chronic granulomatous disease

In general, they fall into 2 large categories, mycobacterial infections and deep mycoses. Of the former, by far the most important is tuberculosis, whereas the latter consists of several prominent examples, most of which are endemic to certain geographic locations.

Additional Reading

Morgan, W. K. C. Coal workers pneumoconiosis. Am. Indus. Hygiene J. 32:29, 1971

Scadding, J. C. Tuberculin sensitivity in tuberculosis. Postgrad. Med. J. 47:694, 1971

Wyatt, J. P. Occupational lung diseases and inferential relationships to general population hazards. Am. J. Path. 64:197, 1971

PULMONARY NEOPLASMS

LEARNING OBJECTIVE

To be able to discuss primary and metastatic tumors of the lung, mentioning the following:

  a) epidemiology and pathogenesis of bronchogenic carcinoma
  b) liability of the lung to metastatic tumor and examples of tumors that commonly metastasize to the lung.

Over 90 per cent of neoplasms primary to the respiratory system are malignant and the most common by far is bronchogenic carcinoma. Although other kinds of tumors are seen, the overwhelming predominance of bronchogenic carcinoma renders all others comparatively rare. This tumor is now the leading cause of cancer death in the United States.

Another common tumor of the respiratory system is a malignancy that has metastasized from some other site (Illustration 16-15).

Bronchogenic carcinoma is a malignant tumor originating in the epithelium of the bronchial tree (Illustration 16-16). A number of histologic varieties are recognized, but the cell of origin for all of these is thought to be the basal cell of respiratory epithelium.

Quite unlike carcinoma of the stomach, bronchogenic carcinoma has shown an absolute increase in incidence over the past few decades. There is a striking statistical correlation between cigarette consumption and bronchogenic carcinoma and some authorities accept recent evidence of a direct causal relationship between

---

16-15. NEOPLASMS OF THE RESPIRATORY SYSTEM

1) PRIMARY

   most neoplasms primary to the respiratory system are malignant

   the most common is bronchogenic carcinoma

2) SECONDARY

   the lung is a common site for tumor metastasis, particularly sarcoma

---

16-16. BRONCHOGENIC CARCINOMA

1) ORIGINATES IN RESPIRATORY EPITHELIUM

2) MOST COMMON CAUSE OF CANCER DEATH IN U.S.: INCREASING INCIDENCE

3) PRIMARILY AFFECTS MALES OF MIDDLE AGE

4) LOW CURE RATE

---

smoking and the development of this tumor. Whatever the reason, the incidence of bronchogenic carcinoma continues to increase at an alarming rate.

Males of middle age are primarily affected with the peak incidence occurring between 50 and 60. The tumor is usually discovered late in its clinical course and cure rates are discouragingly small.

Additional Reading

Hems, G. Factors associated with lung cancer. Brit. J. Cancer XXII:466, 1968

Ashley, D. C. et. al. Cancer of the lung, histology and biological behavior. Cancer 20:165, 1967

Ochsner, A. Bronchogenic carcinoma, a largely preventable lesion assuming epidemic proportions. Chest 59:358, 1971

Rigdon, R. H. Cigarette smoking and lung cancer: A consideration of this relationship. South. Med. J. 62:232, 1969

part 5

systems review — b

chapter 17
MALE AND FEMALE GENITAL SYSTEMS

VENEREAL DISEASE

LEARNING OBJECTIVE

To be able to discuss the concept of venereal disease, developing a detailed comparison between gonorrhea and syphilis as examples. Mention (where applicable):
- a) characteristics of the infecting agent
- b) pathogenesis of the infection
- c) stages of the disease
- d) clinical signs and usual course
- e) possible complications
- f) epidemiology, prophylaxis, treatment and residual immunity

---

17-1. VENEREAL DISEASE
(In order of decreasing incidence in U.S.)
1) GONORRHEA
2) SYPHILIS
3) CHANCROID
4) LYMPHOGRANULOMA VENEREUM
5) GRANULOMA INGUINALE
Gonorrhea and syphilis account for more than 99 per cent of all venereal disease reported in the U.S.

A venereal disease is one that is spread principally by sexual contact. The 5 diseases listed in Illustration 17-1 are all venereal: however, only the first 2 are of any public health significance in the United State and most of Europe: In the United States, gonorrhea and syphilis account for more than 99 per cent of all reported cases. Because of their comparatively overwhelming importance our discussion of venereal disease will be limited to these 2 diseases.

1. Gonorrhea

Gonorrhea is the most prevalent of all venereal diseases; the ratio of gonorrhea to syphilis reported today in the United States is about 20:1. An estimated 2 million new cases of gonorrhea occurred in America in 1970, a record that places the dynamics of this disease within the limits of an epidemic.

Recently failure to control gonorrhea is based on many factors, among which are urban blight, and the rapid collapse of traditional value systems. However, no small part is due to the highly infectious nature of *Neisseria gonorrheae*, the causative organism (Illustration 17-2). Gonorrhea exhibits a very short incubation period (2 to 6 days), it does *not* leave its victim immune to future infection and there is now reason to believe that a large reservoir of asymptomatic female carriers exists, particularly in areas of high prevalence. Young adults (20 to 24 years old) rank first in incidence and it occurs with much greater frequency in the United States among the unmarried and black residents of urban ghettos.

In the male, gonorrhea is usually localized to urothelial surfaces and begins as a purulent urethritis (90 per cent of purulent urethritis in

---

17-2. NEISSERIA GONORRHEAE

---

1) DISCOVERED BY ALBERT NEISSER IN 1879

2) GRAM NEGATIVE DIPLOCOCCUS

3) EXCLUSIVELY HUMAN PATHOGEN: PYOGENIC

4) PENICILLIN-SENSITIVE
    in recent years a slowly develop-
    ing penicillin resistance has been
    noticed

---

males is caused by gonorrhea). There is pain on urination (dysuria), but no other complication in early mild infections. Repeated or persistent infections may spread up the genital tract involving prostate, seminal vesicles and epididymes. Complications include sterility and urethral stricture.

In the female, gonorrhea is a considerably different disease from that in the male. The woman may harbor the organism, but be essentially asymptomatic for long periods. In time, however, the organism may traverse the urethra and spread up the birth canal to involve the fallopian tubes, ovaries and peritoneal cavity. These developments give rise to severe pelvic inflammatory disease (PID) or life-threatening peritonitis. Other complications include pyosalpinx (fallopian tube sealed and distended with pus) and sterility (Illustration 17-3).

Gonococcal bacteremia may result in suppurative arthritis or endocarditis, but these severe complications have grown more rare with the general use of antibiotics. Also rare today is the formerly common gonococcal ophthalmia neonatorum that can occur when the eyes of an infant become infected by passing through the birth canal of an infected mother. Gonorrhea in the male and female is reviewed in Illustration 17-3.

2. Syphilis

Syphilis is an infectious disease characterized by long duration, widespread systematic involvement and a confusing variety of signs and symptoms. The causative agent, *Treponema pallidum*, is an exquisitely delicate organism that has proven to be unfailingly sensitive to a variety of antibiotics (see Illustration 17-4). Yet despite its ease of treatment, syphilis is the third most frequently reported infectious disease in the United States today, outstripped by only gonorrhea and the ubiquitous streptococcal infections.

Acquired Syphilis

Like gonorrhea, syphilis is most prevalent among the young (62 per cent of cases occur between the ages of 15 and 25), the unmarried and black residents of urban ghettos. Control of syphilis is impeded by the same factors that frustrate control of gonorrhea.

Unlike gonorrhea which is usually localized to the urethra, *syphilis is always a generalized, systemic infection.* It is seen as either an acquired or congenital disease (Illustration 17-5).

Although most syphilis is transmitted sexually (about 95 per cent) there is the distinct possibility for extra-sexual spread of this disease (Illustration 17-6). Wherever a living spirochete comes in contact with a body surface there is the potential for its penetrating and initiating an infection. The spirochete will not survive dessication, however, so an effective

---

17-3. GONORRHEA

---

1) MALE
    purulent urethritis (may be asymp-
    tomatic)
    retrograde spread may involve
    prostate, seminal vesicles, epi-
    didymes (but rarely testicles)
    sterility, urethral stricture may re-
    sult

2) FEMALE
    purulent urethritis (may be asymp-
    tomatic)
    retrograde spread may cause sal-
    pingitis, PID, fatal peritonitis
    sterility may result

17-4. *TREPONEMA PALLIDUM*

1) THREE GENERA OF SPIROCHETES CAUSE HUMAN DISEASE
   Treponema
   Borrelia
   Leptospira

2) GENERAL FEATURES OF SPIRO-CHETOSIS
   widespread dissemination of organism within body
   relatively mild reaction
   usual absence of necrosis
   difficulty in isolating culturing and staining organism
   persistence of infection

3) *T. PALLIDUM* IS SINGLE-HOST HUMAN PATHOGEN

4) SENSITIVE TO A NUMBER OF ANTIBIOTICS

17-6. SPREAD OF SYPHILIS

1) SEXUAL EXPOSURE
   contact with moist effusion of primary or secondary lesion is usually required

2) ACCIDENTAL DIRECT INOCULATION
   any contact (sexual or nonsexual) with moist effusion of any primary or secondary lesion is potentially infective (tertiary lesions are not infective)

3) TRANSFUSION
   rare today—
   spirochetes die in banked blood

4) INTRAUTERINE INFECTION
   congenital form

17-5. SYPHILIS (LUES)

1) ACQUIRED
   contracted during extrauterine life, usually as an adult
   about 95 per cent is transmitted sexually

2) CONGENITAL
   contracted in utero through maternal infection
   in recent years there has been a rise in congenital cases

inoculation requires more or less direct contact with contaminated fluid. Saliva or effusate from a weeping lesion make an ideal medium for transmission.

The clinical course of syphilis follows 3 (or 4) stages (Illustration 17-7). The primary stage begins after an incubation period of 1 to 10 weeks with the appearance of a chancre at the point of inoculation. The chancre is the primary lesion of syphilis and the hallmark of the primary stage.

The secondary state usually becomes manifest 1 to 3 months after the beginning of the primary. In a small percentage of cases, primary and secondary lesions may co-exist, but in most instances the chancre will have healed before the appearance of secondary signs (Illustration 17-8).

With resolution of secondary lesions, the infected individual appears to be cured: however, in many cases the disease has merely entered a more occult phase known as the latent stage. Patients within the latent stage are not infectious, but are still personally affected by the disease in that they harbor the organism within their body for varying lengths of time.

About one-third of all untreated cases progress to the tertiary stage (Illustration 17-9), where permanent damage to the cardiovascular and nervous systems may occur. Tertiary lesions may appear at any time 1 to 30 years following early stages of the disease.

17-7. CLINICAL STAGES OF SYPHILIS

1) PRIMARY

appearance of chancre 1 to 10 weeks after exposure

2) SECONDARY

appearance of any one or combination of a variety of skin and mucosal eruptions 1 to 3 months after the chancre is noticed

LATENT:

Interpretation varies but usually taken to mean the stage following disappearance of secondary lesions and preceding the appearance of tertiary

3) TERTIARY (⅓ of untreated cases)

irreversible lesions primarily affecting CV and nervous systems appearing 1 to 30 years following early stages

17-8. SIGNS OF EARLY SYPHILIS

1) PRIMARY

chancre

2) SECONDARY

rash
alopecia
lymphadenopathy
condylomatous lesions
annular skin lesions
split papule
mucous patch

17-9. SIGNS OF TERTIARY SYPHILIS

1) CARDIOVASCULAR LESIONS

syphilitic aortitis
aortic aneurysm (thoracic)

2) CNS DEFICIT

paresis
tabes dorsalis

3) GUMMA

4) MISCELLANEOUS

hepar lobatum

Congenital Syphilis

Congenital syphilis is a form in which the developing fetus is involved as a complication of maternal infection (Illustration 17-10). The spirochete of syphilis is one of the few organisms that can consistently cross placental barriers to infect the fetus. Like its acquired counterpart, congenital syphilis has recently shown an alarming increase in incidence.

For reasons yet unexplained spirochetes infecting the mother cannot invade the fetus until approximately 4½ to 5 months of gestation. Treatment of the infected mother at some time previous to the 5th month will usually prevent fetal infection. Untreated congenital syphilis results in a variety of diseases ranging from fetal wastage and perinatal death to a series of stigmatizing lesions which include depression of the bridge of the nose (saddle nose), a tibial deformity characterized by a sharp curving anterior edge (saber shin) and three highly pathogonomic lesions first described by Hutchinson (Hutchinson's triad) which include notched, screwdriver-shaped central incisors, interstitial keratitis and eighth nerve deafness.

In effect, the newborn with congenital syphilis manifests the secondary stage seen in the acquired form. The clinical course of the congenital disease is roughly comparable to that of its acquired form except, of course, the entire primary stage is missing.

THE MALE GENITAL SYSTEM

17-10. CONGENITAL SYPHILIS

1) MATERNAL DISEASE CAUSES FETAL INFECTION

2) SPIROCHETES CANNOT INVADE FETUS UNTIL APPROXIMATELY 4½–5 MONTHS
   - treatment of mother before 5th month prevents fetal infection

3) FETAL INFECTION CAUSES LATE ABORTION, STILLBIRTH, PERINATAL DEATH, OR STIGMATIZING LESIONS:
   - saddle nose
   - saber shin
   - Hutchinson's triad

4) INFECTED CHILD IS BORN MANIFESTING SECONDARY STAGE OF INFECTION

LEARNING OBJECTIVE

To be able to compare and contrast benign prostatic hypertrophy and carcinoma of the prostate mentioning the following:
   a) incidence and prevalence
   b) hormonal dependence
   c) metastatic pattern (where applicable)
   d) clinical signs
   e) complications

Diseases of the male genital system differ markedly from those of the female because of anatomical and functional dissimilarity between corresponding and even analogous structures. Female genital structures are contained almost completely within the body, whereas those of the male are more exterior. In the male the genital viscera are intimately associated with the urinary outflow tract, whereas in the female the 2 are completely separate. We will see that these features and others lend far different implications to genital diseases in the male and female. As our examples of male genital disease we will use benign prostatic hypertrophy and carcinoma of the prostate (Illustration 17-11).

1. Benign Prostatic Hypertrophy

Benign prostatic hypertrophy is actually hyperplasia of the prostate occurring in a

Additional Reading

Ellner, P. D. Diagnosis of gonococcal infection. Clin. Med. 78:16, 1971
Fiumara, N. J. and Lessell, S. Manifestation of late, congenital syphilis. Arch. Dermatol. 102:78, 1970
Lucas, J. B. The national venereal disease problem. Med. Clin. N. Amer. 56:1073, 1972
Robinson, R. C. V. Acquired syphilis. Clin. Med. 79:25, 1972

17-11. PRINCIPAL DISEASES OF THE MALE GENITAL SYSTEM

In addition to venereal diseases (and other infections) which are very common we will consider the following two as representative:

1) BENIGN PROSTATIC HYPERTROPHY

2) CARCINOMA OF THE PROSTATE

17-12. BENIGN PROSTATIC HYPER-TROPHY

1) ACTUALLY AN EXAMPLE OF HYPER-PLASIA
   glandular, fibromuscular, mixed

2) EXTREMELY COMMON
   prevalence in males of advanced age may reach 80 per cent

3) CLINICAL SIGNIFICANCE BASED ON URINARY OBSTRUCTION

17-13. CARCINOMA OF THE PROSTATE

1) OVERALL MOST COMMON CANCER OF THE HUMAN MALE
   most cases do not become clinically apparent during life and are turned up as an incidental finding at autopsy

2) FIRST CLINICAL SIGNS (EXCEPT FOR PALPATION) RESULT FROM EFFECTS OF METASTASIS
   metastatic lesions in bone
   elevated serum acid phosphatase

3) ANDROGEN-DEPENDENT TUMOR
   hormone therapy successful in control (not cure)

---

nodular configuration, however the term, and even its acronym (BPH) are by now so widely used that there is little practical reason to insist on precision (Illustration 17-12).

BPH is an extremely common disorder usually seen in patients over the age of 50 and affecting up to 80 per cent of males of far advanced age. The cellular pattern of the hyperplasia may be fibromuscular, glandular or a mixture of both. There is almost no agreement as to the etiology of this disease: however, it is generally acknowledged to be associated with the changing hormonal constitution of the aging male, perhaps as a response to the fading of androgen secretion and increased relative significance of estrogen. Eunuchs and early castrates do not develop this condition and it does not appear to be in any way antecedent to carcinoma of the prostate.

The clinical significance of BPH derives almost entirely from its effect on the urinary outflow tract. When severe, it raises the floor of the bladder and slows the transurethral passage of urine. This may lead to urine retention, cystitis, pyelonephritis and, in severe cases, actual obstruction of the urethra and hydronephrosis.

2. Carcinoma of the Prostate

Carcinoma of the prostate is usually seen at age 50 and beyond and becomes very common in advanced years. In an *occult form*, it may approach an incidence of 100 per cent in extreme old age. Most examples of prostatic

carcinoma are discovered at autopsy and never become clinically apparent.

Although it is the most common of all malignant neoplasms in the male, cancer of the prostate ranks far below cancer of the lung as a cause of death, because of its tendency to remain confined.

When prostatic carcinoma does leave the prostate, its first signs may result from local invasion and metastases rather than urinary obstruction (Illustration 17-13). Bone metastases are most often seen, occurring in 70 to 80 per cent of clinically apparent cases. Surgery is of little value, but hormonal treatment has proven successful in the control of this tumor, because of its clear-cut androgen dependence (Illustration 17-13).

Additional Reading

Levine, S. Sexual Differentiation: The development of maleness and femaleness. Calif. Med. 114:12, 1971
Steele, R. et. al. Sexual factors in the epidemiology of cancer of the prostate. J. Chron. Dis. 24:29, 1971

THE FEMALE GENITAL SYSTEM

LEARNING OBJECTIVE

To be able to discuss carcinoma of the breast, carcinoma of the cervix and the fibroid tumor as examples of the most prominent neoplasms of female reproductive structures, mentioning each of the following in detail:

a) incidence, prevalence and age distribution
b) causative, predisposing and protective factors
c) relationship to sexual activity and childbearing
d) hormonal dependence
e) clinical signs, clinical course and complications
f) prophylaxis and treatment

Three prominent diseases of female genital structures will serve as our examples, *carcinoma of the breast, carcinoma of the uterine cervix*, and the *uterine leiomyoma* (Illustration 17-14).

1. Carcinoma of the Breast

The female breast consists of a dozen or so lobules each of which is made up of a system of ducts supported by connective tissue in a matrix of fat cells. The duct system begins as a number of blind-end acinar structures, each terminating at the nipple in an independent opening.

Carcinoma of the breast is a malignant tumor arising from some cell within the duct system. If it arises at one of the numerous acinar ends

---

17-14. PRINCIPAL DISEASES OF FE- MALE GENITAL STRUCTURES

1) CARCINOMA OF THE BREAST

2) CARCINOMA OF THE CERVIX

3) UTERINE LEIOMYOMA (FIBROID)

17-15. CARCINOMA OF THE BREAST

1) MOST COMMON MALIGNANCY IN WOMEN

2) MOST COMMON CAUSE OF CANCER DEATH IN WOMEN

Any lump in the breast must be investigated as soon as it is detected

---

of a duct, it is called a *lobular carcinoma*; if it arises elsewhere along the duct system, it is called a *ductal carcinoma* (Illustration 17-15).

About 80 per cent of malignant breast tumors are invasive *ductal* cancers and 70 per cent of these are classified as scirrhous carcinomas, because they elicit an abundance of firm connective tissue. In the following discussion, we will discuss invasive carcinoma of the breast as if it were a single disease. Bear in mind, however, that the clinical course of this tumor varies widely with the histologic type and a finer distinction must be made on diagnosis.

It is estimated that 68,000 new cases of breast cancer will occur in the United States in 1970 and 30,000 women will die as a direct result of this tumor. It is the major cause of cancer death in women in the United States and the single leading cause of death among women between the ages of 40 and 44. The over-all 5-year survival rate has long been recognized as approximately 50 per cent, but this is known to be influenced by the biologic nature of the tumor, the extent of its progress at interception, and more recently, by skilled employment of management therapy (Illustration 17-16).

Although the male has breast structures analogous to those of the female, carcinoma of the breast is clearly a disease of women (male breast cancers occur with 1/100 the frequency of female). This distinct sex preference is known to be based on the strong hormonal dependence of the tumor, a quality often exploited in the treatment of widely disseminated breast tumors.

Carcinoma of the breast occurs with greater frequency among women of higher than middle

---

17-16. HISTOLOGIC   VARIETIES   OF
BREAST CANCER

---

1) LOBULAR CARCINOMA
> originates at secretory terminus
> of duct system accounts for 5 to
> 10 per cent of *infiltrating* cancer

2) DUCTAL CARCINOMA
> originates along duct system: ac-
> counts for approx. 80 per cent of
> *infiltrating* cancer

3) PAGET'S DISEASE
> thought to be carcinoma of duct
> invading epithelium at areola ac-
> counts for balance of *infiltrating*
> cancer

---

that it ranks third behind carcinoma of the colon). On a worldwide basis, it is probably the most common malignant neoplasm of the female. Almost all examples of this disease are squamous cell carcinoma (Illustration 17-17).

The epidemiology and clinical behavior of carcinoma of the cervix differs clearly from those of breast cancer. In fact, a close comparison of the 2 suggests that *cancer of the cervix may actually be a kind of venereal disease of viral etiology whereas cancer of the breast is a neoplasm incited by hormonal variation*. These ideas are highly speculative at present, but are considered fruitful hypotheses for further study and we will explore them as a means of discussing cervical carcinoma.

Herpes simplex virus is known to exist in at least 2 serologic types, *Type 1* and *Type 2*. The Type 1 virus is associated mainly with mouth lesions (it is responsible for the familiar cold sore) whereas Type 2 virus is similarly associ-

socio-economic status. There seems to be a fairly distinct polygenic inheritance pattern in the occurrence of this tumor, in that women in whose family the tumor has appeared have a 2 to 3 times higher risk of contracting it than the population at large. Unmarried women are slightly more liable as are married women who bear no children, when compared to those who have borne 2 or more. A woman who has recovered from a carcinoma of 1 breast has an increased chance of contracting carcinoma of the remaining breast and women experiencing sustained emotional stress appear to be more susceptible than those leading happy, produc- tive lives.

The behavior of the more common examples of this tumor is such that metastatic growth is most often seen in lung, bone and liver. Despite metastasis, however, the judicious use of chemotherapy and endocrine regulation can often result in years of productive life.

2. Carcinoma of the Cervix

Carcinoma of the cervix is a very common (estimated 42,000 new cases in the United States in 1970), very dangerous disease with a number of fascinating aspects. It is the second most common visceral malignancy of United States females, exceeded in frequency only by carcinoma of the breast (some studies suggest

---

17-17. CARCINOMA OF THE CERVIX

**1) SECOND MOST COMMON CANCER
OF WOMEN: MOST ARE SQUAMOUS
CELL CARCINOMA**

**2) PEAK INCIDENCE BETWEEN 40 to
60: SHIFTING TO YOUNGER RANGE**

3) HIGHER INCIDENCE
> early sexual experience
> marriage
> multiparity
> promiscuity
> low socioeconomic status
> serum antibody to herpes simplex
> (type 2)

4) LOWER INCIDENCE
> nuns
> Jewish women,
> nulliparity
> high socioeconomic status

**5) NO APPARENT GENETIC PATTERN OR
ENDOCRINE RELATIONSHIPS**

---

ated with lesions of the genitalia. Several recent reports have shown a high incidence of neutralizing antibody to the Type 2 virus in women with carcinoma of the cervix. This is usually interpreted as suggesting that herpes virus causing genital lesions *may* also be causing cancer of the cervix.

When added to other features of the epidemiology of this disease (Illustration 17-17), the implication of a virus as causative agent suggests that the *induction* of cervical carcinoma by viral infection occurs at a very early age through sexual intercourse, but that the *promotion* of a clinically apparent tumor requires years of sexual and reproductive activity. Further, it would appear that with full maturity the cervical epithelium becomes more resistant to this infection so when sexual experience begins at a later age there is less chance of contracting the infection.

Unlike carcinoma of the breast, cervical cancer exhibits no hormonal dependence or tendency for familial occurrence. It is positively rather than negatively related to parity and is seen with greater frequency among socioeconomic groups lower than middle class.

The incidence of carcinoma of the cervix appears to correlate positively with sexual promiscuity in that it is seen with great frequency among prostitutes and women in prison. It is comparatively rare among Jewish women, a fact often attributed to circumcision of Jewish males, and it is almost never seen in nuns.

As mentioned above practically all carcinoma of the cervix is squamous cell carcinoma. The lesion apparently develops slowly over a period of many years to become clinically evident about the age of 40. Invasion begins as local extension into adjacent structures and metastases usually occurs late in its clinical course.

Because of the rather predictable behavior of early lesions, carcinoma of the cervix is now considered an almost totally preventable disease. When intercepted early, the cure rate is close to 100 per cent.

3. Uterine Leiomyoma (Fibroid)

The uterine leiomyoma or "fibroid" is the most common benign tumor of any significance in the female. Indeed this disease is so common that it may actually occur in more than 20 per

---

17-18. UTERINE LEIOMYOMA (FIBROID)
1) MOST COMMON BENIGN TUMOR (OF SIGNIFICANCE) IN THE FEMALE prevalence may be as high as 20 per cent of all women over 35
2) STRONGLY ESTROGEN DEPENDENT appears after puberty largest during age of greatest ovarian activity regress after menopause
3) MALIGNANT TRANSFORMATION IS KNOWN BUT RARE

---

cent of all women over the age of 35 (Illustration 17-18).

Again, just as in the case of breast cancer, this tumor exhibits strong hormonal dependence in that it grows rapidly during pregnancy and regresses after menopause. Fibroids may be multiple or solitary and occur within or at either surface of the uterine wall. They are the most common cause of intermenstrual uterine bleeding (metrorrhagia) during childbearing years and may interfere with pregnancy, but they are biologically benign and rarely undergo malignant transformation.

Additional Reading

Anderson, D. E. Some characteristics of familial breast cancer. Cancer 28:1500, 1971

Forsberg, J. G. Estrogen, vaginal cancer and vaginal development. Am. J. Obst. Gynec. 113:83, 1972

Stearns, H. C. Uterine myomas: Clinical and pathologic aspects. Postgrad. Med. 51:165, 1972

Zippin, C. and Petrakis, N. L. Identification of high risk groups in breast cancer. Cancer 28:1381, 1971

DISEASES OF GESTATION

LEARNING OBJECTIVE

To be able to outline and briefly discuss diseases of gestation, describing each of the following:

  a) **general characteristics of the placenta including its endocrine functions**
  b) **the hydatidiform mole**
  c) **choriocarcinoma**
  d) **ectopic pregnancy**

The placenta is a tissue that serves a critical but temporary need, following which it is simply discarded. It is a fetal tissue, arising from the fertilized egg and having a genetic constitution identical to the rest of the conceptus. During pregnancy, the placenta serves as both an endocrine organ and a means of nutrient and other transfer between the mother and developing child. It also manages to prevent its own rejection by the constant shedding of cells into the maternal bloodstream, a strategy which results in the eliciting of antibodies that protect the placenta against attack by the cellular immune system (Illustration 17-19).

There are many diseases associated with the very singular condition of being pregnant. Some are largely functional, whereas others give rise to distinct morphologic changes. We will use 3 as our examples, all of which are of the latter type (Illustration 17-20).

1. Hydatidiform Mole

In about 1 out of every 2,000 pregnancies (in the United States), the chorionic villi undergo marked hydropic swelling giving rise to a mass of cysts known as a hydatidiform mole. This is most often discovered in the fourth or fifth month of gestation and is usually associated with markedly elevated serum and urinary levels of chorionic gonadotropins. The hydatidiform mole is particularly significant in that it may be the first stage in a more malignant form of trophoblastic disease such as choriocarcinoma.

2. Choriocarcinoma

Choriocarcinoma is a malignant tumor of the trophoblastic layer of the chorion. It is ex-

---

17-19. FUNCTIONS OF THE PLACENTA

1) ENDOCRINE
    chorionic gonadotropin
    estrogens
    progesterone
        (the last two are synthesized by cooperative effort with fetal adrenal)

2) NUTRIENT
    system of villi and microvilli provides enormous surface for exchange

3) IMMUNOLOGIC
    regular shedding of trophoblastic cells into maternal blood streams thought to prevent rejection

---

17-20. DISEASES OF GESTATION

1) HYDATIDIFORM MOLE

2) CHORIOCARCINOMA

3) ECTOPIC PREGNANCY

---

tremely rare in the United States, most cases developing in association with a hydatidiform mole, spontaneous abortion or other abnormal pregnancy. Choriocarcinoma can also arise from totipotential cells within the gonads and hence is also seen in males.

Probably because the normal trophoblast invades the wall of the uterus and is immunologically well tolerated, this tumor tends to be markedly aggressive and metastasizes early and widely. Also, because the trophoblast secretes chorionic gonadotropin, the presence of this tumor is usually associated with extremely high serum and urinary levels of this hormone.

Recent development of a practical chemotherapeutic regimen has produced a remarkable improvement in survival rate in cases of choriocarcinoma.

3. Ectopic Pregnancy

Ectopic pregnancy is the condition resulting from implantation of the fertilized ovum at a site other than the uterine wall. The great preponderance of cases occur within the fallopian tube and are associated with pre-existing tubal stricture usually secondary to salpingitis.

Tubal pregnancies most commonly rupture into the peritoneal cavity producing a dramatically sudden, life-threatening peritonitis.

Additional Reading

Carr, M. C. Biology of human trophoblast. Calif. Med. 107:338, 1967

Hertig, A. T. Human trophoblast: Normal and abnormal. Am. J. Clin. Path. 47:249, 1967

Hertz, R. Biological aspects of gestational neoplasms derived from trophoblast. Ann. N. Y. Acad. Sci. 172:279, 1971

chapter 18
URINARY SYSTEM

MALFORMATIONS OF THE KIDNEY

LEARNING OBJECTIVE

To be able to discuss the cause, pathogenesis, significance and clinical course of:
- a) the simple renal cyst
- b) congenital polycystic disease (in its infantile and adult form)

The kidney performs an absolutely indispensible service in regulating the internal environment of the body. Its functions are such that the removal or shut-down of both kidneys would result in the slow, but ultimately fatal, accumulation of metabolic waste, while their malfunction causes the loss of vital protein and ions. The functional unit of the kidney is the *nephron*. There are more than 1 million nephrons in each normal kidney, a number considerably in excess of actual need. For this reason, gradual failure of the kidney is not noticed until the process is quite far advanced.

The upper nephron filters the blood, allowing only the smaller solutes to pass the glomerulus. As the glomerular filtrate trickles through the tubular system, more metabolic waste products are secreted and essential solutes are resorbed by tubular epithelial cells; the solution that emerges is urine (Illustration 18-1).

Malformations of the kidney are quite common, particularly when one includes all examples of the solitary and essentially symptomless cyst. They can be conveniently considered as either gross malformations or cystic disease (Illustration 18-2). Since the former is comparatively uncommon, we will confine our attention to the latter.

1. The Simple Cyst

An extremely common cystic disorder of the kidney is the simple cyst. This lesion may be either solitary or multiple, unilateral or bilat-

---

18-1. THE KIDNEY

1) FUNCTIONAL UNIT IS THE NEPHRON

2) 1 TO 1.25 MILLION NEPHRONS PER KIDNEY
   considerable excess

3) FILTER 190 LITERS OF FLUID PER DAY (130 cc/min)
   only one liter excreted

4) GLOMERULAR FILTRATE IS BLOOD WITHOUT CELLS OR PROTEIN

5) 25 PER CENT OF CARDIAC OUTPUT (AT REST) GOES THROUGH KIDNEY
   0.5 per cent total body weight

6) VITAL FUNCTIONS
   secrete H^+ and metabolic waste
      regulate internal ion concentration
   eliminate excess water
   conserve essential solutes

18-2. MALFORMATIONS OF THE KIDNEY

1) GROSS MALFORMATIONS

2) CYSTIC DISEASE
   simple cyst
      solitary
      multiple
   polycystic disease
      infantile
      adult
   congenital polycystic dysplasia

eral. It is usually without significance unless infected. Indeed, the simple cyst is usually present throughout most of a person's lifetime and is often discovered as an incidental finding at autopsy. Simple cysts are more frequent in the adult than the child, suggesting that they are acquired or at least become manifest during the course of a person's life.

2. Congenital Polycystic Disease

Congenital polycystic disease is a condition in which the renal parenchyma is completely displaced by tightly packed cysts of varying size. It occurs in 3 forms, infantile, adult and dysplastic. All are known to be inherited, but in different genetic patterns.

The infantile form is usually not compatible with life beyond the first year, whereas the adult form may not become manifest until middle age or beyond. In both of these, the untreated condition leads to gradual renal failure, uremia and death.

The third form of cystic disease, congenital polycystic dysplasia, is usually not associated with renal impairment.

Additional Reading

Greene, L. F. Cystic disease of the kidney. GP XXXVII:78, 1968

Randolph, J. G. Congenital abnormalities of the urinary collecting system. Pediat. Clin. N. Amer. 12:2, 1965

Schainuck, L. I. et al. Structural-functional correlations in renal disease (Part II). Human Path. 1:631, 1970

Striker, G. E. et al. Structural-functional correlations in renal disease (Part I). Human Path. 1:615, 1970

GLOMERULONEPHRITIS

LEARNING OBJECTIVE

To review information on immune complex injury presented in Chapter 4 and be able to thoroughly compare and contrast the immune complex and nephrotoxic types of glomerulonephritis mentioning the following:

  a) causative factors and associated diseases
  b) pathogenetic mechanisms
  c) signs, symptoms and clinical course
  d) ultimate effect on the kidney

Glomerulonephritis (GN) is an inflammatory disease of the kidney that begins in the glomerulus. Although the lesions of this kind of disease are primarily glomerular, they ultimately involve other structures of the nephron as well. With regard to its distribution within the kidney, GN occurs in 2 types, focal and diffuse (Illustration 18-3). The focal type affects a limited number of randomly distributed glomeruli and is comparatively unimportant. The diffuse pattern is a far more significant disease and our discussion will be limited to this type. Diffuse glomerulonephritis, whatever its cause, is almost always bilateral, since the agent causing it is carried in the bloodstream. Also, the great preponderance of

---

**18-3. CLASSIFICATION OF GLOMERU-
LONEPHRITIS (GN)**

1) FOCAL GN
    embolic
    immunologic (may progress to diffuse form)

2) DIFFUSE GN
    immune complex type
    nephrotoxic type
    immunologic GN of undetermined
        cause
    non-immunologic GN

diffuse glomerulonephritis is based on immunologic injury to the glomerular basement membrane, a feature which will form the basis for our classification of this disease into 4 subgroups (Illustration 18-3).

1. Immune Complex Glomerulonephritis

The most common form of diffuse glomerulonephritis (GN) is that caused by immune complex injury to the glomerular filter. It is usually seen as a secondary complication of a variety of clearly recognizable diseases in which there is widespread formation of immune complexes within the bloodstream (Illustration 18-4), but it may be encountered as an essentially idiopathic primary disease (membranous glomerulonephritis).

In the pathogenesis of this condition, complexes formed in circulating blood are *mechanically trapped* by the glomerular filter. They fix complement and elicit the usual sequence of complement-mediated inflammatory changes (See Chapter 2) culminating in the attraction of neutrophil leukocytes. In most cases these changes are reversible and the condition subsides without lasting effects (Illustration 18-5).

18-4. CLINICAL PATTERNS OF IMMUNE COMPLEX GN

1) **POST STREPTOCOCCAL GN**
   exotoxemia results in the formation of immune complexes

2) **LUPUS NEPHRITIS**
   tissue destruction leads to release of large amounts of intracellular material, immune complexes form

3) **MALARIAL NEPHRITIS**

4) **NEPHRITIS SECONDARY TO CHRONIC VIRAL INFECTION**

5) **MEMBRANOUS GN**
   (idiopathic)

18-5. PATHOGENESIS OF IMMUNE COMPLEX GN

1) **WIDESPREAD FORMATION OF IMMUNE COMPLEXES OCCURS WITHIN THE BLOODSTREAM**

2) **COMPLEXES BECOME PASSIVELY LODGED IN GLOMERULAR FILTER COMPLEMENT IS FIXED**

3) **REVERSIBLE, ACUTE GN OCCURS**
   assuming complexes are not formed continuously or disease does not progress to chronic form

---

Morphologic changes in the glomerulus consistently associated with this kind of glomerulonephritis are listed in Illustration 18-6.

The most common cause of this kind of immune complex glomerulonephritis is glomerular injury following a streptococcal infection. It is characteristically seen in a young individual 10 to 20 days following resolution of a streptococcal infection of the tonsils, throat or middle ear. It appears suddenly as bilateral low back pain and hematuria and is often accompanied by malaise, fever and nausea. Some amount of proteinuria is always seen and, indeed, the loss of protein through damaged glomeruli may in rare instances become so serious as to lead to the nephrotic syndrome (to be discussed below). Paradoxically, even with this apparent "leakage" of the glomerular filter, there is still a tendency for fluid retention and the blood urea nitrogen concentration (BUN) may increase slightly. There is usually some degree of systemic hypertension undoubtedly related to the impairment of blood flow through the kidneys. Most cases of post-streptococcal GN subside without lasting effect.

Other examples of immune complex GN, such as those associated with systemic lupus erythematosus (SLE), malaria and chronic viral infection, will persist as long as the primary disease is active and immune complexes continue to form. If the primary disease is not arrested, the resulting immune-complex GN will

18-6. GLOMERULAR CHANGES IN ACUTE IMMUNE COMPLEX GN

1) PROLIFERATION OF EPITHELIAL AND MESANGIAL CELLS

2) IRREGULAR THICKENING OF GBM
   nodular configuration of deposits demonstrable by immunofluorescence

3) PRESENCE OF PMN's IN LATER STAGES

4) COMPLETE RESOLUTION
   if disease does not go on to chronic form

18-7. CLINICAL COURSE OF IMMUNE COMPLEX GN

1) IMMUNE COMPLEX INJURY TO GLOMERULI RESULTS IN SYNDROME OF *ACUTE* GLOMERULONEPHRITIS
   mild proteinuria
   hematuria
   transient hypertension
   nausea
   fever
   malaise
   usually complete resolution
   nephrotic syndrome is possible but extremely rare

2) A SMALL NUMBER OF CASES OF POST-STREPTOCOCCAL GN GO ON TO *CHRONIC* GN
   thought based on development of sensitivity to GBM either through autosensitization or cross-reactivity with streptococcal products

ultimately destroy the kidney and prove fatal. This is often seen in SLE where renal disease is a prominent cause of death.

On rare occasions, immune-complex GN will undergo transformation to a chronic form which is slowly but relentlessly progressive. Although the reason is unknown, it is generally conceded that a small minority of cases of post-streptococcal GN will somehow progress to chronic glomerulonephritis and renal failure. The clinical course of immune complex GN is reviewed in Illustration 18-7.

2. Nephrotoxic Glomerulonephritis

Far less common than the immune complex type is a kind of glomerulonephritis in which the body actually manufactures antibodies that react with certain antigens of the glomerular basement membrane (GBM). This form of the disease is called *nephrotoxic glomerulonephritis*. Nephrotoxic glomerulonephritis is a true autoimmune disease in contrast to the immune complex type in which kidney involvement is more like that of an innocent bystander.

Although nephrotoxic GN is often seen in association with other diseases (Illustration 18-8), these are not thought causative in the same way as streptococcal infection or SLE causes immune complex GN. The irreducible requirement for nephrotoxic GN is the forma-

18-8. SYNDROMES THAT INCLUDE NEPHROTOXIC GN

1) GOODPASTURE'S SYNDROME
   in association with pulmonary disease based on anti-alveolar basement membrane antibody

2) "RAPIDLY PROGRESSIVE" GN
   unassociated with another prominent lesion, a single affliction confined to the kidney

tion of anti-GBM antibodies, whatever else may be taking place in the same body at this time. See Illustration 18-9 for a summary of this disease mechanism. A review of the discussion of Goodpasture's syndrome present in Chapter 4 might also be helpful as a supplement to this subject.

Certain glomerular changes are highly pathognomonic of nephrotoxic GN and serve to differentiate it from the immune complex type on renal biopsy. These are listed in Illustration 18-10. Note that the thickening of the GBM (as demonstrated by immunofluorescence) assumes a smooth, linear configuration in contrast to the "lumpy-bumpy" shape of the GBM in the immune complex type.

The clinical course of nephrotoxic GN is best described as progressive. The urinary space becomes obliterated by proliferating epithelial cells, the basement membrane becomes markedly thickened and periglomerular inflammatory infiltrate leads to a constricting fibrosis. The predictable effect is ultimate destruction and sclerosis of each glomerulus and rapid renal failure. In the more slowly progressing varieties of this condition, there is generalized fibrosis and pronounced shrinking of the whole kidney

---

18-10. GLOMERULAR CHANGES IN NEPHROTOXIC GN

1) **PROLIFERATION OF EPITHELIAL CELLS**
   formation of capsular crescents
   obliteration of Bowman's space

2) **REGULAR THICKENING OF GBM**
   linear configuration of deposits
   demonstrable by immunofluorescence

3) **PROGRESSIVE GLOMERULAR AND PERIGLOMERULAR FIBROSIS**

4) **OBLITERATION OF GLOMERULUS**

18-11. CLINICAL COURSE OF NEPHROTOXIC GN

1) **ONSET EXTREMELY VARIABLE**
   usually sudden

2) **RAPIDLY DEVELOPING RENAL FAILURE**
   course of disease spans 1 or 2 weeks
   fatal uremia

The above describes the typical case of an idiopathic nephrotoxic GN called "rapidly progressive GN." Variations of this may be seen when nephrotoxic GN occurs as part of another syndrome

---

18-9. PATHOGENESIS OF NEPHROTOXIC GN

1) **THE BODY BECOMES SENSITIZED TO CERTAIN GBM ANTIGENS**
   mechanism is essentially unknown: may be multiple

2) **ANTI GBM ANTIBODIES ARE PRODUCED AND REACT WITH STATIONARY GBM ANTIGENS**
   complement is fixed
   inflammation results

3) **GN IS RELENTLESSLY PROGRESSIVE BECAUSE OF AUTOIMMUNE ETIOLOGY**
   both antigens and antibodies are produced within same body

---

(end-stage kidney). Such a kidney fails completely (renal shut-down) and the patient begins to manifest the effects of metabolic waste intoxication (uremia). See Illustration 18-11 for a summary of the clinical course of nephrotoxic GN.

<table>
<tr><td>

18-12. OTHER FORMS OF GLOMERULO-
NEPHRITIS

</td></tr>
</table>

In addition to immune complex and nephrotoxic GN 2 other types are usually distinguished:

IMMUNOLOGIC GN OF UNDETERMINED
PATHOGENESIS
    glomerular amyloidosis
    diabetic glomerulosclerosis

NON-IMMUNOLOGIC GN
    minimal-lesion GN
    (also called minimal change GN or
    lipoid nephrosis)

RENAL FUNCTION IN GLOMERULAR DISEASE

LEARNING OBJECTIVE

**To be able to compare and contrast the
following 4 renal syndromes and describe their
association with each of the forms of
glomerulonephritis presented in the preceding
objective:**
  a) **mild proteinuria and hematuria with
      some nausea, fever and malaise**
  b) **the nephrotic syndrome**
  c) **uremia**
  d) **renal sclerosis with anuria (end-stage
      kidney)**

3. Other Forms of Glomerulonephritis

The 2 remaining categories of GN are listed
in Illustration 18-12. Neither can be classified
with certainty as regards their pathogenetic
mechanism. The latter of these (minimal-lesion
GN) is the primary cause of the nephrotic
syndrome in children. Neither will be discussed
here.

Additional Reading

Dixon, F. J. Virus-induced, immune-complex-type
    glomerulonephritis. Transplant. Proc. 1:945, 1969
Fish, A. J. et al. Immunologic mechanisms of
    glomerular injury. The Kidney 3:1, 1970
Koffler, D. et al. Systemic lupus erythematosus
    prototype of immune-complex nephritis in man. J.
    Exp. Med. 134:169, 1971
Lewis, E. J. et al. An immunopathologic study of
    rapidly progressive glomerulonephritis in the adult.
    Human Path. 2:185, 1971
Mostofi, F. K. Patterns of glomerular reaction to
    injury. Human Path. 2:233, 1971
Proskey, A. J. et al. Goodpasture's syndrome: A
    report of five cases and a review of the literature.
    Am J. Med. 48:162, 1970

In acute glomerulonephritis, the clinical
effects of glomerular damage are related more
to its severity than its cause. Also, the severity
of glomerular damage does not always correspond to the degree of morphologic change. All
degrees of glomerular damage lead to the loss of
protein in the urine (proteinuria). In most
instances, erythrocytes will also pass the damaged glomerular filter and hematuria (gross or
at least microscopic) will be detectable.

1. The Nephrotic Syndrome

The most severe form of glomerular damage
gives rise to the clinical picture of the *nephrotic
syndrome* (Illustration 18-14). Ironically one of
the most common causes of the nephrotic
syndrome is "minimal lesion" GN, an observation that underscores the lack of reliable
correlation between functional and morphologic changes in early acute glomerulonephritis.

The nephrotic syndrome is seen more frequently in children than adults and is often
fatal. Although the very common post-streptococcal GN is known to cause the nephrotic
syndrome in some cases, when one considers its
high incidence among young people this association is rather rare.

2. Renal Sclerosis and the "End-Stage" Kidney

We have seen that most forms of acute
glomerulonephritis, even the relatively innocu-

18-13. RELATIONSHIP BETWEEN ACUTE AND CHRONIC GN

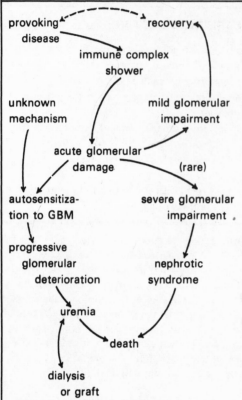

18-14. THE NEPHROTIC SYNDROME

1) MASSIVE PROTEINURIA
   4 gm or more per day

2) HYPOALBUMINEMIA

3) SEVERE EDEMA
   called anasarca
   related to decreased osmotic value
   of serum

4) HYPERLIPIDEMIA
   unknown etiology

18-15. UREMIA

1) COMPLEX RESULT OF METABOLIC WASTE RETENTION: UREA IS CONVENIENT MARKER

2) POLYURIA: PROTEINURIA
   inability to concentrate
   urine   stabilizes   at   s.g.   1.010
   acidosis

ous post-streptococcal kind, can lead to a chronic, progressive form and ultimately to complete renal sclerosis (Illustration 18-14). This is a comparatively rare outcome, except in clear-cut cases of nephrotoxic GN where the course of the disease is sometimes alarmingly short.

The widespread glomerular sclerosis resulting from chronic glomerulonephritis causes irreversible circulatory changes within the kidney and progressive fibrosis of glomeruli tubules and interstitial tissue. The over-all result is an extremely small shrunken, sclerotic kidney called the "end-stage" kidney. Since the end-stage kidney is not functional the patient will suffer from the accumulation of metabolic wastes (uremia), unless regular dialysis is instituted or a grafted kidney is provided.

Additional Reading

Berman, L. The patient who makes no urine. GP XXXVI:106, 1967

Early, L. E. et al. Nephrotic syndrome. Calif. Med. 115:23, 1971

Hamby, W. M. Renal regulation of sodium excretion. Med. Clin. N. Amer. 55:1509, 1971

Hand, W. L. et al. Immunoglobulin synthesis in lower urinary tract infection. J. Lab. Clin. Med. 75:19, 1970

Hulme, B. and Hardwicke, J. Human glomerular permeability to macromolecules in health and disease. Clin. Sci. 34:515, 1968

OBSTRUCTIVE NEPHROPATHY AND PYELONEPHRITIS

LEARNING OBJECTIVE

To be able to discuss the results of obstruction of the urinary outflow tract mentioning the following:
  a) hydronephrosis
  b) acute pyelonephritis (as compared with acute glomerulonephritis)
  c) chronic pyelonephritis (compared with chronic glomerulonephritis)

Simple obstruction of the urinary outflow tract can result in the accumulation of fluid under pressure in the renal pelvis and ureter. This alone is enough to cause severe atrophy of kidney parenchyma, a condition called *hydronephrosis*. See Illustration 18-16. In childhood, the causes of urinary obstruction are nearly always some kind of congenital malformation of the outflow tract. These are commonly found affecting the ureters or ureterocystic junction. In middle age and beyond, the possibilities for obstruction are legion (Illustration 18-17).

Although obstruction alone may destroy a kidney, it is additionally hazardous in that it predisposes the urinary tract to infection. Ordinarily the urinary tract is sterile except for the distal urethra. This is due in no small part to the flushing action of urine passage. When an

---

18-16. HYDRONEPHROSIS

1) OBSTRUCTION OF OUTFLOW TRACT CAUSES ACCUMULATION OF URINE UNDER PRESSURE

2) ABNORMAL PRESSURE RESULTS IN PROFOUND ATROPHY OF RENAL PARENCHYMA

3) ALSO CONSTITUTES SERIOUS PREDISPOSITION TO INFECTION OF URINARY TRACT

18-17. URINARY TRACT OBSTRUCTION IN THE ADULT

1) RENAL OR URETERAL SCAR

2) CALCULI (STONES)

3) TUMORS

4) PREGNANCY

5) PROSTATIC HYPERTROPHY

6) URETHRAL STRICTURE

18-18. PYELONEPHRITIS

1) AN INFECTION OF RENAL PARENCHYMA SECONDARY TO AN ASCENDING (RETROGRADE) INFECTION OF THE URINARY OUTFLOW TRACT
2) ACUTE FORM IS EXTREMELY COMMON, PARTICULARLY IN WOMEN
   second only to respiratory infections in over-all incidence, *E. coli* is most common causative organism
3) CHRONIC FORM MAY LEAD TO END-STAGE KIDNEY
   almost indistinguishable from that resulting from chronic glomerulonephritis

---

obstruction such as a stone or prostatic hyperplasia slows the rate at which urine can be voided and creates irregularities in the urothelial surface, bacteria normally found only in the distal urethra can spread up the urinary tract to involve higher structures. Owing to its local abundance and motility, *Escherichia coli* is the most common cause of such "ascending" urinary tract infections. Ascending infections ultimately reach the renal pelvis from where they spread into the parenchyma. An infection of the kidney that develops in this way is called *pyelonephritis*. The prefix, *pyelo* (pelvis), suggests that all such infections are of the ascending type. In practice, this same word is used in reference to interstitial infections regardless of the route by which they reach the kidney (Illustration 18-18).

Chronic pyelonephritis is often encountered as the predicatble outcome of repeated or persistent acute infections, but many cases of the chronic form of this disease are found without such a history. In the latter cases, the disease seems to begin as a smouldering chronic infection. Chronic pyelonephritis causes progressive fibrosis of the entire kidney and leads to a shrunken, non-functional, "end-stage" kidney, indistinguishable from that caused by chronic glomerulonephritis. The functional impairment is comparable and uremia is the inevitable result.

RENAL VASCULAR DISEASE

LEARNING OBJECTIVE

To review information presented in Chapter 12 regarding embolic disease and be able to discuss renal embolism. Also, to be able to compare and contrast benign nephrosclerosis and malignant nephrosclerosis as examples of renal vascular disease, including the following:

  a) mechanism of the renal regulation of bloodpressure
  b) clinical course of benign and malignant nephrosclerosis
  c) ultimate effect on longstanding benign nephrosclerosis of the kidney

Most kidney disease is attributable to 1 of 3 causes, glomerulonephritis, pyelonephritis or renal vascular disease. Of the last, the most important is benign nephrosclerosis (Illustration 18-19).

18-19. RENAL VASCULAR DISEASE

1) BENIGN NEPHROSCLEROSIS
  idiopathic
  leads to restricted renal blood flow
  associated with hypertension
  rarely progresses to severe functional impairment but a small number go on to end-stage kidney

2) MALIGNANT NEPHROSCLEROSIS

3) RENAL EMBOLISM

18-20. RENAL REGULATION OF SYSTEMIC BLOODPRESSURE

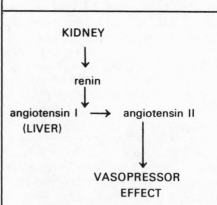

1. Benign Nephrosclerosis

Benign nephrosclerosis is a disease of unknown etiology that is detected as hyaline changes in the walls of small and medium sized renal arteries. The effect is to restrict bloodflow through these vessels and hence through the kidney as a whole.

Any interference with bloodflow through the kidney is always accompanied by an elevation of systemic bloodpressure (Illustration 18-20). In the pathogenesis of this disease, authorities are unsure as to whether renal changes cause the hypertension or the latter is responsbile for vascular changes. Whatever the relationship, benign nephrosclerosis is thought to account for about 10 per cent of all cases of hypertension.

2. Malignant Nephrosclerosis

Malignant nephrosclerosis is the term used to refer to kidney lesions associated with the clinical syndrome of *malignant hypertension.* Malignant hypertension is characterized by a relentless rise in bloodpressure leading ultimately to death by some complication, usually a cerebrovascular accident.

The most consistent and pathognomonic lesion in the kidney of an individual dying of malignant hypertension is fibrinoid necrosis of the walls of arterioles; it is not known whether the hypertension is the cause or effect of the lesion. Malignant nephrosclerosis may be seen in a formerly normotensive individual or it may be seen superimposed on a condition of benign nephrosclerosis.

3. Renal Embolism

Because the kidneys receive about 25 per cent of the cardiac output at rest and process this blood through the extremely complex glomerular capillaries, they are very susceptible to embolic disease. Emboli arising in the left heart show a pronounced tendency to lodge in the kidneys. The most important of these are the bacterial vegetations of subacute endocarditis and thrombi breaking loose from either the heart wall or the surface of the aorta.

Small septic emboli cause focal suppurative glomerulitis, whereas larger emboli obstruct major blood channels causing infarction. Since the kidney is supplied by a single arterial system, infarcts are ischemic. The infarcted area is rapidly cleared and replaced with scar, leaving a white contricted nodular or depressed area in the kidney parenchyma.

RENAL TUBULAR DISEASE

LEARNING OBJECTIVE

To be able to outline the subject of renal tubular disease and develop a comparison between acute tubular necrosis and toxic (mercuric) nephrosis as examples. Mention the following:
   a) cause and pathogenesis
   b) association with shock (where applicable)
   c) sequellae

All kidney disease originating in the tubular system is called *nephrosis.* This use of the term bears no relationship to the modern day meaning of the term "nephrotic syndrome," which, of course, is a clinical phenomenon seen in some forms of acute glomerulonephritis.

Tubular disease occurs in many varieties; however, we will take this opportunity to mention only 3 (Illustration 18-21).

1. Acute Tubular Necrosis

Acute tubular necrosis is a pattern of tubular cell degeneration resulting from a number of different kinds of injury. The common thread in all these injuries appears to be renal tubular ischemia. The tubules receive their vascular

---

18-21. RENAL TUBULAR DISEASE

1) ACUTE TUBULAR NECROSIS
   necrosis of tubular epithelium secondary to tubular ischemia

2) TOXIC NEPHROSIS
   tubular epithelium is damaged by poison or toxin: commonly caused by Hg^{++}

3) METABOLIC NEPHROSIS
   function of tubular epithelium is impaired by metabolic derangement (Fanconi's syndrome)

supply from efferent glomerular vessels. This means that blood must pass first through the glomerular capillary tuft before it reaches the tubules of that same nephron. Anything that interferes with bloodflow is liable to result in acute tubular necrosis.

The most common cause of acute tubular necrosis is shock. Since tubular cells regenerate readily, part of the treatment of protracted shock must be directed toward compensating for the acute renal failure that will result from tubular necrosis.

2. Toxic Nephrosis (Mercuric)

The mercuric ion is a highly corrosive protein precipitant often used as an agent of suicide. It causes severe irritation wherever it comes in contact with tissue, but principally in the stomach where it is absorbed and in the renal tubules and colon, where it is excreted. Tubular epithelial necrosis is particularly pronounced, leading to early diuresis, dehydration, shock, and possible death. If the patient survives, tubular epithelium regenerates and the condition resolves without residual effects.

3. Metabolic Nephrosis

A variety of metabolic disorders lead to impairment of the activity of the highly differentiated proximal renal tubular epithelial cells. Dysfunction of this particular segment of the renal tubule leads to a syndrome characterized by glucosuria, generalized aminoaciduria, phosphaturia and renal tubular acidosis (Fanconi's syndrome). Among diseases commonly causative of Franconi's syndrome are cystinosis, multiple myeloma, certain forms of drug toxicity, and, of course, the destruction of these cells by mercury poisoning as outlined above.

NEOPLASMS OF THE URINARY SYSTEM

LEARNING OBJECTIVE

To be able to discuss neoplasms of the urinary system comparing the renal cell carcinoma, Wilms' tumor and carcinoma of the bladder as examples. Mention the following:
  a) **relative incidence and age distribution**
  b) **cell of origin and distinguishing features of each tumor**
  c) **prognosis**

Like any complex group of tissues, the urinary system can give rise to a number of different benign and malignant tumors; none are unusually common. Three tumors primary to the urinary tract that are most significant in a comparative sense are those listed in Illustration 18-22.

1. Renal Cell Carcinoma

Renal cell carcinoma is a malignant tumor of renal tubular origin. Even though it accounts for only a fraction of a percentage of all cancer deaths in the United States, it is the most common malignant tumor of the kidney and occurs with only slightly less frequency than all cancer of the lower urinary tract.

Characteristic of this tumor is extreme variability of behavior. When intercepted late in its clinical course, it has often invaded the renal vein, a complication that drastically reduces the possibility of cure.

Although a single tumor may be made up of a variety of different-appearing cells, the most strikingly pathognomonic is the clear cell. In its natural state, this cell is filled with lipid-containing vacuoles, which in section are clear and vacant. Because of the prominence of these lipid-ladened cells, this tumor was once thought to originate from adrenal cells trapped in the kidney. This theory, no longer generally accepted, gave rise to the term *hypernephroma,* which is still used with great frequency.

2. Wilms' Tumor

Wilms' tumor is an embryonal tumor of renal origin (nephroblastoma), which ranks second

18-22. PRINCIPAL NEOPLASMS OF THE URINARY SYSTEM

1) RENAL CELL CARCINOMA

2) WILMS' TUMOR

3) CARCINOMA OF THE BLADDER

only to medulloblastoma and neuroblastoma in frequency among children under the age of 1. Even so, it occurs at a rate of only about 1 per 100,000 population per year.

The typical Wilms' tumor consists of at least 2 very different kinds of tumor cells and on that basis was once called an adenosarcoma or carcinosarcoma. It tends to be aggressive, but in recent years therapy has improved to the point where recovery is common.

3. Carcinoma of the Bladder

Carcinoma of the bladder is a malignant tumor of urothelium (almost 90 per cent are transitional cell carcinomas) that is usually seen in older men and causes about 4 per cent of all cancer deaths. It is known to be associated with industrial carcinogens (particularly β-napthylamine), heavy cigarette smoking and infestation with *Schistosoma hematobium,* a parasite common in the Far East.

Survival rates vary with the anaplasticity of the tumor cell and the degree of contiguous spread and metastases at the time of interception.

Additional Reading

Skinner, D. G. et al. Renal cell carcinoma. Am. Fam. Phys. 4:89, 1971
Black, W. C. and Ragsdale, E. F. Wilms' tumor. Am. J. Roent., Rad. Ther. Nuc. Med. CIII:53, 1968
Hurlburt, W. B. Carcinoma of the bladder. Am. Fam. Phys. 2:109, 1970
Cole, P. et al. Smoking and cancer of the lower urinary tract. N. Engl. J. Med. 284:129, 1971

chapter 19
LIVER, PANCREAS AND THE DIGESTIVE TRACT

HEPATITIS

LEARNING OBJECTIVE

To be able to compare and contrast infectious and serum hepatitis mentioning the following:
- a) modes of transmission
- b) epidemiology and clinical picture of both forms
- c) the Australia antigen as it relates to both
- d) complications and residual effects of hepatitis

Hepatitis is an infectious disease which is generalized in its distribution within the body, but has its primary and most conspicuous effect on the liver; it is now known to be caused by at least 2 different viruses (Illustration 19-1). Infection with a hepatitis virus can result in a range of effects from massive liver destruction and death to mild, subclinical discomfort. The clinical course of an infection in any single case will depend upon many poorly defined factors, among which are the age and defense status of the host. In the relatively brief time since World War II, hepatitis has become increasingly important as a public health problem, not only domestically but throughout the world. The origin of hepatitis, like that of other exclusively human infections, is lost in antiquity, but its first description is thought to have been recorded some 2,000 years ago by Hippocrates. Since that time, there have been numerous epidemics, many of which have been associated with wars.

1. Infectious Hepatitis and Serum Hepatitis

Hepatitis is seen as 2 clinical syndromes, *infectious hepatitis* and *serum hepatitis* (Illustration 19-2). Infectious hepatitis (Illustration 19-3) is the form that results when the virus is transmitted via the fecal-oral route. It begins as an infection of the gastrointestinal tract and

---

19-1. HEPATITIS

1) SYSTEMIC VIRAL DISEASE
   principal damage to liver

2) SINGLE-HOST HUMAN PATHOGEN(S)
   no known animal reservoir

3) WORLDWIDE DISTRIBUTION

4) AT LEAST 2 ANTIGENICALLY DIFFERENT AGENTS CAUSE 2 CLINICAL FORMS OF THE DISEASE
   IH: Virus A (fecal-oral transmission)
   SH: Virus B* (parenteral and oral transmission)

   * Virus B is associated with and perhaps identical to "Australia Antigen"

19-2. INFECTIOUS HEPATITIS

1) FAR MORE COMMON THAN SH

2) FECAL-ORAL TRANSMISSION
   a disease of filth and poor sanitation
   spreads readily in areas of dense population
   often epidemic
   begins as intestinal infection

3) CAUSED BY (PERHAPS) 2 ANTIGENICALLY DIFFERENT AGENTS

19-3. SERUM HEPATITIS

1) PARENTERAL TRANSMISSION (DI-RECT INOCULATION) *USUALLY*
    transfusion
    vaccination
    tattoo
    injection
    taking of blood samples
    drug addiction

2) CAUSED BY (PERHAPS) 2 ANTIGENI-CALLY DIFFERENT AGENTS
    Australia antigen is found in most cases (in acute phase)

19-4. CLINICAL COURSE OF VIRAL HEPATITIS

1) HISTORY OF EXPOSURE
    IH: contact with active case or carrier
    SH: inoculation

2) INCUBATION PERIOD (approximate)
    IH: 37 days (abrupt onset)
    SH: 55 days (insidious onset)

3) ACUTE PHASE
    (comparable in IH and SH)
    weakness
    prostration
    lymphadenopathy
    splenomegaly
    jaundice (in most clinically apparent cases)
    pronounced anorexia

4) RESOLUTION
    6 to 8 weeks: adult
    1 to 3 weeks: child

Cases of SH tend to be more protracted

goes on to cause varying degrees of liver damage, ranging from massive necrosis (acute yellow atrophy of the liver) to mild, diffuse cord cell destruction. Infectious hepatitis can be epidemic and is often spread by contaminated drinking water or food, particularly shellfish collected at sites where contaminated rivers flow into the ocean. Conditions favoring the rapid spread of infectious hepatitis are found in institutions and army camps where people are obliged to live in compact quarters.

Serum hepatitis (Illustration 19-3) is the form that results when the virus is acquired by the parenteral route. It most often occurs as the result of blood transfusion, vaccination, tattooing, injection, the taking of blood samples or the practices of drug addiction. It is said to cause a higher number of fatalities than infectious hepatitis, although this feature is highly suspect since serum hepatitis is often contracted by patients suffering from some other disease.

The clinical course of hepatitis (Illustration 19-4) depends to some extent upon whether it was transmitted via the fecal-oral route and shows up as infectious hepatitis or by the parenteral route and is seen as serum hepatitis. In the latter, the median incubation time is somewhat longer (55 days as compared to 37 days in IH). Also, the carrier state is more persistent in SH, sometimes lasting for a number of years, whereas patients recovering from IH may become non-infectious within a year or less.

Aside from the incubation period and carrier state persistence, both forms of the disease are roughly comparable as outlined in Illustration 19-4. The actual amount of time required for resolution of the acute phase varies with the age of the patient. Fulminating cases (acute yellow atrophy of the liver), which are rare in the healthy subject, may prove fatal in as little as 10 days or up to 8 weeks. Immune-complex renal disease may develop as a result of the abundance of immunologic activity, but protection against recurrence is not certain. This is probably due to the limited immunologic identity between agents causing this disease.

Although most cases undergo resolution without residuum, some give rise to chronic hepatitis which, when not directly fatal, may lead to cirrhosis, a condition which will be discussed later.

2. Australia Antigen

Australia antigen [abbreviated Au(1)] and sometimes called hepatitis-associated antigen (HAA) is a virus or virus antigen associated with, and almost certainly one of the etiologic agents of, hepatitis in humans. Its peculiar designation derives from its having been first detected in the serum of an Australian aborigine (Illustration 19-5).

Among the general population of the United States, the frequency of serum-borne Au(1) is something like 0.1 per cent. However, it is detectable in nearly 50 per cent of patients with *acute* viral hepatitis. It is not associated with other kinds of liver disease and disappears from hepatitis serum (in most cases) when the acute phase of the disease passes.

In a few kinds of patients, Au(1) persists in the serum even after the acute phase of hepatitis is over. The foremost example of this type of patient is the child with Down's syndrome. Infection with Au(1) in Down's syndrome leads to a chronic, anicteric hepatitis that persists for many years. In addition to Down's syndrome, it seems that other disorders (leukemia lepromatous leprosy, and the need for dialysis) predispose to chronic Au(1) infection. The common feature in all of these cases is thought to be immunologic deficiency, particularly that of the cellular immune system.

Turning our attention back to the acute stage, you will remember that only 50 per cent of patients with acute hepatitis show Au(1) in their serum. The others have a similar disease, but no corresponding bloodborne antigen. This suggests that there are at least 2 viral agents capable of producing hepatitis, but that only 1 carries (or is) Australia antigen. With regard to clinical manifestations, the length of the incubation period and the possibility for fatal outcome, there appears to be some difference between the disease associated with Au(1) and that in which it is absent. Thus the older concepts of infectious versus serum hepatitis appear to be breaking down and may even be misleading. Either agent can be transmitted by either means and the nature of the disease will be determined by whether or not the virus is introduced directly into the bloodstream (SH) or begins its infection as a disease of the gastrointestinal tract (IH).

Additional Reading

McCollum, R. W. The natural history of hepatitis. Bull. N.Y. Acad. Sci. 45:127, 1969

Mosely, J. W. Viral hepatitis: A group of epidemiologic entities. Canad. Med. Assn. J. 106:427, 1972

Moseley, J. W. and Kendrick, M. A. Hepatitis as a world problem. Bull. N.Y. Acad. Sci. 45:143, 1969

Shulman, N. R. Hepatitis-associated antigen. Am. J. Med. 49:669, 1970

Widmann, F. K. The Australia antigen: Where do we stand? Postgrad. Med. 50:167 and 51:130 (two parts) 1971 and 1972

19-5. THE AUSTRALIA ANTIGEN (HEPATITIS-ASSOCIATED ANTIGEN)

1) A VIRUS ANTIGEN FIRST NOTED IN THE SERUM OF THE AUSTRALIAN ABORIGINE

2) FOUND IN SERUM OF 50 PER CENT OF PATIENTS IN *ACUTE* STAGE OF VIRAL HEPATITIS

3) MORE CLEARLY ASSOCIATED WITH SERUM HEPATITIS

CIRRHOSIS

LEARNING OBJECTIVE

To be able to discuss cirrhosis and its complications including the cause, pathogenesis, hepatic changes and clinical course of the following:

    a) portal cirrhosis and its relationship to alcohol abuse

    b) postnecrotic cirrhosis

    c) biliary cirrhosis

    d) portal hypertension

Cirrhosis is a condition in which fibrous scar is formed throughout the liver, partitioning its cells into mutually isolated groups or nodules. It always results in some disruption of the normal lobular architecture and may interfere with intrahepatic blood circulation. In far advanced cases, it causes gradual failure of liver function. The incidence of this disease has increased significantly since World War II, establishing cirrhosis as one of the most prominent causes of death in the adult male. This is due in part to a corresponding increase in the incidence of hepatitis, but more significantly to an enormous increase in the abuse of alcohol. *Alcoholism is the single most important cause of cirrhosis today* (Illustration 19-6).

Cirrhosis occurs in several characteristic patterns, the specifications of which will be determined by its cause and pathogenesis. We will examine only the most prominent of these (Illustration 19-7).

1. Portal Cirrhosis

Portal cirrhosis (Laennec's cirrhosis) is a particular pattern of cirrhosis caused by the abuse of alcoholic beverages. A similar pattern is seen in severe protein deprivation (kwashiorkor) and so portal cirrhosis is also called nutritional cirrhosis or fatty nutritional cirrhosis (Illustration 19-8).

The exact relationship between alcohol abuse and portal cirrhosis is not known, but *there is no doubt about a clear and unmistakable*

19-7. PRINCIPAL PATTERNS OF CIRRHOSIS

1) PORTAL CIRRHOSIS
 alcohol abuse or severe protein deficiency
 fine nodules
 portal hypertension
 some predisposition to hepatoma

2) POSTNECROTIC CIRRHOSIS
 hepatitis or hepatotoxic drugs
 coarse nodules
 portal hypertension plus predisposition to malignancy

3) BILIARY CIRRHOSIS
 obstruction of biliary outflow tract
 fine nodules
 portal hypertension rare

Other, less common patterns are seen but will not be discussed

---

19-6. CIRRHOSIS

The diffuse formation of fibrous repair tissue (scar) within liver parenchyma

1) CAUSES (APPROXIMATE DISTRIBUTION)
 alcohol abuse: 50 per cent
 liver necrosis (hepatitis, drugs): 20 per cent
 biliary obstruction: 20 per cent
 other: 10 per cent

2) EFFECTS
 hepatic deficiency in far advanced stages
 portal hypertension
 predisposition to liver malignancy

19-8. PORTAL CIRRHOSIS

1) MOST COMMON PATTERN OF CIRRHOSIS

2) PRINCIPAL PATHOGENESIS
 alcohol abuse with fatty degeneration
 diffuse necrosis and regeneration
 fine nodular cirrhosis

3) ALSO SEEN IN SEVERE PROTEIN DEFICIENCY

4) LIVER FAILURE AND PORTAL HYPERTENSION ARE USUAL OUTCOME

association between excessive alcohol intake and portal cirrhosis. The first change in the liver caused by alcohol is the gradual accumulation of fat within hepatic parenchymal cells. There is still a great deal of discussion of the matter, but most authorities now agree that *ethanol (beverage alcohol) exerts a direct toxic effect on the liver cell.* The fat that accumulates does so either as a protective reaction to the overloading of the liver cell with an easily oxidized substrate (ethanol) or because the function of the liver cell is so impaired that it is no longer able to effect the normal transport of this fat to the lipid storage tissue. In addition, however, there is always the possibility that the person who consumes excessive amounts of alcoholic beverages is neglecting his diet and failing to take in enough protein to provide a sufficient quantity of lipotropic agents (choline and methionine) that are needed for the proper transport of fat. A dietary insult may complicate the condition, but the principal cause of liver damage in alcoholic liver degeneration is now thought to be the direct toxic effect of the ethanol on the hepatocyte.

Uncomplicated fatty degeneration of the liver as might be seen in early alcoholism, is reversible and very few cases of this relatively benign condition ever go on to cirrhosis. Grossly the liver is enlarged, fragile and greasy-appearing and may be functionally deficient because of the encumbering effect of the large mass of lipid.

In those instances where the habit of alcohol ingestion persists and particularly where it becomes more and more severe, something (it is not known for sure what does it) may occur to tip the whole process in favor of widespread hepatic scar formation. Even with the onset of mild cirrhosis, however, there is agreement that abstinence from alcohol would arrest the progress of the disease. But, again, in those cases where the habit persists and worsens, the cirrhosis becomes more and more severe leading ultimately to portal hypertension, hepatic parenchymal deficiency and death. The actual cause of death will usually be acute liver failure or massive hemorrhage from a ruptured esophageal varix (to be discussed later under the effects of portal hypertension).

In far advanced cases, thick fibrous bands will have formed at the periphery of many lobules partitioning the parenchyma into fine nodules. These nodules may enlarge somewhat due to regenerative activity as the liver attempts to replace damaged cells. One of the hallmarks of advanced portal cirrhosis is that the substance of the liver appears to consist of tightly packed nests of degenerating and regenerating liver cells encased in thick fibrous capsules. On this basis the condition is often called "fine nodular cirrhosis." In its final stages, the liver is shrunken, hard and almost devoid of normal parenchyma.

2. Postnecrotic Cirrhosis

Any condition, such as viral hepatitis or the direct damaging effect of poisons such as chloroform or carbon tetrachloride that cause massive, indiscriminate destruction of liver parenchymal cells, can lead to a kind of cirrhosis known as *postnecrotic cirrhosis.* The pattern of this kind of cirrhosis is dependent upon the distribution of the antecedent necrosis and is usually not regular in either size or distribution (Illustration 19-9).

The gross picture of postnecrotic cirrhosis is one of large and small degenerative nodules surrounded and partitioned by scar and interspersed with normal hepatic parenchyma. Progressive liver deterioration leading to death from hepatic insufficiency may occur, if liver destruction continues. Hemorrhage from a ruptured esophageal varix is also a hazard.

A peculiar feature of postnecrotic cirrhosis is that it appears to predispose the patient to the occurrence of a primary malignant neoplasm of the liver. This is seen to a somewhat less degree in portal cirrhosis also.

19-9. POSTNECROTIC CIRRHOSIS

---

1) PATHOGENESIS
    liver destruction (hepatitis or hepatotoxins)
    patchy necrosis and regeneration
    large nodular cirrhosis

2) LIVER FAILURE AND PORTAL HYPERTENSION ARE USUAL OUTCOME

3) PREDISPOSITION TO HEPATIC MALIGNANCY

19-10. BILIARY CIRRHOSIS

---

1) PATHOGENESIS
   biliary obstruction (stone or stricture)

   diffuse necrosis—bile staining of
   liver

   fine nodular cirrhosis

2) PORTAL HYPERTENSION IS RARE
   malabsorption (mild) steatorrhea
   and early jaundice result from
   obstruction

---

of the portal system is dependent upon free flow through the liver, anything that distorts liver parenchyma will obstruct portal blood flow.

Pressure in the portal system is normally very low when compared to that of the systemic circulation. With any degree of obstruction, this pressure rises significantly, causing a number of very characteristic clinical signs that are conveniently studied as the syndrome of *portal hypertension* (Illustration 19-11).

Portal hypertension is one of the most frequent complications of cirrhosis, particularly portal cirrhosis. Conversely, although other things may cause portal hypertension, portal cirrhosis is its most common antecedent condition.

The signs of portal hypertension are quite characteristic. The most hazardous of these changes is the occurrence of esophageal varices in which veins coursing just beneath the epithelial surface of the esophagus dilate and

3. Biliary Cirrhosis

Liver cell destruction that begins around the bile ducts gives rise to a pattern of cirrhosis known as biliary cirrhosis (Illustration 19-10). The most common cause of biliary cirrhosis is posthepatic biliary obstruction. Stasis of bile causes its accumulation within the hepatic substance and the deterioration of parenchymal cells. Fibrous bands begin forming around the periphery of the lobule as in the case of portal cirrhosis, but rarely do these bands transect a lobule as in the portal pattern. Jaundice is always an early and prominent part of this syndrome, as is malabsorption and steatorrhea (see Chapter 11). Portal hypertension is uncommon.

4. Portal Hypertension

The portal system is the only large venous network that begins and ends with capillary-size blood vessels; it starts as the venous side of the splanchnic capillary bed and terminates as the hepatic sinusoids. Whereas most other venous pathways grow succeedingly larger as they approach the heart, the portal pathway grows abruptly smaller and more ramified, because of its need to traverse the liver. Since the patency

---

19-11. PORTAL HYPERTENSION

**1) OBSTRUCTION OF PORTAL VENOUS
   SYSTEM RAISES PORTAL PRESSURE**
   distortion of hepatic parenchyma
   (gradual onset)

   ————————

   thrombosis of portal vein (sudden
   onset)

**2) COLLATERAL VENOUS ROUTES BE-
   COME DISTENDED**
   esophageal varices

   ————————

   hemorrhoidal varices

   ————————

   congestive splenomegaly

**3) EXTREME DANGER OF RUPTURED
   ESOPHAGEAL VARIX AND FATAL
   HEMORRHAGE**

---

protrude into the esophageal lumen. With rising pressure, these varices often rupture leading to massive hemorrhage into the stomach, and subsequent hematemesis. Ruptured esophageal varices are the second most common cause of death in patients with advanced cirrhosis, exceeded only by hepatic failure.

Additional Reading

Brick, I. B. and Palmer, E. D. One thousand cases of portal cirrhosis of the liver. Arch. Int. Med. 113:501, 1964

Bebee, G. W. and Simon, H. Cirrhosis of the liver following viral hepatitis, a twenty-year mortality follow-up. Am. J. Epidemiol. 92:279, 1970

Dykes, M. H. M. et al. Halothane and the liver: A review of the epidemiologic, immunologic and metabolic aspects of the relationship. Canad. J. Surg. 15:1, 1972

Lieber, C. S. and Rubin, E. Alcoholic fatty liver. N. Engl. J. Med. 280:705, 1969

Lombardi, B. Effects of choline deficiency on rat hepatocytes. Fed. Prac. 30:139, 1971

19-12. NEOPLASMS OF THE LIVER (MALIGNANT)

1) PRIMARY
   hepatoma
   cholangiocarcinoma

2) METASTATIC
   liver is most common site of metastatic tumor growth (except nodes in region of primary tumor)

This is particularly true of malignancies of the gastrointestinal tract, but many others (pancreas, breast and lung) also show this tendency.

Additional Reading

Misugi, K. et al. Classification of primary malignant tumors of the liver in infancy and childhood. Cancer 20:1760, 1967

NEOPLASMS OF THE LIVER

LEARNING OBJECTIVE

To be able to discuss malignant tumors both primary and metastatic to the liver, mentioning the following:
   a) **the hepatoma and cholangiocarcinoma**
   b) **primary site of tumors that show the highest incidence of liver metastases**

Neoplasms primary to the liver are quite rare, except in those areas in which parasitic infestation of the biliary tract serves as a predisposing factor. In the United States, most malignant tumors arising in the liver are seen in association with cirrhosis.

Malignant tumors primary to the liver arise from either parenchymal cells or bile duct epithilium. The former is known as hepatoma or hepatocarcinoma whereas the latter is called cholangiocarcinoma (Illustration 19-12). Both have rather poor prognoses.

The most common tumor of the liver is a malignant neoplasm metastatic from some other site. In over 50 per cent of cancer deaths, some metastatasis to the liver can be detected.

JAUNDICE (ICTERUS)

LEARNING OBJECTIVE

To be able to discuss jaundice as a sign of disease emphasizing the following:
   a) **normal process of bilirubin excretion**
   b) **hemolytic jaundice**
   c) **hepatocellular jaundice**
   d) **cholestatic jaundice**
   e) **congenital abnormality of bilirubin metabolism**

Jaundice or icterus is the condition in which tissues throughout the body become discolored by the abnormal accumulation of bile pigment. This same bile pigment (bilirubin) accumulates in the serum and hence an associated sign is hyperbilirubinemia. Four general types of jaundice are recognized (Illustration 19-13).

Bile pigment is the excretory product of the heme portion of the hemoglobin molecule. In normal body function, the molecule is broken down and eliminated as shown in Illustration 19-14. The 4 types of jaundice listed in Illustration 19-13 are actually 4 different causes for the failure of the bilirubin elimination process.

Bilirubin that has not been conjugated to gluconurate is detected as "indirect reacting bilirubin" using the Van den Bergh reaction (Illustration 19-15), while that which has been conjugated is manifested as "direct reacting bilirubin" (Illustration 19-16).

1. Hemolytic Jaundice

Hemolytic jaundice results when the rate of breakdown of red blood cells exceeds the rate at which a normal liver can process bilirubin for excretion. Processing by the liver includes the conjugation of bilirubin to the glucuronate ion, a step that renders it more soluble and easily excreted. When erythrocytes are destroyed too rapidly, such as might occur in a hemolytic

---

19-13. JAUNDICE (ICTERUS)

1) HEMOLYTIC
   erythrocytes are destroyed at too rapid a rate for normal liver to process bilirubin

2) HEPATOCELLULAR
   liver damage prevents processing of bilirubin even with normal rate of erythrocyte turnover

3) CHOLESTATIC
   biliary obstruction of drug-induced failure of bile ejection prevents bilirubin excretion

4) CONGENITAL ABNORMALITIES OF BILIRUBIN METABOLISM
   transient or permanent deficiency of liver enzyme necessary for bilirubin excretion

---

19-14. ELIMINATION OF BILIRUBIN

PHAGOCYTE — RBC → IRON
transported to marrow

PORPHYRIN CONVERTED TO
BILIRUBIN-PROTEIN COMPLEX
transported to liver

conjugated to glucuronate
BILIRUBIN DIGLUCURONIDE

excreted

19-15. USE OF THE VAN DEN BERGH REACTION

VAN DEN BERGH REACTION

INDIRECT	DIRECT
BILIRUBIN (linked to serum protein)	BILIRUBIN DIGLUCURONIDE
SOLUBILIZED IN ALCOHOL	

REACTION WITH DIAZOTIZED SULFANILIC ACID TO YIELD COLOR

---

crisis, the *unconjugated* form of bilirubin accumulates in plasma and tissues.

2. Hepatocellular Jaundice

Hepatocellular jaundice is the kind that results from hepatitis or cirrhosis. The damaged liver cannot conjugate bilirubin at a pace rapid enough to accommodate even a normal rate of erythrocyte destruction nor can it eject the

<table>
<tr><td>

19-16. DIRECT AND INDIRECT REACT-ING BILIRUBIN

BILIRUBIN (unconjugated)
  (Van den Bergh indirect reacting)

$+$

UDP-GLUCURONATE

    ⟶ UDP-glucuronyl transferase
           (liver)

BILIRUBIN DIGLUCURONIDE (conjugated)
  (Van den Bergh direct reacting)

</td><td>

19-17. ICTERUS OF THE NEWBORN

---

1) FETUS DOES NOT HAVE FUNCTIONAL CONJUGATING ENZYME (UDP-GLU-CURONYL TRANSFERASE)

2) UNCONJUGATED BILIRUBIN AC-CUMULATES IN TISSUES UNTIL EN-ZYME BECOMES ACTIVE

3) USUALLY NOT EXTENSIVE OR SERI-OUS, EXCEPT IN ERYTHROBLASTO-SIS FETALIS WHERE SERIOUS BRAIN DAMAGE MAY RESULT
    kernicterus

</td></tr>
</table>

conjugated form into biliary spaces. As a result *both* forms of bilirubin accumulate.

3. Cholestatic Jaundice

In cholestatic jaundice, the excretion of bile is prevented by either obstruction of the outflow tract or a drug-induced defect in the cellular ejection of conjugated bilirubin. There is an accumulation of *both conjugated and unconjugated forms* of bilirubin, since both conjugation and ejection are ultimately impaired.

4. Congenital Abnormality of Bilirubin Metabolism

The final cause of jaundice is congenital abnormality of the bilirubin metabolic system. This is commonly seen in the neonate as a transient form that results from a lag in the development of conjugating enzymes in the liver cell (jaundice of the newborn). Because of this lag, many babies are born more or less jaundiced, but the condition clears up rapidly as the enzymes are generated. Jaundice of the newborn is characterized by the accumulation of *unconjugated* bilirubin (Illustration 9-17).

More permanent forms of inherited conjugating enzyme defects and bile ejection defects are also seen, but they are very rare and will not concern us here.

THE GALLBLADDER

LEARNING OBJECTIVE

To review information in Chapter 3 regarding deposits and infiltration and to outline the problem of cholelithiasis and associated cholecystitis mentioning:
    a) epidemiology
    b) composition of the gallstone
    c) complications of cholelithiasis

The gallbladder is heir to a number of the usual kinds of diseases: however, from the standpoint of frequency, the 2 most prominent are stone formation (cholelithiasis) and an associated chronic inflammation (cholecystitis). In fact the 2 are so commonly associated that they will be discussed here as 1 condition (Illustration 19-18).

Gallstones (cholelithiasis) are unusually common in the United States. It has been estimated that perhaps 10 to 20 per cent of the adult population may be affected (Robbins and Angell). The typical gallstone is of mixed composition, containing variable proportions of cholesterol, bilirubin and calcium salts. Stones

19-18. COMMON DISORDERS OF THE GALLBLADDER
1) CHOLELITHIASIS
↓ continued mechanical irritation
2) CHRONIC CHOLECYSTITIS

of pure composition are seen with far less frequency: however, hemolytic disease is known to predispose an individual to the formation of bilirubinate stones.

The etiology of cholelithiasis is not completely understood: however, the most important predisposing factors appear to be abnormalities in bile composition, hemolytic anemia bile stasis and gallbladder infection. Gallstones are more common in women and are usually found after the age of 40. Presence of stones within the gallbladder causes chronic inflammation and fibrous thickening of the normally delicate wall, hence the common association between the 2 processes.

Additional Reading

Small, D. Gallstones. N. Engl. J. Med. 279:588, 1968

THE PANCREAS

LEARNING OBJECTIVE

To review the information on diabetes mellitus (Chapter 10) and be able to discuss the following diseases of the pancreas:
   a) pancreatitis
   b) carcinoma of the pancreas

The range of diseases of the pancreas is unusual in that this organ functions as both an exocrine and endocrine gland. Further, the exocrine products of the pancreas are potent digestive enzymes which have pronounced secondary effects, if liberated by cellular disruption. We will do little more than mention pancreatic diseases here, since anything approaching a thorough discussion would be far too lengthy (Illustration 19-19).

1. Pancreatitis

Pancreatitis is a mysterious disease occurring in acute and chronic forms that appears to have some association with the abuse of alcohol. Disruption of pancreatic acinar cells and release of enzymes causes a complicated pattern of destruction within pancreatic substance and, in severe cases, within adjacent organs as well. Hemorrhage is always a prominent local sign. Pancreatitis is more common in males and an acute attack is seemingly provoked by an alcoholic spree.

2. Carcinoma of the Pancreas

Carcinoma of the pancreas is a reasonably common tumor (approximately 19,000 new cases in 1970) arising in either the head or tail of this organ. Most are adenocarcinomas of bile duct epithelium. Those arising in the head will usually obstruct the biliary tract, causing a palpably enlarged gallbladder and jaundice, whereas those in the tail often remain "silent" until dangerously far advanced and difficult to

19-19. DISEASES OF THE PANCREAS

1) PANCREATITIS
    acute and chronic
    hemorrhage is prominent
    associated with alcohol abuse

2) CARCINOMA OF THE PANCREAS
    head of pancreas (early detection)
    tail of pancreas (late detection)

3) PANCREATIC ENDOCRINE DISORDERS
    diabetes mellitus (review Chapter 10)
    overproduction of endocrine agents

treat. The ease with which the former are detected usually leads to their discovery as small, discrete tumors.

3. Endocrine Disorders of the Pancreas

Endocrine disorders of the pancreas occur as either hypofunction or hyperfunction of islet tissues. Syndromes of the former are known as diabetes mellitus and have been discussed in Chapter 10; those of the latter are quite complex and will not be discussed here.

THE STOMACH

LEARNING OBJECTIVE

To review information on atrophic gastritis presented in Chapter 11 and to be able to discuss the following diseases of the stomach (and duodenum) in some detail:

a) gastritis
b) peptic ulceration of the stomach and duodenum
c) carcinoma of the stomach

The stomach, like other organs, exhibits a somewhat unique constellation of diseases based on its location and function. We will mention only a few of these, again selecting the most prominent or those that best illustrate a pathogenic mechanism (Illustration 19-20).

1. Gastritis

Gastritis is a rather vague term meaning, of course, inflammation of the stomach. The most common form is acute gastritis, which results from the swallowing of any of a number of gastric irritants, most notably alcoholic beverages and, in some cases, aspirin (or both in sequence). The acute form usually resolves quickly, once the irritant is withdrawn.

Atrophic gastritis is a far more serious condition thought to result from an autoimmune attack on some component of the gastric wall. Irreversible atrophy of glandular structures occurs and the patient is deprived of

---

> **19-20. PRINCIPAL DISEASES OF THE STOMACH**
>
> **1) GASTRITIS**
>   acute
>   atrophic
>
> **2) PEPTIC ULCERATION**
>   acute and chronic: more common in duodenum than stomach
>
> **3) CARCINOMA OF THE STOMACH**

---

pepsin, acid and intrinsic factor. We have encountered atrophic gastritis once before (Chapter 11) and have discussed its importance in pernicious anemia. At this point the student would do well to return to Chapter 11 and re-read this section.

2. Peptic Ulceration

Peptic ulcers are lesions of the gastrointestinal tract complicated by acid-pepsin digestion of the gut wall (Illustration 19-21). The overwhelming majority occur in the proximal duodenum and stomach; however, a very small number are seen in the esophagus and elsewhere along the digestive tract.

Peptic ulcers of the duodenum are far more common than those of the stomach. They occur with great frequency among young adults and males are affected far more than females. Peptic ulcers of the stomach occur in an older age group, but still affect men more often than women.

Peptic ulceration among young males seems to be a highly complex, multifactorial disease. Predisposition to ulcer formation undoubtedly consists of an hereditary component (individuals with type O blood are more prone), a hormonal component and, perhaps, even a component that derives from the quality of a person's gastric mucin. But the fact remains that careful elucidation of the predisposing factors does not explain the disease. All in all, it seems that the ulcer, itself, results from either failure of the enteric mucosa to repair itself after local injury or to renew its sloughed cells at a rate sufficient to prevent spontaneous interruption of its surface. With a break in the

19-21. PEPTIC ULCERATION

1) GASTRIC ULCERS MORE COMMON IN OLDER MALES—DUODENAL ULCERS IN YOUNGER MALES

2) MULTIFACTORIAL DISEASE
   heredity
   quality of gastric mucin
   physical or psychic stress acts as precipitating factor (Curling's ulcer is example)

surface, peptic digestion of subjacent tissues can occur and the ulcer becomes more extensive and chronic.

If this initial step is accepted, the most important missing piece to the puzzle becomes the reason for failure of the mitotic rate of epithelial cells. What is it that slows the reproduction of gastric and duodenal epithelium to the point where it can no longer keep up with the rate at which cells are sloughed or needed for repair of an incidental scratch? The answer, of course, is not available. But it seems certain that one of the most important factors in any explanation of ulcerogenesis will be stress, either physical or psychic.

Ulceration is one of the most predictable reactions of the entire gastrointestinal tract to various kinds of serious and sustained stress. Ulceromembranous gingivitis, apthous ulcers of the mouth, erosive esophagitis, peptic ulceration and ulcerative colitis are some of the more prominent examples of the diseases now suspected to result from this phenomenon.

Perhaps the most clear-cut example of gastrointestinal ulceration secondary to stress is Curling's ulcer, in which one or more serious ulcers of the stomach and duodenum are often seen following a severe burn.

3. Carcinoma of the Stomach

Carcinoma of the stomach is a highly dangerous malignancy of reasonably important incidence (estimated 17,000 new cases in United States in 1970) that enjoys the singular distinction of declining in its over-all significance. Although it was once the most frequent cause of cancer death in the American male,

carcinoma of the stomach has shown an absolutely decreasing incidence over the past 40 years. The reason is unknown.

Carcinoma of the stomach is principally a disease of the older male. The risk of contracting this cancer shows both hereditary and geographic components. It is more common in Japan than in the United States, but Japanese immigrants to the United States take on the risk of the adopted country within a short time. It occurs with great frequency among the males of certain familial groups and is more common among individuals of blood group A.

Most examples of stomach cancer are adenocarcinoma: however, the gross appearance and clinical behavior of this tumor varies widely among cases. As it is usually intercepted late in its clinical course, the recovery rate is disappointingly small.

Additional Reading

Bralow, S. P. Current concepts of peptic ulceration. Am. J. Digest. Dis. 14:655, 1969
Skillman, J. J. and Silen, W. Acute Gastroduodenal "stress" Ulceration: Barrier disruption of varied pathogenesis. Gastroenterology 59:478, 1970

SMALL INTESTINE

LEARNING OBJECTIVE

To review infectious diseases of the gastrointestinal tract and to be able to discuss the following:

   a) incidence of malignancy of the small intestine
   b) the cause, pathogenesis, clinical course and complications of regional enteritis (Crohn's disease)

The small intestine is an unusual segment of the gastrointestinal tract in many respects: however, from the standpoint of pathology its most commendable attribute is that *it rarely gives rise to a malignant tumor*. Principal diseases of the small intestine are largely infectious or inflammatory. We will mention only 2 examples of these in our discussion (Illustration 19-22).

19-22. PRINCIPAL DISEASES OF THE SMALL INTESTINE	**19-23.** INFECTIOUS DISEASES OF THE GASTROINTESTINAL TRACT

19-22. PRINCIPAL DISEASES OF THE SMALL INTESTINE

1) INFECTIOUS DISEASES
    (not confined to the small intestine)

2) REGIONAL ENTERITIS
    (Chrohn's disease) also not confined to small intestine
– – – – – – – – –
The small intestine is a comparatively rare site for the origin of a malignant tumor

19-23. INFECTIOUS DISEASES OF THE GASTROINTESTINAL TRACT

1) FOOD POISONING
    enterotoxin-producing   bacteria

2) SALMONELLA INFECTIONS

3) SHIGELLA INFECTIONS

4) CHOLERA

5) AMEBIC COLITIS

– – – – – – – – – – – –

Given alteration of gut flora by the use of broad spectrum antibiotics the G.I. tract becomes susceptible to infection with staphylococci and other unusual pathogens

1. Infectious Diseases

Infectious diseases of the gastrointestinal tract usually affect both the small and large bowel, but we will cover them in summary here. Although many infectious agents use the gastrointestinal tract as a portal of entry (poliovirus, hepatitis virus, etc.), only a select few infectious diseases can be considered primary to the gut and fewer yet usually remain confined there. The most prominent of these (Illustration 19-23) are caused by organisms which usually invade superficially or not at all.

Most of these agents have been discussed elsewhere (Chapters 7 and 8) and should be reviewed at this time.

2. Regional Enteritis (Crohn's Disease)

Regional enteritis or Crohn's disease is an inflammatory disease of the small (and large) intestine that is closely related in both etiology and clinical course to ulcerative colitis. It usually affects the terminal ileum, but can be found in other segments of the gastrointestinal tract as well. It is most often seen in young adults, but no age group is exempt; its incidence is equally divided between the sexes, but it tends to occur with less frequency among members of the black race.

Characteristics of Crohn's disease is a granulomatous induration of the entire thickness of the wall of a segment of the gut (transmural involvement), which may also be detectable in surrounding lymph nodes. The affected seg-

ment can become rigid and non-functional, if the process worsens or continues, and surgical intervention is often necessary. The prognosis is considered more favorable than that of ulcerative colitis.

Additional Reading

Baeza, M. Carcinoid tumors of the gastrointestinal tract. Dis. Colon Rectum 12:147, 1969

McGuigan, J. E. Immunology in gastrointestinal research and patient care. Am. J. Surg. 119:111, 1970

Rogers, A. I. Steatorrhea. Postgrad. Med. 50:123, 1971

COLON AND RECTUM

LEARNING OBJECTIVE

To be able to discuss the following 2 colorectal diseases mentioning cause, pathogenesis, clinical course and complications:
- **a) ulcerative colitis**
- **b) carcinoma of the colon and rectum**
- **c) interrelationship**

Diseases of the colon and rectum will be considered as a unit and of these only 2 new examples will be introduced (Illustration 19-24).

1. Ulcerative Colitis

Ulcerative colitis is an increasingly common, chronic, relapsing disease of the colon (and sometimes the distal ileum) in which there is widespread superficial ulceration of the mucosa. It occurs in a range of severity from mild and chronic to fulminant and rapidly fatal. The etiology of ulcerative colitis is poorly understood, but autoimmunity is thought to play some part and emotional stress is known to precipitate exacerbations of the acute stage.

Longstanding ulcerative colitis is dangerous in that repeated attacks may lead to intestinal perforation or hemorrhage. A small percentage of patients with ulcerative colitis of very long duration develop carcinoma of the colon.

2. Carcinoma of the Colon and Rectum

Carcinoma of the colon and rectum is an extremely prominent malignancy (75,000 new cases in 1970), causing a very significant proportion of cancer deaths in the United States. The peak incidence occurs between 50 and 65 years of age, but it is now seen with greater frequency among younger individuals. There is a slight female preponderance among tumors originating in the colon: however, the distribution between sexes is reasonably equal.

These tumors are almost invariably adenocarcinomas and are usually detected because of their effect on bowel habits or because they lead to the presence of blood in the stool. Although they may grow in situ for some time, metastasis to the liver is a frequent occurrence (Illustration 19-25).

19-24. PRINCIPAL DISEASES OF THE COLON AND RECTUM

1) INFECTIOUS DISEASES

2) ULCERATIVE COLITIS

3) POLYPS

4) CARCINOMA OF THE COLON AND RECTUM

19-25. COLORECTAL CANCER

1) EXTREMELY PROMINENT MALIGNANCY

2) ALMOST INVARIABLY ADENOCARCINOMAS

3) USUALLY DETECTED BECAUSE OF:
   effect on bowel habits
   presence of blood in stool

4) CARCINOEMBRYONIC ANTIGEN MAY PROVE TO BE PRACTICABLE MEANS OF DETECTING EARLY, OPERABLE CASES

5) METASTASIS TO LIVER IS COMMON

Additional Reading

Cole, W. H. Cancer of the colon and rectum. Surg. Clin. N. Amer. 52:871, 1972

Griffen, W. O. and Meeker, W. R. Colon carcinoma and immunologic phenomena. Surg. Clin. N. Amer. 52:839, 1972

Hagihara, P. F. and Griffin, W. O. Physiology of the colon and rectum. Surg. Clin. N. Amer. 52:797, 1972

Schachter, H. et al. Ulcerative and "granulomatous" colitis—validity of differential diagnostic criteria. Ann. Int. Med. 72:841, 1970

chapter 20
FUNCTIONAL DIS-ORDERS OF THE MIND

THEORIES OF PSYCHOPATHOLOGY

LEARNING OBJECTIVE

To be able to compare concepts of the mind as promulgated by the 2 principal schools of psychology ("behavioral" and "dynamic") with regard to:
   a) behavioral determinism
   b) innate factors (such as basic drives)
   c) learned factors
   d) principles of psychotherapy

We have seen in Chapter 15 that the brain, like most other organs, is liable to a variety of infectious, neoplastic and degenerative diseases. We must now turn our attention to functional disorders, a group of diseases the prevalence of which far overshadows any of those based on organic change. In fact, with the exception of dental caries and the common cold, functional disorders of the mind are perhaps the most common of all diseases in nations where urban concentration and industrial technology have progressed farthest. In the United States alone, 600,000 persons are now admitted to psychiatric hospitals each year, while many more are treated by private physicians.

Characteristic of these diseases is the absence of any demonstrable change in the structure or chemistry of the brain. This lack of tangible evidence makes it practically impossible to discuss functional disorders of the mind in terms of pathogenetic mechanism presented in previous chapters. In fact, to institute any discussion, we must first invoke a new set of principles and, to some extent, even a new language. It seems apparent, however, that, regardless of the difficulty, one must not simply overlook an area as important as the mind in a summary of the subject of human disease.

A concept of diseases of the mind must be based on a description of its normal function, but, since reasoning about the function of the mind is done through introspection or inference from the behavior of others, there is very little agreement on key theories. One is actually obliged to select among a number of mature and equally plausible systems of psychology to explain higher functions of the central nervous system. These systems actually exist in a spectrum-like distribution from the behavioral theories at one extreme to those based on Freudian principles at the other. Rather than use a single example as representative of these divergent opinions, we will develop a parallel comparison between theories situated at both extremes of this spectrum. We will use the terms *behavioral* and *dynamic* to designate these theories. Bear in mind, however, that these terms denote 2 contrasting points of view rather than 2 closed systems of doctrine. Many practitioners, for example, would subscribe to elements and ideas from both ends of the spectrum.

1. Determinants of Behavior

Behavior, of course, is the product of the mind. It represents the only *objective* manifestation of mental function. And, as such, it is held to be the only trustworthy subject for study in the behavioral school. Access to mental function is also gained through introspection: however, the introspective approach can only center around the study of mood changes observed in one's self or reported by others. Where the behavioral school would emphasize objectivity, the dynamic school places comparable importance on introspection and the study of affect. As shown in Illustration 20-1, the behavioral school would dismiss the functions of the mind as complex but essentially unknown processes and concentrate study on the response to a stimulus (behavior), whereas the dynamic school considers the response incidental to the operation of what is

312

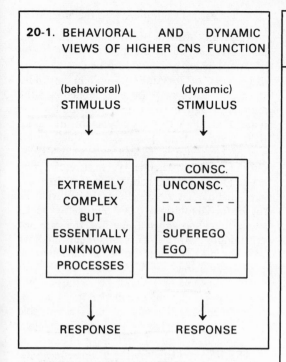

20-1. BEHAVIORAL AND DYNAMIC VIEWS OF HIGHER CNS FUNCTION

(behavioral)   (dynamic)
STIMULUS   STIMULUS

CONSC.

| EXTREMELY COMPLEX BUT ESSENTIALLY UNKNOWN PROCESSES | UNCONSC. - - - - - - ID SUPEREGO EGO |

RESPONSE   RESPONSE

20-2. OPERATIONAL ORGANIZATION OF THE MIND (BEHAVIORAL)

1) MIND IS A PRODUCT OF COMPLEX NEURAL CIRCUITRY AND CHEMICAL REACTION

    we know little of how it works and we are not able to postulate definite functional compartments

2) STRICT OBJECTIVITY MUST BE MAINTAINED IF PROGRESS IS TO BE MADE

    behavior is the product of the mind: it must be studied as objectively as saliva or pancreatic fluid

3) CONDITIONED BEHAVIOR IS AN OBJECTIVELY VALID, UNIVERSALLY ACCEPTED PHENOMENON AND REPRESENTS A TENABLE BASIS FOR A SCIENCE OF THE MIND

seen as a highly structured intrapsychic mechanism that leads first to a feeling and only then to an element of behavior.

Further contrasts between the 2 schools are drawn in Illustrations 20-2 and 20-3. Again emphasis is placed on the uncompromising quest for objectivity on the part of the behavioral school as opposed to the dynamic school's emphasis on intrapsychic structure and the interaction among the components of this structure in generating moods which, in turn, determine behavior.

2. Innate Components of the Mind

In lower animals, many fundamental needs are satisfied by a kind of automatic behavior. For example, they seek food, mate and protect themselves without specific training in such tasks. These patterns of behavior are predetermined and are actually inherited as part of the animals' nervous systems; they are said to be *instinctive*.

In the human being, most instincts are weak and vestigial. One has only to think of the years of training required to equip the infant for adulthood to be impressed at how little behavioral competence is built into the human

being at birth. The years of dependency are not without meaning, however. The adaptive success of the human species is based in large part on precisely this quality of freedom from pre-ordained ways of doing things. He enjoys an ability to override many natural motives by volition. He can elect to defer or even frustrate the satisfaction of basic needs, if it becomes expedient to do so.

With rare exceptions the instincts of his progenitors are present in the human being as *basic drives*. Drives *urge* a man to act in certain ways, but do not normally *compel* him. Satisfaction of drives are rewarded by the experience of pleasure, but, although eagerly anticipated, pleasure can be declined. This remarkable freedom from instinctive compulsion allows the human to actually design his behavior to meet the needs of each situation. Clearly, this amounts to a potent selective advantage in that the human species is not locked into a set pattern of behavior that would equip it conveniently (but exclusively) for a given set of environmental features. The human individual is at least potentially capable of

---

20-3. OPERATIONAL ORGANIZATION OF THE MIND (DYNAMIC)

---

1) ID

     psychic representation of the basic drives: unreasoning, non-integrative

2) SUPEREGO

     psychic representation of the imprint of culture on the mind: unreasoning, non-integrative

3) EGO

     source of reason and mental integration

     executive function:

          mediates day-to-day living

     synthetic function:

          develops more complete independence from non-integrative mental processes and extrapersonal influences

---

20-4. INNATE COMPONENTS OF THE MIND (BOTH SCHOOLS)

---

1) INVOLUNTARY INSTINCTUAL BEHAVIOR OF LOWER ANIMALS IS RESIDUAL IN MAN AS BASIC DRIVES

2) BASIC DRIVES CONSTITUTE A STRONG MOTIVE FORCE IN DETERMINING BEHAVIOR

---

adapting his behavior to changes in the environment and can even seek new environments into which he can fit by simply modifying his habits. There is little doubt that this extreme degree of behavioral flexibility contributes to the fact that, considering higher animals, the human species is the most successful and widely distributed in the world.

3. Learned Components of the Mind

Although both schools would accept the importance of innate components of the mind as determinates of mood and behavior, severe divergence of opinion occurs in attitudes toward acquired or learned components of the mind (Illustration 20-5). The behavioral school holds that all patterns of behavior are essentially learned, even those used in the carrying out of basic drives. Indeed, according to this outlook, human personality consists of a rich collection of various habits. Some of these are good habits, i.e. they allow the individual's successful adaptation to his physical or social situation; others are maladaptive, they are not harmonious with elements of his surroundings and are the constant source of travail in his day-to-day living.

In the dynamic school, of course, such emphasis on learning and habit would be unacceptable. Adherents of this school hold that patterns of behavior are simply manifestations of their antecedent feelings. That is, all behavior is motivated by the feelings that result from the interaction of intrapsychic structures.

4. Principles of Psychotherapy

As might be expected from the foregoing discussion, principles of psychotherapy differ radically between the 2 schools (Illustration 20-6). According to the behavioral school, the correction of disordered behavior is best

---

20-5. LEARNED COMPONENTS OF THE MIND

---

1) BEHAVIORAL

     patterns of behavior are largely learned

     re-learning of "better" patterns is the key to correcting behavior

2) DYNAMIC

     patterns of behavior are motivated by unconscious desires

     insight into motivation is the key to correcting disordered behavior

---

20-6. PRINCIPLES OF PSYCHOTHER-
APY

---

1) BEHAVIORAL SCHOOL
   correction of disordered behavior
   can be achieved through behavioral modification

   the patient must be retrained in
   patterns of behavior that have
   more adaptive valve

2) DYNAMIC SCHOOL
   correction of disordered behavior
   follows insight into the antecedents of distorted feelings
   the patient must be led to a realization of his own sentiments
   ("talking cure")

---

achieved by replacing bad or maladaptive habits with patterns of behavior that have more adaptive value. The person exhibiting confused behavior must be re-trained, his habits must be altered in such a way that they fit better with his situation.

Quite in contrast, the dynamic school proposes that the correction of disordered behavior can only follow insight into the distortion of feelings that is causing them. Since the sentiment is antecedent to the behavior, the patient must be led to an understanding of his confused feelings and behavioral modification will follow automatically. This has come to be known as the "talking cure".

Additional Reading

Campbell, B. A. and Misanin, J. R. Basic drives. Ann. Rev. Psychol. 20:57, 1969

Ford, D. H. and Urban, H. B. Systems of Psychotherapy. New York, John Wiley & Sons, Inc., 1965

Gazzaniga, M. S. One brain—Two minds. Am. Scientist 60:311, 1972

Marmor, J. Dynamic psychotherapy and behavior therapy, are they irreconcilable? Arch. Gen. Psychiat. 24:22, 1971

McGur, P. The chemistry of mind. Am. Scientist 59:221, 1971

Rutter, M. Concepts of autism: A review of research. J. Child Psychol. Psychiat. 9:1, 1968

Ulrich, R. et al. (ed.) Control of Human Behavior. Glenview Ill., Scott Forseman and Co., 1965

CLASSIFICATION OF DISEASES ASSOCIATED WITH MENTAL DYSFUNCTION

LEARNING OBJECTIVE

To be able to outline a system for the classification of diseases associated with mental dysfunction and describe the boundaries of each category

Regardless of one's outlook on the mechanism of higher functions of the central nervous system (the term *mind* is actually unacceptable to the strict behaviorist), diseases of mental dysfunction are classified according to a generally accepted scheme. The first order of this classificaion is seen in Illustration 20-7. These categories correspond to diseases originating in the mind, diseases of the body occurring secondary to mental disease and diseases of the mind occurring secondary to organic diseases elsewhere in the body. We will consider each of these major categories of diseases of the mind and mind-body relationship in succeeding learning objectives.

20-7. DISEASES OF THE MIND (AND MIND-BODY RELATIONSHIP)

---

1) MENTAL DISEASE
   disturbances of:
      thought processes
      perception
      feelings
      behavior (social, personal)

2) PSYCHOSOMATIC DISEASE
   disturbances of body function
      caused by a disease primary
      to the mind

3) REACTIVE MENTAL DISEASE (SO-
   MATOPSYCHIC DISEASE)
   disturbances of mental function
      caused by a disease primary
      to the body

20-8. MENTAL DISEASE

1) PSYCHOTIC DISORDERS

profound mental disorder, patient has no contact with reality and no insight into his own state of illness: utterly misrepresents his personal situation

2) PERSONALITY (NEUROTIC) DISOR-DERS

patient has reasonable contact with reality: realizes his own illness and (in most instances) will accurately represent his personal situation

The first major category, mental disease (or diseases primary to higher functions of the central nervous system), is usually further subdivided into psychosis and neurosis (Illustration 20-8). Our discussion will be confined to the second of these, since psychoses are generally considered to be examples of organic (as opposed to functional) disorders of the central nervous system. Again it must be pointed out that the clear distinction between functional and organic disorders is not an acceptable dichotomy in the behavioral school. Most behaviorists hold that functional disorders represent those in which an organic lesion, although present, is so subtle as to be beyond detection.

Additional Reading

Berkman, P. L. Measurement of mental health in a general population survey. Am. J. Epidermiol. 94:105, 1971

ROOTS OF MENTAL DYSFUNCTION

LEARNING OBJECTIVE

To be able to outline the mechanism of the conflict using examples. To be able to explain attitudes of both the behavioral and dynamic schools of psychotherapy toward this phenomenon

Another point of commonality between the behavioral and dynamic schools of psychology is that most mental dysfunction has its roots in the *conflict*. The 2 schools would define the concept and pathogenesis of the conflict quite differently, however.

In the behavioral school, a conflict is conceived as the practicing of techniques of behavior that have poor adaptive value (Illustration 20-9). Since these patterns of behavior failed to adapt an individual to his surroundings, they lead to a constant distortion of his mood or feelings. His behavior is maladaptive; hence, he lives in conflict with his physical or societal environment.

Quite in contrast, the concept of the conflict held by the dynamic school is one of psychic malfunction; it exists within the mind, rather than as a failure of fit between an individual and his environment. In the *intrapsychic conflict*, 1 element of the unconscious mind is pitted against another (Illustration 20-10). This usually involves the superego in contest with the id, the result being to distract the ego and

20-9. ROOTS OF MENTAL DYSFUNCTION (BEHAVIORAL SCHOOL)

1) PSYCHOPATHOLOGY IS CAUSED BY THE LEARNING OF BEHAVIOR TECHNIQUES THAT HAVE POOR ADAPTIVE VALUE

"bad habits"

2) THE PRACTICE OF THESE BAD HABITS LEADS TO A DISTORTION OF MOOD OR FEELINGS

20-10. ROOTS OF MENTAL DYSFUNC-
TION (DYNAMIC SCHOOL)

---

1) THE SUPEREGO ABHORS A SENTI-
MENT ORIGINATING IN THE ID

2) RESULTING *INTRAPSYCHIC CON-
FLICT* OCCUPIES EGO WITH DIS-
TRACTING EFFORT WEAKENING ITS
EXECUTIVE ABILITIES AND PREVENT-
ING ITS FURTHER DEVELOPMENT

3) PATIENT RESORTS TO NON-INTEGRA-
TIVE PATTERNS OF BEHAVIOR AND
AFFECT

4) RESULTING MENTAL CONFUSION
LEADS TO A DISTORTION OF MOOD
OR FEELING

---

prevent its proper function and further development. Such turmoil of the mind, of course,
leads to a distortion of mood or feeling.

It is important to recognize that the concept
of the conflict is consistent with basic tenets of
both schools. In the behavioral school, the
conflict is objectified as an improper relationship between an individual's habits and his
situation; in the dynamic school, the conflict is
intrapsychic. The unconscious mental confusion resulting from a contest between 1
compartment of the mind and another cannot
be viewed objectively, it must be reported by
the patient and only incidentally leads to
disordered behavior.

Additional Reading

Calhoun, J. B. A "Behavioral Sink," in Bliss, E. L.
(ed.), Roots of Behavior. Hagerstown, Harper &
Row, 1962

MANIFESTATIONS OF MENTAL DYSFUNCTION

LEARNING OBJECTIVES

To be able to discuss the clinical manifestations
of mental disorder engendered by conflict and
describe principal patterns of the following:
   a) disorders of affect, particularly as
      regards the signs and sequellae of
      anxiety and depression
   b) disorders of behavior, used as adjustive
      techniques.

In the previous learning objective, we saw
that the existence of a conflict generated
confusion within higher functions of the central
nervous system. It must be borne in mind, of
course, that a solitary conflict would be more
the exception than the rule. The picture one
sees in a single individual is usually that of
multiple conflicts of mixed quality and intensity. When something happens in a person's
life that exacerbates a conflict the experience
leads directly to a *disorder of affect*. Disorders
of affect are usually so intolerable that in order
to avoid or neutralize them an individual will
adopt certain patterns of behavior or thought.
Thus, he practices disorders of behavior to
avoid disorders of affect (Illustration 20-11).

Stated in another way, disorders of affect
lead to disorders of behavior. The individual in
conflict has learned that, by thinking in a

20-11. MANIFESTATIONS OF CONFLICT

---

1) DISORDERS OF AFFECT
   (anxiety or depression)
   highly unpleasant feelings of mental disturbance, roughly analogous to the experience of pain
   in malfunction of the body

2) ADJUSTIVE TECHNIQUES
   techniques of avoiding or neutralizing the exacerbation of a conflict and thereby preventing the
   experience of a *disorder of affect*

20-12. DISORDERS OF AFFECT

1) ANXIETY
    unfocused fear: emotional hyper-
    reactivity
 	
2) DEPRESSION
    unreasoning despair: emotional
    lethargy

20-13. ADJUSTIVE TECHNIQUES

1) PHOBIA, AVOIDANCE, EVASION, RE-
    ACTION FORMATION, REPRESSION,
    RATIONALIZATION
 	
2) OBSESSION, COMPULSION
 	
3) SEXUAL DISORDERS
 	
4) SELF-DESTRUCTIVE PRACTICES
    alcoholism
    smoking to excess
    drug abuse
    overeating
 	
5) MISCELLANEOUS
    stuttering
    enuresis
    thumbsucking

certain way or by adopting ritual-like patterns of unusual behavior, he can avoid exacerbating his conflict and suffering the far more punishing experience of a disorder of affect (Illustration 20-12). He desperately practices mechanical patterns of reasoning or behavior as *adjustive techniques.* A thorough analysis of adjustive techniques would be far beyond the scope of this discussion: however, a list is provided in Illustration 20-13 that will give some idea of the types of practices that could be considered in this category. When an individual is unable to devise patterns of thought or behavior that would allow adjustment to his conflicted situation, he must live with the disorder of affect that results. These are usually seen as 1 of 2 basic types, *anxiety* or *depression*.

1. Anxiety

Anxiety is a kind of mental pain. It bears approximately the same relationship to illness of the mind as the experience of conventional pain bears to organic disease. It warns us that we have not adapted to a situation (behavioral school) or that the ego is failing (dynamic school), and that this shortcoming is not being compensated.

Like fever and anemia, anxiety is not a disease, but rather a sign of disease. The experience of anxiety, like that of pain, is extremely unpleasant, but it serves to warn us of a deeper, more grievous condition. A person experiencing anxiety will make every attempt to neutralize the feeling. Because of the efficacy of adjustive techniques, anxiety will rarely be intercepted in an easily interpretable form unless an attack of acute distress is provoked by a particular situation. This is often the case when anxiety becomes manifest under such circumstances as a visit to the dentist's office, an encounter with a snake, or when called upon to speak before an audience.

Chronic anxiety is the form that leads to psychosomatic disease. Chronic anxiety is anxiety that does not relent. It warns us that something is maladaptive in the very style of our lives (Illustration 20-14).

The behavioral and physiologic changes that accompany anxiety are widespread and obvious. A list of such changes is provided in Illustration 20-15: however, not all of these will be seen in every case of anxiety.

2. Depression

Depression is the experience of despair. If anxiety could be considered a syndrome of emotional hyper-reactivity, then depression is its counterpart in emotional lethargy (Illustration 20-16).

Freud and most subsequent authorities, recognizing the great prevalence of depression, considered it as occurring in a range of severity from normal grief or discouragement to a

20-14. ANXIETY

1) SUBJECTIVELY EXPERIENCED QUALITY OF FEAR DIRECTED TOWARD THE FUTURE WITH NO RECOGNIZABLE THREAT OR A THREAT OUT OF PROPORTION TO THE EMOTION IT EVOKES

    also described as terror, horror, alarm, fright, panic, trepidation, dread, scare, apprehension

2) EMOTIONAL HYPER-REACTIVITY: INTENSITY VARIES FROM MILD TO OVERWHELMING

3) MANIFEST BODILY CHANGES THAT CAN LEAD TO PSYCHOSOMATIC DISEASE IF PROTRACTED

20-15. BEHAVIORAL AND PHYSIOLOGIC CHANGES ASSOCIATED WITH ANXIETY

1) "NERVOUS" BEHAVIOR
    irritability
    tremor
    disturbance of sleep

2) SWEATING PALMS

3) HEADACHE, NAUSEA, BLURRED VISION

4) CHEST PAIN, PALPITATION, DYSPNEA

5) CHILL, WEAKNESS, PARESTHESIA

6) HYPERTENSION

20-16. DEPRESSION

1) SUBJECTIVELY EXPERIENCED QUALITY OF DESPAIR

    also described as helplessness, hopelessness, abandonment, passivity

2) INTENSITY VARIES FROM MILD TO OVERWHELMING

3) MANIFEST BODILY CHANGES THAT CAN LEAD TO PSYCHOSOMATIC DISEASE IF PROTRACTED

20-17. BEHAVIORAL AND PHYSIOLOGIC CHANGES ASSOCIATED WITH DEPRESSION

1) DIFFICULTY IN CONCENTRATION

2) CHRONIC EXHAUSTION, LACK OF ENTHUSIASM, UNDERACHIEVEMENT

3) IDEAS OF SELF DESTRUCTION

4) PREOCCUPATION WITH SOMATIC SYMPTOMS
    hypochondriasis

persistent mood of hopelessness. Its less severe (normal or neurotic) forms are periodic and transient, whereas in the psychotic it may take the form of absolute passivity with catatonia. The etiology of depression is a matter of continuing controversy. Despite the fact that it accounts for the greatest bulk of psychiatric hospital admission, its cause is unknown and treatment is still based on empiricism. There is little doubt that depression is actually a group of diseases all giving rise to a similar clinical picture. The more severe and intractable of these are thought to be based on the inheritance of a so-called "endogenous factor," which predisposes a person to the experience of depressive illness, whereas milder neurotic depressions are thought to be psychogenic or functional in etiology. Whatever its cause, depression, like anxiety, is most unpleasant and might be considered another variety of mental pain. Also, like anxiety, depression is recognized by characteristic behavioral and physiologic changes (Illustration 20-17) and can lead to psychosomatic disease.

PSYCHOSOMATIC DISEASE

LEARNING OBJECTIVES

To be able to describe the pathogenesis of psychosomatic disease and cite several examples of diseases that are thought to have a strong psychosomatic component. Also, to be able to compare and contrast:
   a) psychophysiologic disease
   b) hysteria or conversion

Emotional disorder is, of course, a disease in its own right. The afflicted person is forced to endure great mental discomfort. His behavior often works against his own welfare and he may be incapacitated by anxiety or depression.

In many cases, however, emotional disease, in addition to its effect on the mind, leads to either somatic symptoms or actual organic signs or lesions. When the mind affects the body in this way, the condition is known as *psychosomatic disease*.

Psychosomatic disease is usually subdivided into 2 basic kinds, psychophysiologic disease and hysteria (Illustration 20-18). Since these 2 are quite different in both cause and effect, we take time to look briefly at each.

1. Psychophysiologic Disease

Psychophysiologic disease is a morbid change in the body caused by sustained emotional stress. It most often results from longstanding anxiety or depression, both of which elicit comparable kinds (Illustration 20-19).

The link between mind and body is carried out through the general adaptation syndrome in

---

20-18. PSYCHOSOMATIC DISEASE

1) PSYCHOPHYSIOLOGIC DISEASE
   a morbid change in the body caused by sustained emotional stress

2) HYSTERIA (CONVERSION)
   the conversion of emotional stess to a physical symptom

20-19. PSYCHOPHYSIOLOGIC   DISEASE

SUSTAINED   ANXIETY
EMOTIONAL   ←   OR
STRESS   DEPRESSION

GENERAL ADAPTATION
SYNDROME

↓

PSYCHOPHYSIOLOGIC DISEASE
   asthma and allergy
   gastrointestinal disturbance
   hypertension and sequelae
   immunologic impairment and sequelae
   others

---

which the body reacts to mental stress as if it were meeting an actual physical threat. Adrenocortical hormones are secreted in unusual amounts, giving rise to a number of rather characteristic physiologic alterations.

The specific kind of disease that will result will depend to a large measure on the nature and severity of the emotional disorder and on other more individual qualities of the patient. Those most often seen are listed in Illustration 20-19.

The real importance of emotional factors in physical disease is still not totally appreciated.

The now well defined effect of sustained emotional stress on the function of immunologic defenses opens whole new areas for investigation. For centuries, physicians have vaguely recognized and often reported the association between personality types and disease patterns: however, the accumulation of unqualified evidence to support such contentions has been difficult and only recently accepted as a legitimate area of research.

2. Hysteria (Conversion)

Hysteria is psychosomatic disease in which emotional stress is dealt with by its unconscious conversion to a physical symptom. For this reason it is also frequently called a *conversion reaction*. The term, hysteria, derives from the ancient belief that the symptom was somehow caused by a displacement or disorder of the uterus.

The person manifesting hysteria can simulate any kind of major disease or physical change from pain to pregnancy. The symptom will usually be symbolic of the underlying emotional disorder and can be made convincingly real to the diagnostician.

A detailed discussion of hysteria is beyond the scope of this discussion and it is mentioned only for the sake of completing the perspective of psychosomatic disorders.

20-20. REACTIVE MENTAL DISEASE (SOMATOPSYCHIC DISEASE)

1) MENTAL DISORDER ASSOCIATED WITH SLE

2) MENTAL DISORDER ASSOCIATED WITH VARIOUS STATES OF HORMONAL IMBALANCE
    hypothyroidism
    hyperparathyroidism
    pheochromocytoma

Additional Reading

McKegney, P. Psychosomatic gastrointestinal disturbances. Postgrad. Med. 47:109, May, 1970
Ziegler, F. J. Hysterical conversion reactions. Postgrad. Med. 47:174, 1970

REACTIVE MENTAL DISEASE

LEARNING OBJECTIVE

To be aware of the potential for mental disease represented by certain kinds of illness that take origin in the body.

Just as diseases of the mind can give rise to secondary disorders of body function, so can certain diseases originating in the body cause secondary mental disease. It has been known for some time, for example, that hypothyroidism is associated with a kind of mental disorder that appears to clear up without residual effect when adequate levels of thyroid hormone are restored. More recently, certain psychiatric symptoms have been described as a concomitant of systemic lupus erythematosus. Also, it has recently become apparent that a form of emotional disorder (but not mental retardation) will almost always accompany polysomy of sex chromosomes.

These examples clearly demonstrate the potential for a kind of mental disease which is seemingly secondary to illness taking origin in the body. Mental disease arising in this manner is termed *reactive mental disease* or *somatopsychic disease*. Presumably, the condition of the mind obtains directly from the condition of the body and, at least in the case of hormonal imbalance, can be shown to improve when the primary disease is corrected.

Additional Readings

Asher, R. Myxedematous madness. Brit. Med. J. 2:555, 1949
Gurland, B. J. et al. The study of the psychiatric symptoms of systemic lupus erythematosus, a critical review. Psychosomat. Med. XXXIV:199, 1972

INDEX